RNA INTERFERENCE

RNA INTERFERENCE
Application to Drug Discovery
and Challenges to Pharmaceutical
Development

Edited by

PAUL H. JOHNSON
PhaseRx, Inc.
Seattle, Washington

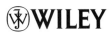

A JOHN WILEY & SONS, INC., PUBLICATION

Published by John Wiley & Sons, Inc., Hoboken, New Jersey.
Published simultaneously in Canada.

For general information on our other products and services or for technical support, please contact our
Customer Care Department within the United States at (800) 762-2974, outside the United States at
(317) 572-3993 or fax (317) 572-4002.

Wiley also publishes its books in a variety of electronic formats. Some content that appears in print may
not be available in electronic format. For more information about Wiley products, visit our web site at
www.wiley.com

Library of Congress Cataloging-in-Publication Data

RNA interference : application to drug discovery and challenges to pharmaceutical development /
edited by Paul H. Johnson.
    p. ; cm.
Includes bibliographical references and index.
ISBN 978-0-471-77151-7 (cloth)
1. RNA.   2. Small interfering RNA.   3. Drug development.   I. Johnson,
Paul H., 1943-
[DNLM: 1. RNA Interference.   2. Drug Discovery. QU 475]
QP623.R573 2011
572.8′8–dc22

                                                        2010030999

Printed in Singapore

10   9   8   7   6   5   4   3   2   1

CONTENTS

CONTRIBUTORS

ROGER ADAMI, mdRNA, Inc., 3830 Monte Villa Parkway, Bothell, WA 98021

MARK BEHLKE, Integrated DNA Technologies, Inc., 1710 Commercial Park, Coralville, IA 52241

RODERICK L. BEIJERSBERGEN, The Netherlands Cancer Institute, Division of Molecular Carcinogenesis, Plesmanlaan 121, 1066 CX Amsterdam, The Netherlands

JAMES A. BIRCHLER, Division of Biological Sciences, Tucker Hall, University of Missouri, Columbia, Missouri 65211

KUNYUAN CUI, Agave Pharma, Inc., 1124 Columbia St., Seattle, WA 98104

DIANE FRANK, AVI BioPharma, Inc., 3450 Monte Villa Parkway Suite 101, Bothell, WA 98021

YANLIN GUO, Department of Biological Sciences, University of Southern Mississippi, 118 College Dr. #5018, Hattiesburg, MS 39406

ADAM N. HARRIS, Life Technologies Corporation, 1600 Faraday Avenue, Carlsbad, CA 92008

FAQING HUANG, Department of Chemistry and Biochemistry, University of Southern Mississippi, 118 College Dr. #5043, Hattiesburg, MS 39402

MICHAEL HOUSTON, mdRNA, Inc., 3830 Monte Villa Parkway, Bothell, WA 98021

PAUL H. JOHNSON, PhaseRx, Inc., 410 West Harrison St., Suite 300, Seattle, WA 98110

ADAM JUDGE, Tekmira Pharmaceuticals Corporation, 100-8900 Glenlyon Parkway, Burnaby, BC, Canada V5J 5J8

IAN MACLACHLAN, Tekmira Pharmaceuticals Corporation, 100-8900 Glenlyon Parkway, Burnaby, BC, Canada V5J 5J8

STEVEN C. QUAY, Atossa Genetics, Inc., 4105 E Madison St., Suite 320, Seattle, WA 98112

MARJORIE ROBBINS, Tekmira Pharmaceuticals Corporation, 100-8900 Glenlyon Parkway, Burnaby, BC, Canada V5J 5J8

ALIASGER K. SALEM, Division of Pharmaceutics, College of Pharmacy, University of Iowa, Iowa City, IA 52242

OLIVER C. STEINBACH, Department Bio-Molecular Engineering, Sector Molecular Medicine, Philips Research Laboratories, High Tech Campus 11, NL-5656 AE Eindhoven, The Netherlands

STEPHEN MARK TOMPKINS, Department of Infectious Diseases, 111 Carlton St., University of Georgia, Athens, GA 30602

RALPH TRIPP, University of Georgia, Department of Infectious Diseases, 111 Carlton St., Athens, GA 30603

HARRY WANG, mdRNA, Inc., 3830 Monte Villa Parkway, Bothell, WA 98021

KRISTIN A. WIEDERHOLT, Life Technologies Corporation, 1600 Faraday Avenue, Carlsbad, CA 92008

C. J. YU, Beckman Institute, M/C 139-74, California Institute of Technology, 1200 E. California Blvd., Pasadena, CA 91125

PREFACE

RNA interference (RNAi) is a form of posttranscriptional gene silencing within cells involved in the control of gene expression. The RNAi pathway is found in many eukaryotes including animals and humans. It is initiated by the enzyme Dicer, which cleaves long double-stranded RNA molecules into short fragments of about 20 base pairs. The products of this reaction, small interfering RNA (siRNA) and microRNA (miRNA) molecules, bind to other homologous RNAs (transcripts) and affect their activity (protein expression) *via* degradation or translational inhibition. RNAi functions in defending cells against parasitic genes—viruses and transposons—and also in directing development as well as gene expression in general. The specific and potent effect of RNAi on gene expression makes it a valuable research tool in both cell culture and animal models to systematically shut down each gene in the cell to help identify the components necessary for a particular function/cellular process. RNAi may also be exploited in humans by introducing synthetic siRNA into cells and suppression (silencing) of disease-causing genes.

Exploitation of the RNAi pathway is a promising approach to treat a variety of diseases. Of great importance is the current view that 80% of the genome is not drugable by small molecules (10%) or biologics (10%), but is potentially drugable by gene silencing technologies. RNAi is seen as a promising way to treat cancer by silencing genes differentially upregulated in tumor cells or genes involved in cell division. Other proposed clinical applications include antiviral therapies to treat infection by herpes simplex virus type 2 and the inhibition of viral gene expression in cancerous cells, knockdown of host receptors and coreceptors for HIV, the silencing of hepatitis A and hepatitis B genes, silencing of influenza gene expression, and inhibition of measles viral replication. Potential treatments for neurodegenerative diseases include muscular dystrophy and polyglutamine diseases such as Huntington's disease.

A key area of research in the use of RNAi for clinical applications is the development of safe and effective delivery systems that permit targeting to specific cell types and tissues with efficient cell uptake and release into the cytoplasm, the site of action. The goal of this book is to bring together a series of critical review and analysis chapters by leading scientists in the RNAi field that assess the key issues in the development of RNAi-based drugs for clinical applications.

The first section of the book covers the biology of RNAi. Chapter 1 discusses the origins and overview of RNAi. Chapter 2 describes nucleic acids as regulatory molecules including the artificial modulation of gene expression using antisense technology, triplex-forming oligonucleotides, nucleic acid decoys, aptamers, ribozymes and DNAzymes, and RNAi by siRNAs and miRNAs. Chapter 3 examines the use of siRNA oligonucleotides to study gene function including siRNA design strategies, target specificity, chemical modification, delivering siRNA in cell culture, and the experimental design and detection of gene silencing (knockdown). Chapter 4 explains genome scanning by RNAi, dissection of physiological and pathological processes with genetic screens, large-scale RNAi-based screens in mammalian cells, and the design and practical implementation of high-throughput RNAi screens.

The second section of the book deals with the development of siRNA for therapeutic applications. Chapter 5 discusses the discovery of siRNA delivery agents, focusing on issues and challenges related to cellular uptake mechanisms and tight junction dynamics, peptide-based delivery, targeting specific cell types, and high-throughput screening approaches. Chapter 6 describes the potential for use of delivery systems for synthetic siRNAs to overcome the limitations of siRNAs and enhance therapeutic efficacy including current limitations to delivery of siRNAs *in vivo*, interferon induction and the innate immune system, siRNA administration without delivery assistance, nonviral delivery vehicles for siRNAs, physical delivery, synthetic siRNA delivery systems, pegylation of siRNA delivery vehicles, cell targeting ligand conjugation to siRNA delivery vehicles, and the rational design of modular multicomponent siRNA delivery systems. Chapter 7 focuses on immunologically based *in vivo* toxicities including the mechanisms of nucleic acid-mediated immune stimulation, Toll-like receptors, TLR-independent mechanisms and protein kinase R, factors influencing immune stimulation, and the implications for pharmaceutical product development. Chapter 8 discusses synthetic siRNA drug development and therapeutic applications for respiratory syncytial virus and influenza viruses and describes the application of RNAi to viral diseases focusing on proofs of concept for therapeutic RNAi treatment of virus infection, viral countermeasures for RNAi, translating siRNA delivery to the clinic, and RNAi versus traditional antiviral drugs.

Currently, there are more than 80 gene silencing therapeutics in clinical trials (http://clinicaltrials.gov/). They have the potential to provide a new class of broadly applicable therapies with clinically relevant efficacy and safety. Efficient delivery and cost-effective manufacturing are major challenges that must be met to achieve success. While current manufacturing processes are not yet cost-effective, they are likely to show significant improvement over time. No current delivery system appears to have the desired efficiency, cell selectivity, and safety profile necessary for an RNAi therapeutic to have a clear clinical advantage over other classes of drugs. However, on the basis of recent results and promising new systems under development, there is reason to believe that this will change in the near future.

RNAi therapeutics, a new class of drugs with unprecedented specificity, efficacy and safety, have the potential to revolutionize drug development and the future of medicine by providing broadly applicable therapies against targets that are currently undrugable.

PAUL H. JOHNSON

Seattle, WA
July 2010

FOREWORD

RNA interference (RNAi) has rapidly progressed from an intriguing scientific discovery to a powerful tool for studying gene function. In addition to the use of RNAi in the research laboratory, many investigators and commercial ventures are exploiting its potential as a sequence and gene-specific therapeutic agent. The idea that an oligonucleotide could be used to block gene function by virtue of Watson–Crick base pairing is not new, but was described over three decades ago by Paul Zamecnik and colleagues. The original antisense oligonucleotides were largely composed of DNA with various backbone modifications to stabilize the oligos or alter their Watson–Crick binding stability. For various reasons, with a few minor exceptions, the potential of antisense oligos to serve as functional genomic tools or therapeutic agents has never been fully realized. Since RNAi is in effect a form of antisense, why is it so much more potent than the conventional oligonucleotide approaches? Perhaps the biggest difference between RNAi and the antisense DNAs is that RNAi engages a specific set of cellular proteins that have evolved over millions of years for regulating gene expression. In contrast, antisense DNA approaches relied upon diffusion of the oligo to the target mRNA sequence wherein RNAseH is recruited to cleave the RNA. The two phenomena are similar in that the major mammalian Argonaute protein effecter of RNAi, Ago2, has an RNAseH-like cleavage domain at the active site. The association of Ago2 with other components of the RNAi machinery provides efficient target recognition and results in target destruction following Ago2-mediated cleavage. Thus, it is fair to state that RNAi is the most powerful sequence specific inhibitor of gene expression available for both functional genomics and therapeutic applications.

The chapters in this volume cover a large swath of the applications and challenges of using RNAi in drug discovery and as a therapeutic modality. A couple of chapters review the use of siRNAs for therapeutic target identification and gene function analyses. There are several chapters that focus on strategies and issues of concern for using siRNAs as therapeutic agents. Of particular importance are strategies for delivery of therapeutic small RNAs. A number of clever approaches ranging from conjugation of ligands to siRNAs through encapsulation of siRNAs in nanoparticles have been published in the literature. Many of these are reviewed in the chapters of this volume. There are also applications in which siRNAs are not packaged, but backbone modified versions are applied directly, such as intraocular injection for macular degeneration treatment, or inhalation for treatment of RSV or influenza infections. Other chapters address the major concerns of systemic delivery, which are rapid clearance through the kidney and liver versus desired uptake into tumors or other tissues. Some of the delivery strategies and vehicles that are being developed can circumvent rapid kidney clearance, but the liver still remains as a major receptacle for systemic RNAs, even when the siRNAs are taken up by other tissues or tumors. That being said, there is a need to ensure that the siRNAs are not creating toxicities by triggering downregulation of targeted mRNAs in tissues other than those that are diseased. Other concerns are off-target effects caused by siRNAs functioning on nontargeted mRNAs to block translation or even direct cleavage. Thus, bio-informatics' analyses of siRNA design along with backbone modifications to block miRNA-like function or preventing passenger strand activity need to be carefully evaluated. Additional off-targeting is achieved by siRNAs engaging Toll-like receptors in immune cells, and triggering of interferon responses. A chapter is devoted to this problem with recommended strategies to abrogate interferon responses.

Overall, this volume covers the major areas of siRNA application to date. The authors of each chapter are experts in the respective topic area of the chapter, so the reader should gain valuable insight and information about the promises and pitfalls of RNAi. It is rather amazing that only 12 years ago the scientific world had no clue that such a powerful, sequence specific mechanism of gene regulation existed, yet already many clinical trials are well underway employing RNAi triggers. This volume captures the excitement and momentum of the field of siRNA applications, and should serve a useful purpose in years to come.

JOHN J. ROSSI

Duarte, CA
July 2010

PART I

BIOLOGY OF RNA INTERFERENCE

CHAPTER 1

RNA INTERFERENCE: WHAT IS IT?

JAMES A. BIRCHLER

WHAT IS RNAi?

In its most simple incarnation, it is the technique in which double-stranded RNA (dsRNA) is used to target the destruction of the homologous messenger RNA (mRNA). The first indication that such was the case involved studies of the use of antisense RNA to block the translation of specific proteins in the nematode *Caenorhabditis elegans* [1]. The concept at the time was that the introduction of antisense RNA would show base pair complementarity to the mRNA and block the progression of translation. This technique had shown some level of success in a variety of species. Interestingly, with the use of a control of the sense RNA, the same level of inhibition of protein synthesis was achieved as using the antisense. Thus, the technique of RNA interference (RNAi) was born.

Shortly thereafter, the basis of the effectiveness of both sense and antisense RNAs for RNA silencing became known [2]. This seminal contribution established that the active ingredient in RNAi was indeed a dsRNA and that the direct usage of dsRNA was very effective in eliminating the homologous mRNA. This realization ignited great interest in the use of RNAi as a reverse genetic technique throughout eukaryotic organisms.

While the technique of RNAi caused a revolution in genetics, we should drop back and review a body of work that preceded its development and that we now understand is related in mechanism. This work involves gene silencing by the introduction of transgenes into various plant species. The first example involved antibiotic resistance genes transformed into tobacco [3]. When one transgene was introduced its expression was robust. A second antibiotic resistance gene was transformed and found to be well expressed. Both

RNA Interference: Application to Drug Discovery and Challenges to Pharmaceutical Development, Edited by Paul H. Johnson
Copyright © 2011 John Wiley & Sons, Inc.

types used the same promoter. When the two transgenes were crossed together into the same plants, they both became inactive. Subsequent outcrossing to separate the two types of transgenes resulted in the recovery of the activity of both in the following generation. This type of transgene silencing was established to work at the transcriptional level.

At about the same time, experiments were underway in two laboratories to attempt to make petunia flowers darker than normal by adding an extra copy of the chalcone synthase gene, which encodes the first step of anthocyanin pigment biosynthesis, by transformation of petunias [4, 5]. However, the result found was that the extra copy of the chalcone synthase gene produced white flowers rather than darker ones. This phenomenon was referred to as cosuppression and was found to operate at the posttranscriptional level.

As the literature developed about cosuppression and additional examples were described, it was realized that a similar mechanism was operative against many plant viruses. Such viruses typically have an RNA genome and it was demonstrated that transgenes expressing a homologous RNA would serve to target the viral RNA for destruction [6].

Thus, the concept arose that this process was a defense mechanism against transposable elements and viruses [7]. Indeed, the virulence genes of plant viruses were found to inhibit the process of posttranscriptional silencing [8]. This fact strengthens the argument that host cells use this silencing mechanism against viruses and that viruses have evolved ways to circumvent such silencing. RNAi as a viral defense has also been observed in the animal kingdom [9].

After the discovery that RNAi had a basis in dsRNA, elegant experiments were performed that produced dsRNA homologous to promoters of the original transcriptionally silenced antibiotic resistance genes [10]. The formation of these RNAs was effective in silencing the target transgene. However, when separated during meiotic segregation, the transgene could regain its activity. The demonstration that dsRNA was involved with transcriptional transgene silencing drew a connection between the two types of silencing. If aberrant RNAs were produced with homology to the promoter, then transcriptional silencing would result whereas aberrant RNAs with homology to mRNAs would produce posttranscriptional silencing.

Transgene cosuppression was found in *Drosophila*, which extended this type of silencing to the animal kingdom [11, 12]. A hybrid transgene with the promoter from the *white* eye color gene was fused to the structural portion of the *Alcohol dehydrogenase* gene showed successively less expression with increased copy number. In this case, the silencing was not as strong as usually found in plants but was progressively stronger with increased number of transgenes. The transgenes that were silenced became associated with the Polycomb repressive complex of chromatin proteins implying a transcriptional level silencing, which was later directly confirmed.

The silencing of the *Drosophila* I retroelement, which is responsible for one type of hybrid dysgenesis, possesses many characteristics of a similar mechanism to cosuppresion in that the silencing is homology dependent [13, 14]. Transgenes of a portion of the element are capable of silencing all copies in the genome. The ability to silence is transmitted only through the maternal parent to the progeny—a characteristic that is similar to the process of hybrid dysgenesis.

The posttranscriptional basis of cosuppression suggested that an RNA moiety was involved in recognizing the homologous RNAs for destruction. A search for the entity involved led to the discovery of very small RNAs that were a mere 21–23 base pairs (bp) in length [15]. This discovery together with a developing literature about RNAi inspired biochemical studies of the molecular mechanism.

In *C. elegans* and plants, the RNAi process can spread through the organism in a systemic manner [16,17]. The small RNAs likely act as primers to serve as a substrate with the homologous mRNA for RNA-dependent RNA polymerase to generate additional quantities of dsRNAs that then are acted upon by Dicer. This forms a self-perpetuating cascade that can continue via spread through the organism and at least in *C. elegans* into the next generation [18]. Such systemic spread has not been observed in *Drosophila* or mammals [19].

Much of the biochemistry of RNAi has been performed using *Drosophila* extracts. The enzyme that catalyzes the conversion of dsRNAs to single-stranded short interfering RNAs was sought. This protein was identified and was referred to as Dicer, a ribonuclease III type enzyme [20]. Further analysis of the machinery involved led to the description of the RNA interference silencing complex, which incorporates the small RNAs as guides to target the destruction of homologous mRNAs [21–27]. Parallel studies identified several genes that were required for RNAi processes, which include several RNA helicases and members of the Argonaute family of proteins. The Argonaute family of proteins supplies the "slicer function" to cleave the mRNA [28].

Further connections between the small RNA silencing machinery and transcriptional silencing were observed in *Drosophila* and fission yeast. The Polycomb-dependent transgene gene silencing in flies was established to act on the transcriptional level via run-on transcription assays [29]. A separate type of transgene silencing was also described for *Drosophila* that was post-transcriptional, namely, for a dosage series of the full-length *Alcohol dehydrogenase* gene [29]. Both types of silencing were blocked by the piwi mutation, which encodes an Argonaute family protein. The transcriptional silencing was also partially blocked by another Argonaute mutation, aubergine.

In fission yeast, the centromere repeats are silenced by the RNAi machinery [30]. In this species, there is only a single Dicer, RNA-dependent RNA polymerase and Argonaute, which facilitated the analysis. The silencing machinery generates small RNAs, which attract the histone methyltransferase that methylates lysine 9 of histone 3 (H3-K9). This modification serves to foster silenced chromatin by attracting Swi6, the yeast homologue of Heterochromatin Protein 1. In *Drosophila*, genes required for RNAi in embryos [31] suppress heterochromatic silencing and reduce the histone modifications of H3-K9 [32].

Transcriptional silencing in fission yeast is associated with a separate protein effector complex referred to as the RITS complex [33]. Furthermore, interaction with RNA polymerase II is implicated in that mutations in the largest and second largest subunit of polII disrupt the formation of small RNAs involved with centromeric silencing [34]. Indeed in plants, a separate RNA polymerase has evolved that is required for silencing functions [35–37].

While Dicer is involved with the production of small interfering RNAs (siRNAs), other classes of small RNAs, studied most thoroughly from the germline of flies and mammals, are generated in a Dicer-independent mechanism [38–40]. These RNAs are referred to as piRNAs because they are associated with the Argonaute family protein, piwi, or its mammalian homologues. The Argonaute family of proteins possess a "slicer" function capable of endonucleolytic cleavage of RNA [39,40]. The piRNAs are slightly larger than siRNAs being about 24 bp in length. The piRNAs are heavily involved with the control of transposons in the germline but other classes of genes have also been found among the piRNA sequences [41–46]. Interestingly, there are "loci" in *Drosophila* that consist of retrotransposon fragments that are transcribed and feed into the metabolism of piRNAs that act to silence the homologous transposons [40].

While the piRNAs are presumed to operate posttranscriptionally and mainly in the germline, numerous reports of mutant effects on chromatin level phenomena have been made for the gene products involved with piRNAs. These include transcriptional transgene silencing [29], heterochromatic silencing [32], pairing sensitive silencing [47,48], chromatin insulator function [49], nucleolar integrity [50], centromere function [51], and telomere chromatin [52]. The full understanding of the function of the Argonaute family and its involvement in Dicer-dependent and -independent small RNA biology is not yet understood.

In addition to the siRNA and piRNAs, a third major class of small RNAs are called microRNAs (miRNAs) [53–55]. These originate from endogenous loci that have a foldback structure interrupted by a spacer region. These small RNAs function to block the translation of mRNAs with which they share close but not identical homology [56]. In some cases, they serve to trigger the destruction of the mRNA. Thus, they act as a modulation mechanism for gene expression that is posttranscriptional. In vertebrates, the miRNAs are generated by the same Dicer enzyme as siRNAs given that there is only one such enzyme encoded in the genome [57]. Because miRNAs are the prevalent small RNA in mammals, it was once thought that no endogenous siRNAs were produced, but recent deep sequencing projects have found them, thus illustrating an overlapping enzyme specificity. However, in *Drosophila*, there are two Dicer genes with a diverged preference for generating either miRNAs or siRNAs [58].

As the knowledge of small RNA silencing processes continues to grow the involvement in a variety of both posttranscriptional and transcriptional silencing (or activation) processes is increasingly evident. While "RNAi" was originally recognized as a powerful reverse genetic technique, its basis obviously rests on a biological phenomenon that the scientific community has yet to fully grasp. The interrelationship of posttranscriptional and transcriptional silencing mechanisms is far from clear and the occasional overlap of gene products involved with the generation of si, pi, and miRNAs suggests connections that are yet to be revealed [41–46]. The number of chromatin level processes affected by gene products involved with the generation and processing of small RNAs continues to expand suggesting that small RNAs might have quite prevalent roles in many mechanisms in the cell. The vast number of antisense transcripts also suggests a level of gene regulation that is yet to be fully understood [59]. Thus, the phenomenon of RNAi as a revolutionary genetic technique is likely a reflection of a much deeper and pervasive RNA biology of which we still have much to learn.

REFERENCES

1. Guo, S. and Kemphues, K. J. (1994). par-1, a gene required for establishing polarity in *C. elegans* embryos, encodes a putative Ser/Thr kinase that is asymmetrically distributed. *Cell* **81**: 611–20.
2. Fire, A., Xu, S., Montgomery, M. K., Kostas, S. A., Driver, S. E., and Mello, C. C. (1998). Potent and specific genetic interference by double-stranded RNA in *Caenorhabditis elegans*. *Nature* **391**: 806–11.
3. Matzke, M. A., Primig, M., Trnovsky, J., and Matzke, A. J. M. (1989). Reversible methylation and inactivation of marker genes in sequentially transformed tobacco plants. *EMBO J* **8**: 643–9.
4. Napoli, C., Lemieux, C., and Jorgenson, R. (1990). Introduction of a chimeric chalcone synthase gene in Petunia results in reversible co-suppression of homologous genes in trans. *Plant Cell* **2**: 279–89.

5. Van Der Krol, A. R., Mur, L. A., Beld, M., Mol, J. N. M., and Stuitje, A. R. (1990). Flavanoid genes in Petunia: addition of a limited number of gene copies may lead to a suppression of gene expression. *Plant Cell* **2**: 291–9.

6. Lindbo, J.A., Silva-Rosales, L., Proebsting, W. M., and Dougherty, W. G. (1993). Induction of a highly specific antiviral state in transgenic plants: implications for regulation of gene expression and virus resistance. *Plant Cell* **5**: 1749–59.

7. Flavell, R. B. (1994). Inactivation of gene expression in plants as a consequence of specific sequence duplication. *Proc Natl Acad Sci USA* **91**: 3490–6.

8. Anandalakshmi, R., Pruss, G. J., Ge, X., Marathe, R., Mallory, A. C., Smith, T. H., and Vance, V. B. (1998). A viral suppressor of gene silencing in plants. *Proc Natl Acad Sci USA* **95**: 13079–84.

9. Li, H., Li, W. X., and Ding, S. W. (2002). Induction and suppression of RNA silencing by an animal virus. *Science* **296**: 1319–21.

10. Mette, M. F., Aufsatz, W., Van Der Winden, J., Matzke, M. A., and Matzke, A. J. (2000). Transcriptional silencing and promoter methylation triggered by double-stranded RNA. *EMBO J* **19**: 5194–201.

11. Pal-Bhadra, M., Bhadra, U., and Birchler, J. A. (1997). Cosuppression in Drosophila: gene silencing of *Alcohol dehydrogenase* by white-Adh transgenes is Polycomb dependent. *Cell* **90**: 479–90.

12. Pal-Bhadra, M., Bhadra, U., and Birchler, J. A. (1999). Cosuppression of non-homologous transgenes in Drosophila involves mutually related endogenous sequences. *Cell* **99**: 35–46.

13. Chaboissier, M. C., Bucheton, A., and Finnegan, D. J. (1998). Copy number control of a transposable element, the I factor, a LINE-like element in Drosophila. *Proc Natl Acad Sci USA* **95**: 11781–85.

14. Jensen, S., Gassama, M. P., and Heidmann, T. (1999). Taming of transposable elements by homology-dependent gene silencing. *Nat Genet* **21**: 209–12.

15. Hamilton, A. J. and Baulcombe, D. C. (1999). A species of small antisense RNA in posttranscriptional gene silencing in plants. *Science* **286**: 950–2

16. Palauqui, J. C., Elmayan, T., Pollien, J. M., and Vaucheret, H. (1997). Systemic acquired silencing: transgene-specific post-transcriptional silencing is transmitted by grafting from silenced stocks to non-silenced scions. *EMBO J* **16**: 4738–45.

17. Tabara, H., Grishok, A., and Mello, C. C. (1998). RNAi in *C. elegans*: soaking in the genome sequence. *Science* **282**: 430–1.

18. Grishok, A., Tabara, H., and Mello, C. C. (2000). Genetic requirements for inheritance of RNAi in *C. elegans*. *Science* **287**: 2494–7.

19. Roignant, J.-Y., Carré, C., Mugat, B., Szymczak, D., Lepesant, J. A., and Antoniewski, C. (2003). Absence of transitive and systemic pathways allows cell-specific and isoform-specific RNAi in Drosophila. *RNA* **9**: 299–308.

20. Bernstein, E., Caudy, A. A., Hammond, S. M., and Hannon, G. J. (2001). Role for a bidentate ribonuclease in the initiation step of RNA interference. *Nature* **409**: 363–6.

21. Caudy, A. A., Ketting, R. F., Hammond, S. M., Denli, A. M., Bathoorn, A. M., Tops, B. B., Silva, J. M., Myers, M. M., Hannon, G. J., and Plasterk, R. H. (2003). A micrococcal nuclease homologue in RNAi effector complexes. *Nature* **425**: 411–4.

22. Caudy, A. A., Myers, M., Hannon, G. J., and Hammond, S. M. (2002). Fragile X-related protein and VIG associate with the RNA interference machinery. *Genes Dev* **16**: 2491–6.

23. Elbashir, S. M., Lendeckel, W., and Tuschl, T. (2001). RNA interference is mediated by 21- and 22-nucleotide RNAs. *Genes Dev* **15**: 188–200.

24. Elbashir, S. M., Martinez, J., Patkaniowska, A., Lendeckel, W., and Tuschl, T. (2001). Functional anatomy of siRNAs for mediating efficient RNAi in *Drosophila melanogaster* embryo lysate. *EMBO J* **20**: 6877–88.

25. Ishizuka, A., Siomi, M. C., and Siomi, H. (2002). A Drosophila fragile X protein interacts with components of RNAi and ribosomal proteins. *Genes Dev* **16**: 2497–508.

26. Tomari, Y., Du, T., Haley, B., Schwarz, D. S., Bennett, R., Cook, H. A., Koppetsch, B. S., Theurkauf, W. E., and Zamore, P. D. (2004). RISC assembly defects in the Drosophila RNAi mutant armitage. *Cell* **116**: 831–41.

27. Tomari, Y., Matranga, C., Haley, B., Martinez, N., and Zamore, P. D. (2004). A protein sensor for siRNA asymmetry. *Science* **306**: 1377–80.

28. Okamura, K., Ishizuka, A., Siomi, H., and Siomi, M. C. (2004). Distinct roles for Argonaute proteins in small RNA-directed RNA cleavage pathways. *Genes Dev* **18**: 1655–66.

29. Pal Bhadra, M., Bhadra, U., and Birchler, J. A. (2002). RNAi related mechanisms affect both transcriptional and post-transcriptional transgene silencing in Drosophila. *Mol Cell* **9**: 315–27.

30. Volpe, T. A., Kidner, C., Hall, I. M., Teng, G., Grewal, S. I., and Martienssen, R. A. (2002). Regulation of heterochromatic silencing and histone H3 lysine-9 methylation by RNAi. *Science* **297**: 1833–7.

31. Kennerdell, J. R., Yamaguchi, S., and Carthew, R. W. (2002). RNAi is activated during Drosophila oocyte maturation in a manner dependent on aubergine and spindle-E. *Genes Dev* **16**: 1884–9.

32. Pal-Bhadra, M., Leibovitch, B. A., Gandhi, S. G., Rao, M., Bhadra, U., Birchler, J. A., and Elgin, S. C. (2004). Heterochromatic silencing and HP1 localization in Drosophila are dependent on the RNAi machinery. *Science* **303**: 669–72.

33. Verdel, A., Jia, S., Gerber, S., Sugiyama, T., Gygi, S., Grewal, S. I., and Moazed, D. (2004). RNAi-mediated targeting of heterochromatin by the RITS complex. *Science* **303**: 672–6.

34. Schramke, V., Sheedy, D. M., Denli, A. M., Bonila, C., Ekwall, K., Hannon, G. J., and Allshire, R. C. (2005). RNA-interference-directed chromatin modification coupled to RNA polymerase II transcription. *Nature* **435**: 1275–9.

35. Onodera, Y., Haag, J. R., Ream, T., Nunes, P. C., Pontes, O., and Pikaard, C. S. (2005). Plant nuclear RNA polymerase IV mediates siRNA and DNA methylation-dependent heterochromatin formation. *Cell* **120**: 613–22.

36. Herr, A. J., Jensen, M. B., Dalmay, T., and Baulcombe, D. C. (2005). RNA polymerase IV directs silencing of endogenous DNA. *Science* **308**: 118–20.

37. Huettel, B., Kanno, T., Daxinger, L., Aufsatz, W., Matzke, A. J., and Matzke, M. (2006). Endogenous targets of RNA-directed DNA methylation and Pol IV in Arabidopsis. *EMBO J* **25**: 2828–36.

38. Vagin, V.V., Sigova, A., Li, C., Seitz, H., Gvozdev, V., and Zamore, P. (2006). A distinct small RNA pathway silences selfish genetic elements in the germline. *Science* **313**: 320–4.

39. Gunawardane, L. S., Saito, K., Nishida, K. M., Miyoshi, K., Kawamura, Y., Nagami, T., Siomi, H., and Siomi, M. C. (2007). A slicer-mediated mechanisms for repeat-associated siRNA 5′ end formation in Drosophila. *Science* **315**: 1587–90.

40. Brennecke, J., Aravin, A. A., Stark, A., Dus, M., Kellis, M., Sachidanandam, R., and Hannon, G. J. (2007). Discrete small RNA-generating loci as master regulators of transposon activity in Drosophila. *Cell* **128**: 1089–103.

41. Ghildiyal, M., Seitz, H., Horwich, M. D., Li, C., Du, T., Lee, S., Xu, J., Kittler, E. L., Zapp, M. L., Weng, Z., and Zamore, P. D. (2008). Endogenous siRNAs derived from transposons and mRNAs in Drosophila somatic cells. *Science* **320**: 1077–81.

42. Czech, B., Malone, C. D., Zhou, R., Stark, A., Schlingeheyde, C., Dus, M., Perrimon, N., Kellis, M., Wohlschlegel, J. A., Sachidanandam, R., Hannon, G. J., and Brennecke, J. (2008). An endogenous small interfering RNA pathway in Drosophila. *Nature* **453**: 798–802.

43. Okamura, K., Chung, W. J., Ruby, J. G., Guo, H., Bartel, D. P., and Lai, E. C. (2008). The Drosophila hairpin RNA pathway generates endogenous short interfering RNAs. *Nature* **453**: 803–6.

44. Kawamura, Y., Saito, K., Kin, T., Ono, Y., Asai, K., Sunohara, T., Okada, T. N., Siomi, M. C., and Siomi, H. (2008). Drosophila endogenous small RNAs bind to Argonaute 2 in somatic cells. *Nature* **453**: 793–7.

45. Tam, O. H., Aravin, A. A., Stein, P., Girard, A., Murchison, E. P., Cheloufi, S., Hodges, E., Anger, M., Sachidanandam, R., Schultz, R. M., and Hannon, G. J. (2008). Pseudogene-derived small interfering RNAs regulate gene expression in mouse oocytes. *Nature* **453**: 534–8.

46. Chung, W.J., Okamura, K., Martin, R., and Lai, E. C. (2008). Endogenous RNA interference provides a somatic defense against Drosophila transposons. *Curr Biol* **18**: 795–802.

47. Pal-Bhadra, M., Bhadra, U., and Birchler, J. A. (2004). Interrelationship of RNA interference and transcriptional gene silencing in Drosophila. *Cold Spring Harb Symp Quant Biol* **69**: 433–8.

48. Grimaud, C., Bantignies, F., Pal-Bhadra, M., Bhadra, U., and Cavalli, G. (2006). RNAi components are required for nuclear clustering of Polycomb Group Response Elements. *Cell* **124**: 957–71.

49. Lei, E. P. and Corces, V. G. (2006). RNA interference machinery influences the nuclear organization of a chromatin insulator. *Nat Genet* **38**: 936–41.

50. Peng, J. C. and Karpen, G. H. (2007). H3K9 methylation and RNA interference regulate nucleolar organization and repeated DNA stability. *Nat Cell Biol* **9**: 25–35.

51. Deshpande, G., Calhoun, G., and Schedl, P. (2005). Drosophila argonaute-2 is required early in embryogenesis for the assembly of centric/centromeric heterochromatin, nuclear division, nuclear migration, and germ-cell formation. *Genes Dev* **19**: 1680–5.

52. Yin, H. and Lin, H. (2007). An epigenetic activation role of Piwi and a Piwi-associated piRNA in Drosophila melanogaster. *Nature* **450**: 3173–9.

53. Lee, R. C., Feinbaum, R. L., and Ambros, V. (1993). The *C. elegans* heterochronic gene lin-4 encodes small RNAs with antisense complementarity to lin-14. *Cell* **75**: 843–54.

54. Wightman, B., Ha, I., and Ruvkun, G. (1993). Posttranscriptional regulation of the heterochronic gene lin-14 by lin-4 mediates temporal pattern formation in *C. elegans*. *Cell* **75**: 855–62.

55. Reinhart, B. J., Slack, F. J., Basson, M., Pasquinelli, A. E., Bettinger, J. C., Rougvie, A. E., Horvitz, H. R., and Ruvkun, G. (2000). The 21-nucleotide let-7 RNA regulates developmental timing in *Caenorhabditis elegans*. *Nature* **403**: 901–6.

56. Grishok, A., Pasquinelli, A. E., Conte, D., Li, N., Parrish, S., Ha, I., Baillie, D. L., Fire, A., Ruvkun, G., and Mello, C. C. (2001). Genes and mechanisms related to RNA interference regulate expression of the small temporal RNAs that control *C. elegans* developmental timing. *Cell* **106**: 23–34.

57. Bernstein, E., Kim, S. Y., Carmell, M. A., Murchison, E. P., Alcorn, H., Li, M. Z., Mills, A. A., Elledge, S. J., Anderson, K. V., and Hannon, G. J. (2003). Dicer is essential for mouse development. *Nat Genet* **35**: 215–7.

58. Lee, Y. S., Nakahara, K., Pham, J. W., Kim, K., He, Z., Sontheimer, E. J., and Carthew, R. W. (2004). Distinct roles for Drosophila Dicer-1 and Dicer-2 in the siRNA/miRNA silencing pathways. *Cell* **117**: 69–81.

59. Carlile, M., Nalbant, P., Preston-Fayers, K., McHaffie, G. S., and Werner, A. (2008). Processing of naturally occurring sense/antisense transcripts of the vertebrate Slc34a gene into short RNAs. *Physiol Genomics* **34**: 95–100.

CHAPTER 2

NUCLEIC ACIDS AS REGULATORY MOLECULES

FAQING HUANG, C. J. YU, and YANLIN GUO

2.1 GENE EXPRESSION AND ITS REGULATION

2.1.1 Genes, Chromosomes, and Genomes

The basic nature of the gene was defined by Mendel more than a century ago. Summarized in his two laws—the Law of Segregation and the Law of Independent Assortment, the gene was recognized as a "particulate factor" that passes unchanged from parent to progeny. In the 1940s, it was discovered that DNA (deoxyribonucleic acid) is the carrier of genetic information, thereby directly linking genes with DNA. Following the discovery of the double-stranded DNA (dsDNA) structure by Watson and Crick in 1953, it became clear that genetic information may be stored in DNA in the form of specific sequences of nucleotides (A, G, C, and T) and that genetic information can be transmitted by semiconservative replication through Watson–Crick base pairing. The four normal nucleotides are made of two different types—purines (A & G) and pyrimidines (C & T). Today, it is firmly established that, as the genetic material, genes on DNA molecules provide a blueprint that directs the developmental processes of cellular organisms and ultimately controls all aspects of cellular activities. At the molecular level, a gene is defined as a segment of DNA that encodes the information required to direct the synthesis of a gene product—either a particular protein or just an RNA molecule.

DNA can be a very long molecule. For instance, the total length of nuclear DNA in each human cell is about 2 m, while the diameter of the cell nucleus is only 5–8 μm. In order to ensure the equal distribution of DNA between both daughter cells during mitosis and to avoid damage of DNA

RNA Interference: Application to Drug Discovery and Challenges to Pharmaceutical Development, Edited by Paul H. Johnson
Copyright © 2011 John Wiley & Sons, Inc.

molecules, DNA molecules form complexes with proteins and are orderly packaged into chromosomes in eukaryotic cells. Every eukaryotic species has a characteristic number of chromosomes in each cell nucleus. For example, human somatic cells (all body cells except the reproductive cells) contain 23 pairs of chromosomes. Each chromosome contains one DNA molecule that carries several hundred to a few thousand genes. The complete set of genetic information carried by DNA in chromosomes of an organism is called its genome. The complete genome sequences of several model organisms including humans have been deciphered as a result of the Human Genome Project. Genome sequencing projects have revealed that in higher organisms there is a considerable amount of DNA that does not encode proteins. Therefore, the noncoding DNA is commonly referred to as nonfunctional DNA. For instance, the human genome consists of $\sim$3.1 billion base pairs. Less than 2% of the genome actually codes for genes, which corresponds to 20,000–25,000 proteins. It is apparent that, in order to selectively express these genes from the vast majority of nonfunctional DNA in the genome and to express different genes differentially, cells must have a well-controlled gene expression system.

2.1.2   An Overview of Gene Expression

One of the central questions of molecular cell biology is how the genetic information encoded in a gene is translated into specific cellular activities. In other words, how does the information encoded by a gene contribute its particular role to the properties and functions of the cell? To exert a gene's function, the information encoded by the nucleotide sequence of a gene is used to yield a specific gene product—a functional protein or a functional noncoding RNA [1]. In this chapter, we will limit our discussion to protein as the gene product. In most cases, it is the protein that actually performs the task of that particular gene in the cell. In multicellular organisms, each cell type is programmed to express specific subsets of protein-encoding genes that determine the biochemical and phenotypic properties of that cell type. Whether it is a neuron for the transmission of neuronal signals or a lymphocyte for immune responses. Although differences between a neuron and a lymphocyte are extreme in both morphology and function, they still have the same DNA. Therefore, cells of an organism differ not because they contain different genes, but rather because they have turned on/off a specific set of genes for their specialized cellular functions.

Most cells in multicellular organisms are developmentally programmed to perform their specialized cellular functions. However, they must also be able to alter their patterns of protein synthesis to meet the needs of cells in response to environmental changes. For instance, the synthesis of several proteins is dramatically increased in liver cells when the cells are exposed to a glucocorticoid hormone. This is because the glucocorticoid is released in the body during starvation and signals the cell the need for increased glucose production. In response to this stimulus, liver cells will turn on a set of genes that are required for the synthesis of glucose from amino acids or other small molecules. This example underscores the basic principle of gene expression in multicellular organisms. Different types of cells must selectively express the genes for their functions, and they must modify the expression patterns of certain genes in response to extracellular signals.

2.1.3   Gene Expression—from Genes to Proteins

The protein-encoding genes of an organism contain all the necessary instruction for protein synthesis. However, DNA itself does not directly participate in protein synthesis. Instead, the information in a gene is converted into the sequence of a messenger RNA (mRNA) in a process called transcription. Transcription is a general term for the DNA-templated synthesis of any RNA (including mRNA, transfer RNA—tRNA, ribosomal—rRNA, and other non-coding RNAs). An mRNA molecule with a defined sequence of A, G, C, and U is a faithful transcript of the DNA sequence of a gene. The mRNA molecule then acts as a template to direct the synthesis of a protein by the protein synthesis machinery—the ribosome (consisting of several rRNAs and tens of ribosomal proteins) through a process known as translation. During translation, tRNAs play important roles as the adapter molecules, specific amino acid carriers, and specific codon recognition. Therefore, the genetic information in the cell is first transcribed from DNA to RNA and then to protein. The entire process of genetic information flow from an information-containing gene to a functional protein product is commonly referred to as gene expression. All cells, from bacteria to human, follow the same pattern of gene expression—this principle is so fundamental that it is called the *central dogma* of molecular biology. However, the central dogma says nothing about the regulation of gene expression. Thus, obvious questions arise as to what determines the types and amounts of the proteins that characterize a particular cell type, or what factors allow the cell to modify the gene expression pattern in response to changes in its environment. These are the central questions of gene expression regulation in current molecular cell biology.

2.1.4   Gene Structure

A eukaryotic gene contains both coding and noncoding regions. The non-coding regions include the promoter, transcriptional regulatory sequences, and polyadenylation signals. The promoter is the sequence where an RNA polymerase and transcription factors bind and start transcription. Transcriptional regulatory sequences—or *cis*-regulatory elements such as enhancers, either distal or proximal to the promoter, are the sequences for the binding of transcription factors that are critical for transcription regulation. The polyadenylation signal encodes for the polyadenylation sequence in the mRNA transcript. In many eukaryotic genes, the sequence of nucleotides that codes for the protein is not continuous; rather, gene sequences are split into segments by noncoding DNA. The DNA segments that do not encode amino acids are called introns, and the coding regions are called exons. Introns may occupy a large portion of a gene sequence. The terms intron and exon are used for both the RNA sequences and the DNA sequences that encode them.

2.1.5 Transcription and RNA Processing

In eukaryotic cells, transcription takes place in the nucleus. During transcription, RNA polymerases and transcription factors initiate the transcription process by binding to the promoter and enhancer of the gene and polymerize ribonucleoside triphosphates (ATP, GTP, CTP, and UTP) complementary to the DNA coding strand. The newly synthesized mRNA is released shortly after RNA polymerase passes the polyadenylation signal sequence. Eukaryotes possess three types of RNA polymerases named I, II, and III. RNA polymerase II is used for mRNA synthesis, while the other two RNA polymerases transcribe rRNA, tRNA, and other RNAs. Transcription is a highly complex process that may involve numerous transcription factors to achieve a desired level of transcription.

Eukaryotic mRNAs have to be transported to the cytoplasm where translation takes place. Primary mRNA (pre-mRNA) transcripts from transcription undergo several modifications in the nucleus to produce functional mRNAs before they are exported to the cytoplasm. These modifications are collectively referred to as RNA processing that usually includes the following: (1) 5' capping—addition of a methylated guanylate (G) cap at the 5' end, (2) 3' polyadenylation (poly(A) tailing)—addition of 100–250 adenylates (A) at the 3' end, and (3) RNA splicing—the process of removing introns and joining exons. It is proposed that 5' capping and 3' poly(A) tailing may facilitate the nuclear export of mature mRNAs and protect them from degradation. RNA splicing is perhaps the most remarkable step of RNA processing by a large complex called the spliceosome that involves a group of small nuclear RNAs (snRNAs). During transcription, RNA polymerase II transcribes both introns and exons from a protein-coding gene. Introns are then precisely cut out from pre-mRNA and exons are correctly joined together, forming an mRNA molecule with a continuous coding sequence.

2.1.6 Translation

Translation is the biosynthesis of a polypeptide using mRNA as a template, a process that takes place on ribosomes. Ribosomes are huge complexes consisting of rRNAs and ribosomal proteins. The ribosome acts as an assembly factory where amino acids are polymerized to form polypeptide chains. During translation, a set of three-consecutive nucleotides on an mRNA molecule, known as a codon, specifies one amino acid. A tRNA molecule brings the specific amino acid to its correct positions through the interaction between the anticodon on the tRNA and a cognate codon on the mRNA.

As in the case of transcription, translation is a complex process that proceeds in an ordered and coordinated manner, including initiation, elongation, and termination phases. It requires the assistance of numerous protein factors at each step. The above discussion represents an oversimplified version of gene expression. The entire process of gene expression in eukaryotic cells is illustrated in Figure 2.1.

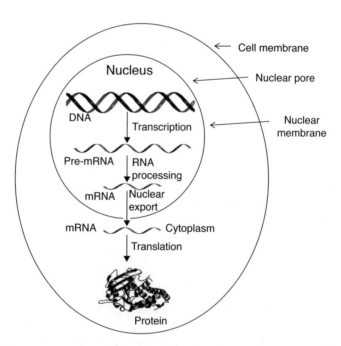

FIGURE 2.1   Processes involved in eukaryotic gene expression. Transcription and RNA processing (splicing, capping, and polyadenylation) occur in the nucleus; translation and posttranscriptional modification (not shown) take place in the cytoplasm.

2.1.7 Regulation of Gene Expression

The primary purpose of gene control in multicellular organisms is to ensure the precise expression of genes in proper cells at the right time during growth and development. Gene expression can be controlled at each level in the pathway from DNA to protein. In principle, gene expression can be regulated by (1) the frequency and the rate of transcription, (2) the processing of pre-mRNA, (3) the nuclear export of mRNA, (4) the stability of mature mRNA, (5) the selective translation of mRNA, and (6) the posttranslational regulation of protein activity and/or stability. At each step, several mechanisms may be involved.

Theoretically, the regulation of gene expression can take place at each of the aforementioned steps; however, control at the transcription level is by far the most important one. Whether a gene in a multicellular organism is expressed in a particular cell is largely a consequence of the initiation of transcription. This is logical because only transcriptional control can ensure that no unnecessary intermediate molecules (pre-mRNA and mRNA) are produced and accumulated. Using mRNA as the intermediate molecule to direct protein synthesis has several advantages for cells. First, it protects the genetic information by avoiding direct use of DNA since its frequent use may cause DNA damage. Second, many copies of an RNA transcript can be made from one gene and multiple copies of a protein can be made simultaneously from an mRNA molecule. Third, transcription and RNA processing provide cells with additional mechanisms for the control of gene expression. Therefore, the assembly of transcription initiation complexes, regulated by transcription factors, is the most critical step in the control of the initiation of transcription, while the processing of pre-mRNA and the stability of mature mRNA are of central importance for the translation step of gene expression.

2.2 ARTIFICIAL MODULATION OF GENE EXPRESSION

2.2.1 An Overview of Artificial Control of Gene Expression

From the above discussion, it is evident that the expression of a gene in the eukaryotic cell requires multiple processes (Figure 2.1) involving transcription (RNA biosynthesis), pre-mRNA processing (splicing, capping, and polyadenylation), nuclear export of mRNA to the cytoplasm, translation (polypeptide biosynthesis), and posttranslational modifications of the protein products. Interference with any of these processes may lead to a significant change of cellular protein concentrations. Therefore, to artificially regulate the expression activity of a specific gene, an exogenous agent may be introduced into the cell to block one or more of these processes through specific interactions with a target or targets in the gene expression pathway.

Traditionally, small molecules including synthetic organic chemicals, analogs of small biomolecules (sugars, amino acids, nucleobases, nucleosides, metabolic intermediates, etc.), antibiotics, hormones, and small peptides are frequently used to modulate gene expression activities either in basic biological studies or in clinical applications. This situation is well reflected by the fact that the vast majority of clinical drugs on the market are based on small molecules.

Although nucleic acids (DNA and RNA) were recognized as important biomolecules in cellular function early in the history of biosciences, their functional roles were falsely limited to information coding (DNA) and protein biosynthesis (rRNA, mRNA, and tRNA). Since protein seemed to be capable of performing any biological task, it was generally believed that the proteins were the sole class of molecules responsible for the extraordinarily complex biological activities. With the recent advancements in nucleic acid research, however, nucleic acids (especially RNA) have been increasingly recognized as very capable and versatile molecules that possess great potential to act as effective agents for regulating gene expression. In fact, different nucleic acids-based technologies are now available to allow precise control of a specific gene expression level through more than one mechanism along the gene expression pathway.

Figure 2.2 schematically summarizes currently available nucleic acid-based technologies for artificial regulation of gene expression and their mechanisms of action. Since all the technologies result in lowering cellular protein levels, they all belong to the loss-of-function approach, that is, downregulation of gene expression. In contrast, methods of introducing exogenous genes into the cell, such as those achieved through gene therapy, represent the gain-of-function approach, because additional protein molecules are expressed.

The gene regulation technologies depicted in Figure 2.2 can be divided into three categories—antigene, anti-RNA, and antiprotein, according to their targets of action. The antigene approach employs a mechanism to block RNA transcription from its gene (DNA). A triplex-forming oligonucleotide (TFO) may be used to bind a specific double-stranded region of DNA and form a triple helix, blocking transcription initiation and/or elongation. Alternatively, an exogenous DNA or RNA decoy may be introduced into the cell to sequestrate transcription factors that are required for transcription initiation. An anti-RNA effect may be achieved through different mechanisms—pre-mRNA splicing inhibition by antisense oligonucleotides (ASOs), blocking of mRNA nuclear export to the cytoplasm by an RNA decoy, inhibition of translation through DNA–RNA heteroduplex formation by ASOs, ASO-activated mRNA degradation by RNase H, mRNA cleavage by ribozymes (Rz) and DNAzymes

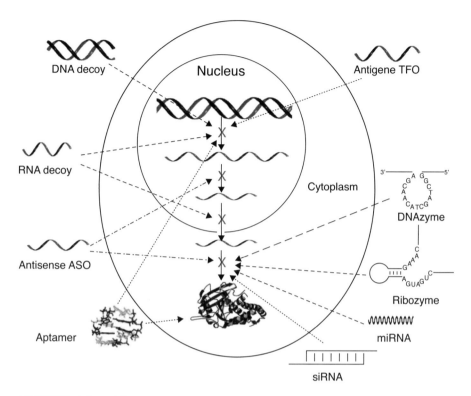

FIGURE 2.2 Different strategies and targeting mechanisms for artificial modulation of gene expression. Double-stranded DNA decoys, single-stranded RNA decoys, DNA/RNA aptamers, and antigene TFOs (triplex-forming oligonucleotides) may be used to block transcription by interacting with either transcription factors or double-stranded DNA. Antisense oligonucleotides (ASOs) may interfere with RNA splicing. An RNA decoy can impair nuclear export of RNA. ASOs, ribozymes, DNAzymes, miRNAs, and siRNAs represent commonly used strategies to target mRNAs, leading to lower levels of cellular proteins through reduced translation. Although RNA/DNA aptamers may be used to target either DNA or RNA, proteins are by far the most favored targets for gene regulation by aptamers. All strategies share the same ultimate results—reduction of cellular concentrations of specific gene products, with no or minimal effects on the expression of other genes.

(Dz), and small interfering (siRNA)- or microRNA (miRNA)-induced mRNA degradation. Finally, RNA/DNA aptamers may be used to remove proteins from cellular activities through specific aptamer–protein binding with high affinities.

These nucleic acid-based gene control technologies are revolutionizing the ways by which scientists conduct research—identifying/validating protein targets and mapping molecular interaction pathways. In a different arena, these technologies are being assessed and exploited for their potentials to act as pharmaceutical agents to fight human diseases. In the rest of this chapter, we will briefly describe the principle of each technology, its applications in gene expression control, and chemistries required for its successful applications.

2.2.2 Antisense Technology

The concept of using ASOs as therapeutic agents to interfere with gene expression was introduced by Zamecnic and Stepheson in 1978 in their pioneering work of inhibition of Rous sarcoma virus infection in chicken fibroblasts by an antisense tridecamer AATGGTAAAATGG [2, 3]. ASOs are small single-stranded deoxyribonucleotides containing ~20 nucleotides (nt). The unique sequence of an ASO allows specific target RNA binding through complementary Watson–Crick base pairing. Upon hybridization with its target mRNA, an ASO may lead to specific inhibition of gene expression by one or more of the three different mechanisms (Figure 2.3)—target mRNA cleavage by the endogenous endonuclease RNase H through activation of the enzyme by the formation of an RNA–ASO heteroduplex [4, 5], prevention of translation by steric blocking [6, 7], and inhibition of pre-mRNA splicing [8, 9]. While mRNA cleavage by ASO-activated RNase H is believed to be the major

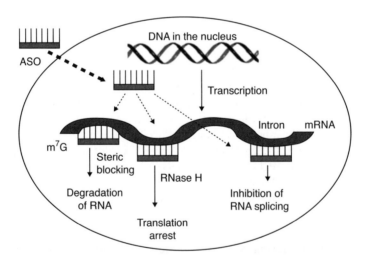

FIGURE 2.3   Three major action mechanisms of ASOs. When an ASO is taken up by the cell, it can hybridize to its target RNA. Formation of an RNA–ASO heteroduplex may induce (1) activation of the ubiquitous cellular RNase H, leading to selective degradation of the target mRNA, (2) steric blocking, resulting in translation arrest, and/or (3) inhibition of pre-mRNA splicing. In principle, ASOs may be used to selectively knock down any target gene expression.

mechanism for downregulation of the target gene expression by most types of ASOs, translation blocking by ASO can be significant as well. Translation blocking may play a major role in gene downregulation for some chemically modified ASOs. On the other hand, inhibition of pre-mRNA splicing by ASOs represents minor cases of ASO applications. Whatever the mechanisms of ASO action, an effective ASO should reduce the mRNA level of a specific gene, leading to reduced biosynthesis of a target protein.

During the past two decades, the perceived high specificity of ASO hybridization with a target RNA sequence, coupled with general availability of synthetic ASOs, has made the antisense strategy an attractive technology to regulate the expression of specific genes that are implicated in diseases, such as cancers and viral infections. Numerous research papers have been published on the subject of gene regulation by ASOs. A recent search of PubMed (http://www.ncbi.nlm.nih.gov/entrez/query.fcgi?CMD=search&DB=pubmed) by the keywords "antisense oligonucleotide" generated a list of ~13,000 publications.

Inhibition of bcl-2 by ASOs   Programmed cell death or apoptosis is a common mechanism used by organisms to remove unwanted cells (such as severely damaged cells). Apoptosis plays an important role in development and the maintenance of homeostasis. Interference with the normal apoptotic process may lead to the development of cancer. The bcl-2 (**B**-**c**ell **l**ymphoma/leukemia-2) protein is one of the regulators of apoptosis in a variety of tissues. Activation of the *bcl-2* gene by the t(14;18) chromosomal translocation in B-cell lymphoma has been implicated in the development of cancers such as breast, prostate, lung carcinomas, and melanoma. Using two versions of a 20-nt ASO (normal phosphodiester backbone (PO) and nuclease-resistant phosphorothioate backbone (PS) with the sequence 5′-CAGCGTGCGCCATCCTTCCC) targeting the start codon region of the human bcl-2 mRNA, Reed et al. [10] demonstrated that both PO and PS ASOs could effectively inhibit the growth of human 697 leukemia cells. Quantitative immunofluorescence analysis showed specific inhibition of bcl-2 expression by both ASOs without affecting expression of HLA-DR (a **m**ajor **h**istocompatibility **c**omplex, MHC, cell surface receptor encoded by the **h**uman **l**eukocyte **a**ntigen class II genes) and other control antigens. The sequence-specificity was further confirmed by a sense oligonucleotide control that showed no effects on bcl-2 expression and cell growth. Similarly, Kitada et al. [11] showed that an ASO (5′-TCTCCCAGCGTGCGCCAT) complementary to the first six codons (ATGGCGCACGCTGGGAGA, the underlined ATG is the initiation codon) of the human bcl-2 mRNA could completely abolish bcl-2 protein translation in a cell free system derived from reticulocyte lysates. Sequence specificity by the ASO was demonstrated by a scrambled oligonucleotide control that resulted in no change in bcl-2 protein expression. Furthermore, the human ASO did not affect the translation of chicken bcl-2, whose first six codons (<u>A</u>TGGC<u>**T**</u>CAC<u>**CC**</u>CGGGAGA, the underlined bold T, C, C are changes from human bcl-2 mRNA) contain three mismatches. Introduction of the ASO to either the NIH-3T3 fibroblast cell line that had been transfected with a recombinant retrovirus containing the human bcl-2 cDNA or the t(14;18)-containing lymphoma cell line SU-DHL-4 resulted in concentration-dependent reductions in the 26-kD human bcl-2 protein analyzed by immunoblotting, while the scrambled oligonucleotide had no effect. At 200 μM, 84–95% inhibition of bcl-2 protein expression was obtained by the ASO, while little effect was observed on the levels of other mitochondrial control proteins, indicating that the inhibitory effects were specifically caused by an antisense mechanism.

Inhibition of Protein Kinase C Alpha   The <u>p</u>rotein <u>k</u>inase <u>C</u> (PKC) family is composed of a number of serine/threonine kinase isoenzymes. These isoenzymes play important roles in cell signal transduction in the regulation of cell cycle, apoptosis, proliferation, invasion, and differentiation in both cancer cells and normal cells. Protein kinase C alpha (PKCα) is a phospholipid-dependent serine/threomine kinase that is involved in signal transduction in response to growth factors, hormones, and neurotransmitters. Altered PKCα expression has been implicated in carcinogenesis and tumor progression.

In a study to demonstrate the effect of ASO on PKCα protein expression in human lung carcinoma (A549) cells [12], multiple ASOs were used to target different sites on PKCα mRNA, including the 5′-untranslated region (5′-UTR), the AUG translation initiation codon region, different regions of the open reading frame (ORF), and the 3′-untranslated region (3′-UTR). All ASOs were nuclease-resistant phosphorothioate oligodeoxynucleotides. The study found considerable differences in the effects of ASOs to inhibit PKCα protein expression that was analyzed by immunoblotting. The most effective ASOs were those that targeted the AUG initiation codon region and the 3′-UTR, while the ORF sequence represented the least effective target for ASOs. An ASO (named ISIS 3522 with the sequence 5′-GGGACCATGGCTGACGTTTT) targeting the AUG initiation codon region represented one of the most potent phosphorothioate oligodeoxynucleotides, reducing PKCα protein levels by 60%. Analysis of PKCα mRNA by Northern blotting revealed a reduction of PKCα mRNA by 80–90%, suggesting that the ASO was most likely acting through the mechanism of mRNA cleavage by RNase H upon mRNA-ASO heteroduplex formation. Through kinetic analysis, it was shown that ASO-induced PKCα mRNA reduction was both rapid (~70% of maximal inhibition occurred within the first 4 h after ASO treatment) and reversible (returned to normal mRNA levels within 72 h after ASO treatment). Repeated applications of the ASO every 48 h were sufficient to maintain 80–90% reduced PKCα mRNA levels and a stable state of reduced PKCα protein by 70–80%. Furthermore, the study showed that the ASO inhibited only PKCα expression without affecting the cellular levels of PKCδ, PKCε, and PKCζ, indicating that the antisense effect was specific for the target sequence.

ASO Specificity and Design   As shown in Figure 2.3, inhibition of protein expression by ASOs may be achieved by three different mechanisms. Early experiments seemed to indicate that ASOs were the "magic bullets" for targeting specific genes. In the early 1990s, the idea of using antisense technology for clinical applications became the basis for the emergence of a number of companies with the optimism of transforming ASOs into therapeutic agents. However, the faith in ASOs soon began to fade because of irreproducibility of and disappointments in numerous *in vitro* and *in vivo* experiments using ASOs. Confidence in ASOs emerging as therapeutic agents tumbled in the late 1990s and hit the bottom late in 1999, when the ASO ISIS 2302 for treating Crohn's disease failed in the human phase 3 clinical trials.

One of the observed problems was that ASO-based therapeutics seemed to work too well and were effective for a variety of diseases ranging from viral infection to tumors. However, thorough investigations indicated that most ASO effects were primarily due to the nonspecific boosting of the immune system by the CpG sequence [13] in ASOs, rather than to specific knockdown of the targeted gene. Another problem was that different ASOs against a specific target mRNA might have varying efficiencies in inhibiting target gene expression. Therefore, rational ASO design is essential to achieving the desired effectiveness and specificity. The following four parameters should be considered in designing ASOs [14]: (i) secondary structure prediction of the target mRNA, (ii) identification of preferable local RNA secondary structures, (iii) motif searching and GC content calculation, and (vi) binding energy ($\Delta G°$) prediction. Accurate secondary structure prediction of target mRNA is critical for designing effective ASOs. Unfortunately, there is no truly reliable algorithm to predict mRNA secondary structures and folding patterns. The following two programs are the most commonly used: the *m*fold program (http://www.bioinfo.rpi.edu/applications/mfold) that predicts all possible optimal and suboptimal structures of a particular RNA sequence [15] and the *s*fold program (http://sfold.wadsworth.org/cgi-bin/index.pl) that predicts only the best secondary structures [16]. Using both programs may help to determine the most frequently occurring secondary structure(s) of a target mRNA. Effective ASO design should focus on the regions where mRNA is accessible for Watson–Crick base pairing. The accessible regions typically include both $3'$ and $5'$ ends, internal loops, and hairpins and bulges of 10 or more consecutive nucleotides. In conjunction with the *m*fold program, another program, MAST (mRNA Accessible Site Tagging) (http://www.bioit.org.cn/ao/targetfinder.htm), may be used to facilitate ASO site selection.

Motifs and GC content may significantly affect ASO activities. Experimental data indicate that ASOs containing CCAC, TCCC, ACTC, GCCA, and CTCT motifs can enhance gene expression inhibition, while GGGG, ACTG, AAA and TAA motifs may reduce the effectiveness of ASOs. It turns out that the target mRNA-cutting activity of RNase H depends on the sequence and thermodynamic stability of mRNA–ASO heteroduplexes [17]. Effective ASOs (20 nt) containing ≥ 11 G/C residues are effective, while ASOs with ≤ 9 G/C residues are associated with poor inhibition of gene expression. ASO binding energy ($\Delta G°$) may be predicted by a program called "OligoWalk" from the package RNA Structure 3.5 (http://rna.urmc.rochester.edu/cgi-bin/server_exe/oligowalk/oligowalk_form.cgi). For a potent ASO, the $\Delta G°$ of an mRNA–ASO heteroduplex should be ≤ -8 kcal/mol and the $\Delta G°$ of the ASO–ASO interaction should be ≥ -1.1 kcal/mol.

Unmethylated CpG dinucleotides have been observed to activate strong immune responses by Toll-like receptor-9 in immune cells, resulting in non-specific expression inhibition of a broad range of genes. The immunostimulatory effects of CpG can be further amplified when the CpG is flanked by two 5' purines and two 3' pyrimidines (such as AACGTT). Therefore, in designing effective ASOs with high target specificities, CpG motifs should be avoided.

Chemical Modifications and Nuclease Stability An unmodified oligonucleotide can be degraded quickly by numerous cellular nucleases. In addition, the net negative charges of an unmodified oligonucleotide prevent the internalization of ASOs across the cell membrane. In order to develop ASOs as effective regulators for gene expression, various modifications of ASO backbones have been performed to increase nuclease stability, enhance circulation time, increase affinity and potency, and decrease nonspecific toxicity, as shown in Figure 2.4.

First-Generation Modification Phosphorothioate (PS) ASOs are considered the first generation of modified oligonucleotide backbones, where the nonbridging oxygen is replaced by a sulfur atom. This modification substantially increases the stability of ASOs against nucleases. In addition, PS ASOs support recognition by RNase H for target mRNA cleavage and prolong the circulation time of ASOs because of their binding to serum proteins. However, PS ASOs have some drawbacks, such as lower binding affinity to target mRNAs ($\Delta T_m = -0.5$ to $-1°C$ per modification) and nonsequence specific interactions with the cell surface and intracellular proteins (i.e., stickiness),

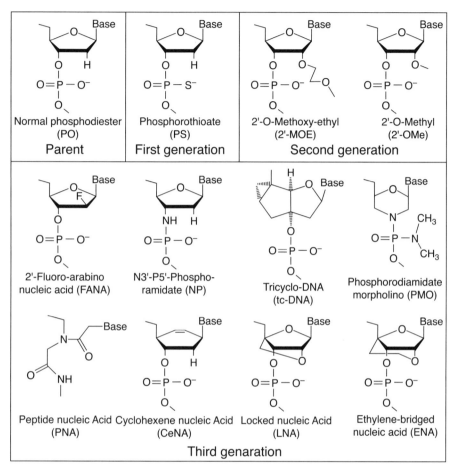

FIGURE 2.4   Structures of some modified oligonucleotide backbones.

which can lead to significant side effects. In spite of these disadvantages, PS ASOs are still the most popular antisense molecules that are widely used in basic research and pharmaceutical development.

Second-Generation Modification   In order to overcome the drawbacks of PS ASOs, modifications at the 2′ position of the ribose ring have led to two types of sugar-modified nucleotides, 2′-MOE (2′-O-methoxy-ethyl) and 2′-OMe (2′-O-methyl) (Figure 2.4), which have been used for the construction of second-generation ASOs. Although the introduction of either 2′-MOE or 2′-OMe greatly enhances the binding affinity ($\Delta T_m = +2°C$ per modification) and the nuclease stability of ASOs, fully substituted ASOs by either 2′-MOE or 2′-OMe result in loss of the ability to recruit RNase H for cleavage of the target mRNA in the mRNA–ASO heteroduplexes. To

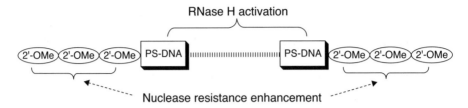

FIGURE 2.5   Structure of a 2′-OMe gapmer.

circumvent this shortcoming, gapmers can be designed and synthesized, as shown in Figure 2.5. The central region contains about 10 PS nucleotides, and both ends are attached to five 2′-MOE or 2′-OMe modified nucleotides. Such chimeric gapmers maintain the enzymatic activity of RNase H, while enhancing the binding affinity and nuclease resistance of ASOs.

Third-Generation Modification   To further improve the properties of ASOs as therapeutics, various modifications on either the phosphodiester backbone and/or the sugar have been made to yield the third-generation ASOs. Among them, 2′-fluoro-arabino nucleic acids (FANAs) and cyclohexene nucleic acids (CeNAs) support the activation of RNase H for the enzymatic cleavage of target mRNA. Peptide nucleic acids (PNAs) represent a class of molecules that is the result of a marriage between peptides and nucleic acids. With a neutral peptide backbone, PNAs can strongly hybridize to DNA or RNA with a high specificity via Watson–Crick base paring. PNAs can even replace one strand of DNA–DNA duplexes by helix invasion due to their greater binding affinities. Since PNAs are neither peptides nor nucleic acids, they are stable against both nucleases and peptidases. On the other hand, PNAs have poor aqueous solubility due to their lack of charges. PNAs do not induce RNase H activity. The action mechanism for PNAs as ASOs is thought to be mainly mediated via steric blocking, resulting in translational arrest. Although extensive studies have shown the effectiveness of PNAs in gene silencing *ex vivo*, the *in vivo* efficacy of PNAs remains to be seen.

Phosphorodiamidate morpholinos (PMOs) are DNA-like oligomers with six-membered morpholino rings and neutral phosphorodiamidate linkages. They have better water solubility than PNAs. Modification by phosphorodi-amidate morpholino also confers the resulting ASOs excellent resistance to nucleases in biological fluids. Like PNAs, PMOs do not activate RNase H for the enzymatic degradation of target mRNA. Because of the poor cellular uptake by mammalian cells, arginine-rich peptides (ARP) are frequently used as delivery vehicles to carry PMOs across the cellular membrane. Antisense efficacy of PMOs in animal models and human clinical trials has been demonstrated.

Locked nucleic acids (LNAs) and the more recent ethylene-bridged nucleic acids (ENAs) have similar structures, in which 2′-O and 4′-C are tethered by either a methylene (strained five-membered ring) or an ethylene bridge (less strained six-membered ring). LNAs or ENAs display very high binding affinity toward RNA ($\Delta T_m = +3$ to $+8°C$ per modification). Like other 2′-modified oligonucleotides, neither LNAs nor ENAs can activate RNase H. However, a similar gapmer strategy as that described in Figure 2.5 can be used to increase their potency for gene downregulation.

Pharmacokinetics and Toxicities of ASOs   All three generation ASOs have gone through preclinical toxicity studies, and some of the promising ASOs are under clinical development for humans. In general, ASOs produce dose-dependent, transient and mild to moderate toxicities, as demonstrated in rodents, primates and humans. The most common acute toxicities associated with the administration of ASOs are the activation of the transient complement cascade and the inhibition of the clotting cascade. These toxic effects are associated with ASO backbone chemistries and are independent of ASO sequences.

ASOs as Therapeutics in Human Clinical Trials   It has been almost three decades since the introduction of antisense strategy for downregulation of gene expression. Extensive research and development efforts from both academia and the pharmaceutical industry, plus billions of dollars in spending, have resulted in only one antisense drug (Vitravene) that was approved by the US FDA in 1998 for treating cytomegalovirus (CMV)-induced retinitis in AIDS patients. Vitravene remains the only antisense drug on the market. With an annual sale of only $157,000 for ISIS Pharmaceuticals (Carlsbad, US) and Novartis (Basel, Switzerland), it is obvious that antisense-based R&D efforts have yielded very disappointing results. Nevertheless, the concept of gene regulation by ASOs remains alive and it is hoped that more antisense-based therapeutics may emerge from the pipeline in the future. Today, a number of antisense-based agents are in clinical trials for patients with cancer, viral infection, diabetics, autoimmune disorders, and allergic asthma. Table 2.1 lists some promising ASOs in human clinical trials. The majority of the listed antisense drug candidates belong to the first-generation phosphorothioate oligonucleotides.

2.2.3 Downregulation of Gene Expression by TFOs

A third strand oligonucleotide can bind the major groove of a DNA duplex to form a triple helix (Figure 2.6), if certain conditions (such as DNA sequence, ionic strength, and media pH) are met. Formation of DNA triplexes was first

TABLE 2.1 Some ASOs as Therapeutics in Human Clinical Trials.

ASO Name	Company Name	Clinical Stage	Lead Indication	Generation of ASO	Gene Target
Vitravene	Isis Pharmaceuticals	FDA approved	Peripheral CMV retinitis	PS	IE1 and IE2 of HCMV
LRrafAON-ETU	NeoPharm	Phase I	Advanced cancer	PS	c-raf-1
Genasense	Genta Inc.	Phase III	Advanced melanoma	PS	Bcl-2
RESTEN-MP	AVI Biopharm	Phase II	Cardiovascular restenosis	PMO	c-myc
AVI-4126	AVI Biopharm	Phase I	Cancer	PMO	c-myc
OGX-011	OncoGenex Technologies,	Phase II	Lung cancer	2'-MOE	Clusterin
GTI-2040	Lorus Therapeutics	Phase II	Kidney cancer	PS	Ribonucleotide reductase
TPI-ASM8	Topigen Pharmaceuticals	Phase II	Asthma	PS	Cytokine receptors
AP 12009	Antisense Pharma	Phase II	Pancreatic cancer	PS	TGF-β2
Alicaforsen	Isis Pharmaceuticals	Phase II	Ulcerative colitis	PS	ICAM-1
ISIS 301012	Isis Pharmaceuticals	Phase II	High cholesterol	2'-MOE	apoB-100
ISIS 113715	Isis Pharmaceuticals	Phase II	Diabetes	2'-MOE	PTP-1 B
ATL1102	Antisense Therapeutics	Phase II	Multiple sclerosis	2'-OMe	VLA-4
LY2181308	Eli Lilly	Phase I	Cancer	2'-OMe	Survivin
LY2275796	Eli Lilly	Phase I	Cancer	2'-OMe	eIF4E

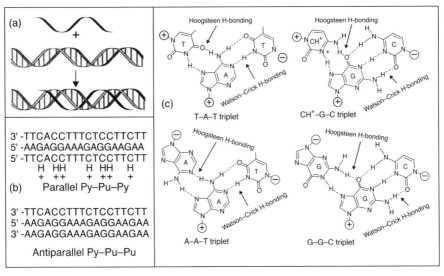

FIGURE 2.6 (a) A schematic diagram showing DNA triplex formation from double-stranded homopurine–homopyrimidine (Pu–Py) DNA and a third strand triplex-forming oligonucleotide (TFO). (b) Two types of common triplex structures, parallel Py–Pu–Py and antiparallel Py–Pu–Pu, are formed by a third strand Py or Pu. The parallel or antiparallel polarity of a triplex refers to the direction of the third strand relative to the central Pu strand. (c) Four common triplet DNA structures that contain two types of hydrogen bonds—the normal Watson–Crick type (A = T & G≡C) and Hoogsteen type (A = T & G = CH+)—that involve the N7 of purines (A & G) of the central strand.

demonstrated by Felsenfeld et al. using homopurine (Pu) and homopyrimidine (Py) nucleic acids [18, 19]. The most common sequence requirements for triplex formation are double-stranded Pu–Py DNA tracts and a third strand of either Pu or Py oligonucleotide, which is termed TFO. The third strand may run either in parallel or antiparallel relative to the central Pu strand depending on whether the third strand is Py or Pu (i.e., to form Py–Pu–Py or Py–Pu–Pu triplex) (Figure 2.6b). As shown in Figure 2.6c, specific sequence recognition is achieved through triplet formation that follows the simple rules of T–A–T and CH+–G–C for a third strand Py and T–A–A and C–G–G if the third strand is Pu. Triplexes are formed through Hoogsteen hydrogen bonding, which uses the N7 of the central strand Pu (A & G) to form hydrogen bonds with the third strand. Other types of DNA triplexes may also form based on different triplet formation rules and varying third strand polarities [20]. Since the triplet CH+–G–C formation requires protonation at the third strand C, formation of parallel triplexes of the type Py–Pu–Py is favored under acidic conditions.

The ability of TFOs to recognize specific sequences containing homopurine/homopyrimidine tracks offers a mechanism for modulating gene expression through triplex formation. Since the target is genomic DNA, triplex-based gene expression interference is often called an antigene approach. Triplex formation may prevent transcription, either by precluding the binding and interaction of various required transcription factors or by blocking transcription initiation and elongation. That is, through triplex formation, a gene may be masked such that it becomes dormant from expression. On the basis of experimental data from gene expression suppression by triplex formation, a minimal oligonucleotide length of around 20 unmodified nucleotides appears to be necessary for a TFO to bind its target DNA duplex with sufficient affinity to achieve biological effects. Chemical conjugation of TFOs with molecular groups such as cholesterol and the intercalating agents acridine and psoralen can increase the binding affinity, thereby reducing the TFO size required to form stable triplexes.

Inhibition of c-Src Expression by TFOs

The human proto-oncogene *c-Src* is a member of a large family of conserved genes, whose products have been shown to participate in many signal transduction pathways and other cellular processes. *c-Src* encodes a tyrosine kinase, $pp60^{c-src}$, which is involved in both the regulation of normal cellular processes and the development of human cancer. Overexpression of *c-Src* has been linked to the development of human tumors—colon, breast, lung, and pancreas.

The promoter region of *c-Src* contains two binding sites (GC1 and GA2) for the transcription factor Sp1, which is essential for full transcriptional activity. In addition, within the promoter region there are three Pu–Py tracts: TC1: 5′-CTTCCTCCTTCCTCCTCCTCCC, TC2: 5′-CTCCCTCCCTCCTCTTC CCCTCCCC, and TC3: 5′-CCTCCTCCTCCTCCTCCTCCCTTTCTCTCTC (only Py strands are shown; the sequences of the corresponding Pu strands can be easily derived from the base-pairing rule of G–C and A–T). These Pu–Py tracts are essential for full activity of the c-Src promoter. Deletion of these tracts significantly reduces transcription activity. A novel factor named SPy (Src pyrimidine binding factor) binds these Pu–Py tracts and coactivates *c-Src* transcription along with transcription factor Sp1 [21]. In an *in vitro* experiment using the *Drosophila* SL2 cell line, individual G-rich polypurine TFOs (TC1Aap: 5′-GAAGGAGGAAGGAGGAGGAGGG, TC2Aap: 5′-GAGGGAGGGAGGGAGAAGGGGAGGGG, and TC3Aap: 5′-GGAGGAGGAGGAGGAGGAGGGAAAGAGAGAG, all can form antiparallel triplexes) designed to target the Pu–Py tracts were shown to inhibit the expression of the reporter gene chloramphenicol acetyltransferase (CAT) under control of the c-Src promoter by up to 70% relative to a control oligonucleotide. The result indicates that Pu–Py tracts (~20 nt) within genomic DNA sequences are potential targets for downregulation of gene expression by TFOs.

A number of other experiments have demonstrated TFOs may be used to knock down the expression of specific genes. For example, a TFO designed to target the Sp1 site in the human *MCP-1* gene promoter has been shown to inhibit the expression of the chemokine MCP-1 (monocyte chemoattractant protein-1), whose expression is activated in response to inflammatory stimuli. Expression inhibition of bcl-2 protein can be achieved by a TFO targeting the 3'-UTR of the *bcl-2* proto-oncogene. Acridine-conjugated TFOs targeting nuclear factor-κB (NF-κB) binding site within the interleukin-2 receptor alpha (*IL-2Rα*) promotor region were shown to inhibit the expression of *IL-2Rα*. TFOs capable of binding to the critical Pu–Py tract in the promoter of the Ki-*ras* proto-oncogene can significantly inhibit reporter gene (CAT) expression in human 293 cells. Chemically modified TFOs can inhibit the expression of intercellular adhesion molecule 1 (ICAM-1) in A549 cells. TFOs designed to target the HIV-1 polypurine tract (PPT) sequence have been shown to inhibit transcriptional elongation in either transient or stable expression systems.

Chemically Modified TFOs   A variety of chemical modifications have been introduced into TFOs to increase their intracellular stability against nucleases and improve their binding affinity. TFO modifications may be divided into two categories—intercalating agents to improve triplex stability and base and sugar-phosphate backbone modifications to increase nuclease resistance. Many modifications can lead to both increased triplex stability and nuclease resistance. Intercalating agents include acridine derivatives and psoralen, which is also a cross-linking agent upon photo irradiation. Examples of base modifications include 5-methyl cytidine and 5-propynyl uridine modifications. Sugar–phosphate backbone modifications include many of those also used in antisense technology. Sugar modifications include 2'-aminoethoxy, LNA, and ENA, while backbone modifications are PS, NP (N3-P5-phosphoramidate), methylphosphonate, PNA, and PMO.

The TFO literature has been expanding rapidly in recent years, indicating significant advances in using TFOs to regulate gene expression. The major advantage of TFOs over ASOs is the strict requirement for homopurine–homopyrimidine (Pu–Py) sequences. In the genome of a given organism, there are not many Pu–Py sequences. Therefore, in principle gene targeting by TFOs should not encounter so-called off-target effects. In addition, compared with other strategies of gene expression modulation at the mRNA and protein levels, the TFO antigene approach has the unique advantage of targeting the sole source coding information for gene expression. Since only one or two copies of a gene normally exist in the cell, the triplex-based antigene approach could in theory effectively silence a gene from expression. However, caution should be exercised when applying TFOs and interpreting results, because oligonucleotides may form alternative structures and achieve downregulation of gene expression by mechanisms other than TFO formation. For example, G-rich TFOs may form G-quartet structures. G-rich oligonucleotides were shown to have a strong antiproliferative activity against a number of cancer cell lines, but the results might be achieved through binding of G-rich oligonucleotides with protein factors, such as nucleolin (a protein involved in cell proliferation) and the transcription factor CNBP (cellular nucleic acid binding protein) required for transcription. Finally, genomic DNA is associated with histones to form nucleosomes that are connected by dsDNA. It has been shown that DNA sequences in the nucleosome region are not accessible for triplex formation by TFOs. Therefore, only the Pu–Py tracts in the spacer regions between neighboring nucleosomes are valid targets for triplex-based gene downregulation.

2.2.4 Gene Regulation by Nucleic Acid Decoys

A nucleic acid decoy is a small dsDNA or single-stranded RNA that mimics the *cis*-regulatory element (enhancer within the promoter region) for gene transcription. Transcription of a specific gene often requires the binding of one or more regulatory proteins (transcription factors) to the *cis*-regulatory element, which is normally located upstream of the transcription initiation site (Figure 2.7a). Introduction of an exogenous nucleic acid decoy can interfere with transcription initiation by sequestration of available transcription factors through specific binding of transcription factors with the decoy (Figure 2.7b).

TAR RNA Decoy The action of a nucleic acid decoy was first demonstrated by Sullenger et al. in 1990 when they introduced an overexpressed 60-nt RNA decoy of the HIV TAR sequence into CD4$^+$ T cells [22]. HIV viral transcription requires the potent viral transcription activator **Tat** (**t**ransactivator of **t**ranscription). Viral transcription activation is achieved (Figure 2.8b) by specific interaction of Tat and cellular cyclin T1 with the viral RNA element called **t**rans-**a**ctivation **r**esponse element (TAR) (Figure 2.8a), which is located at the 5′ end of the viral RNA. The overexpressed TAR decoy was able to sequestrate Tat, resulting in suppression of viral transcription (Figure 2.8c). The effect of the TAR decoy was a dramatic inhibition (>99%) of HIV-1 viral replication. Overexpression of the TAR decoy did not compromise cell viability, indicating that the RNA decoy interacts specifically with Tat and cyclin T1 but not with other essential cellular factors.

RRE RNA Decoy Rev (**re**gulator of **v**iral gene expression) is an essential HIV RNA-binding protein that directs the export of viral mRNA from the

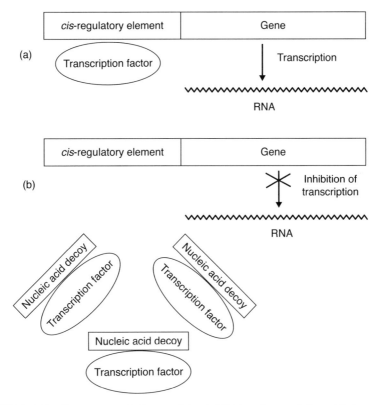

FIGURE 2.7   Gene transcription and its inhibition by nucleic acid decoys. (a) When a gene-specific transcription factor is recruited to the upstream *cis*-regulatory element, transcription of the gene is activated to produce RNA, which gives rise to protein after translation. (b) If a foreign nucleic acid decoy similar to the *cis*-regulatory element is introduced, the decoy binds the transcription factor and makes it unavailable for binding to the *cis*-regulatory element. As a result, gene transcription and subsequent translation are blocked.

nucleus to the cytoplasm, where viral proteins are produced. Rev interacts with viral RNA through the <u>R</u>ev-<u>r</u>esponse <u>e</u>lement (RRE), which includes 234-nt RNA stem-loops located within the envelope coding region of HIV-1 mRNA. Under a tRNA promoter, an expressed 45-nt RNA decoy including RRE stem loops IIA and IIB suppressed HIV-1 replication by >90% in CEM cells (human leukemic cells) [23]. In further experiments with the 13-nt RNA sequence RBE (<u>R</u>ev-<u>b</u>inding <u>e</u>lement) corresponding to the central IIB loop, HIV-1 replication was inhibited even better than by the 45-nt RNA decoy.

E2F dsDNA Decoy   Transcription factor E2F plays a critical role in the regulation of cell cycle and cell proliferation. In quiescent cells, E2F is

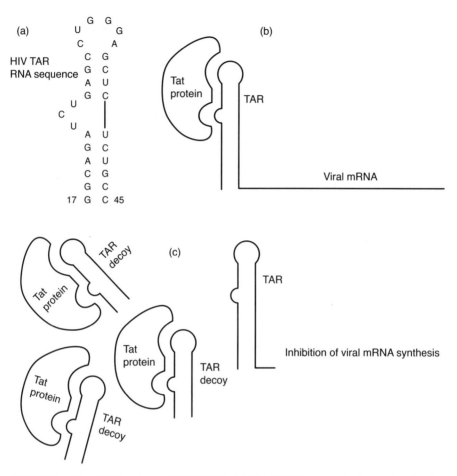

FIGURE 2.8   (a) Structure of HIV TAR. (b) Viral RNA transcription activation by HIV Tat protein. (c) Introduction of TAR decoy RNA leads to the sequestration of Tat through Tat-RNA decoy binding. As a result, viral RNA transcription is inhibited.

sequestered by forming a complex with cyclin A, cdk 2, and Rb. During cell proliferation, E2F dissociates from the complex and trans-activates the expression of multiple cell cycle regulatory genes, including c-*myc*, c-*myb*, cdc 2 kinase, PCNA (Proliferating Cell Nuclear Antigen), and thymidine kinase. Upregulation is achieved by specific binding (Figure 2.9a) of E2F to a *cis*-regulatory element with the consensus sequence TTTCGCGC within the promoter [24]. It is believed that restenosis after angioplasty results, in part, from vascular smooth muscle cell proliferation and migration induced by E2F-activated expression of cell cycle genes.

The essential interaction between E2F and the *cis*-regulatory element TTTCGCGC for cell cycle gene activation provides an excellent target for gene control by applying a dsDNA decoy strategy (Figure 2.9b). A synthetic

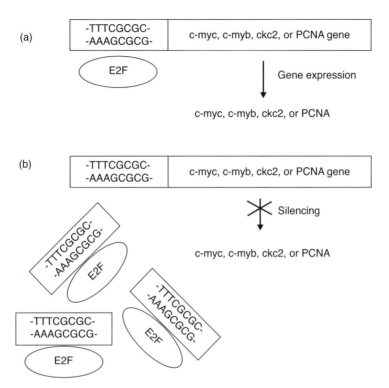

FIGURE 2.9 (a) Interaction of E2F with the *cis*-regulatory element of a number of genes is required for their transcription activation. (b) A dsDNA decoy containing the sequence of the *cis*-regulatory element binds E2F and block transcription of c-*myc*, c-*myb*, cdc 2 kinase, and PCNA.

double-stranded 14-nt DNA containing the consensus sequence can effectively compete for E2F with its binding site, as demonstrated by gel mobility shift assays [25]. Transfection of the decoy into rat balloon-injured carotid arteries achieved almost complete inhibition of neointimal formation at two weeks after balloon injury, while a similar but mismatched dsDNA had no effect on neointimal hyperplasia. It was shown that the E2F decoy specifically reduced both PCNA and cdc 2 kinase mRNA levels. The experiment demonstrated that *in vivo* delivery of a double-stranded E2F DNA decoy can specifically inhibit the expression of certain cell cycle genes, which may lead to the suppression of smooth muscle proliferation and restenosis.

The promising experimental results described above have led to the concept of using the E2F DNA decoy to reduce human bypass vein graft failure, which is characterized by neointimal hyperplasia and accelerated atherosclerosis. Autologous vein grafting is the primary method for surgical revascularization in patients suffering from occlusive coronary disease. However, the procedure has a long-term failure rate of $\sim 50\%$. Failures are contributed by the formation of a neointimal layer during the postoperative remodeling of the initially thin-walled vein. In an experiment with rabbits, vein grafts were transfected with an E2F DNA decoy during the operation. Long-term inhibition of neointimal hyperplasia and preservation of endothelial function were achieved for at least 6 months after the operation. On the basis of these experimental data, a clinical program was initiated using *ex vivo*, pressure-mediated E2F decoy transfection to improve human bypass vein grafts. Results indicated that the E2F decoy was able to reduce target cell cycle gene expression and to inhibit vascular cell proliferation. While graft failures occurred in the patient group that had not received the E2F decoy treatment, no failures were observed in the decoy-treated patients after 6 months, indicating that the E2F decoy was functioning as expected in blocking neointimal hyperplasia. A phase III clinical trial with Edifoligide (E2F decoy) was launched by Corgentech, Inc (San Francisco, US). However, the trial was terminated because of its failure to meet the trial's primary and secondary endpoints, although Edifoligide was generally well tolerated in the 3014-patients that participated in the trial.

NF-κB dsDNA Decoy   NF-κB is a transcription factor essential for the inflammatory and immunological responses. Through coordinated transactivation, NF-κB upregulates expression of chemokines, interferons, MHC proteins, growth factors, and cell adhesion molecules, whose activation is believed to play a role in diseases such as myocardial infarction and glomerulonephritis.

In a rat cardiac ischemia-reperfusion model, rat coronary artery transfection with a double-stranded NF-κB DNA decoy containing the consensus sequence for NF-κB binding was shown to markedly reduce the damaged area of myocytes 24 h after reperfusion compared with the effect of a scrambled DNA sequence and untransfected rats [26]. The specificity of the NF-κB DNA decoy for the inhibition of cytokine and adhesion molecule expression was confirmed by *in vitro* experiments. Introduction of the NF-κB DNA decoy significantly reduced levels of cytokines IL-6 and IL-8 and of adhesion molecules VCAM (vascular cell adhesion molecule)and ICAM, while scrambled control sequences had no effect. Further studies with the NF-κB DNA decoy demonstrated its *in vivo* effectiveness in myocardial protection, abolishing glomerular inflammation, and attenuating neuronal damage following brain ischemia.

CRE dsDNA Decoy   A number of genes involved in cell growth and differentiation have the <u>c</u>yclic AMP <u>r</u>esponse <u>e</u>lement (CRE) with the consensus palindromic sequence TGACGTCA in their enhancer regions. Through specific interaction with CRE, transcription factors CRE-<u>b</u>inding (CREB) protein and <u>a</u>ctivation <u>t</u>ranscription <u>f</u>actor-2 (ATF-2) trans-activate gene expression.

Sequestration of CREB and ATF-2 via complexation by other agents may therefore interfere with cell growth and tumor progression.

A CRE DNA decoy consisting of the consensus palindromic sequence TGACGTCA was shown to compete with CRE enhancers for binding transcription factors and interfered with CRE- and AP-1-directed transcription. The decoy could enter the cell, inhibit transcription of specific CRE-directed genes, and inhibit tumor cell growth both *in vitro* and *in vivo* [27]. Noncancerous cells were not affected by the decoy.

In a microarray (a signal transduction pathway array containing 1152 genes) experiment [28] with the CRE DNA decoy treatment on tumors, ~10% of the genes on the array showed altered expression of >2-fold. Genes that define cell cycle signatures were either significantly stimulated or suppressed in decoy-treated tumors. The CRE decoy, but not the scrambled control DNA, inhibited "cell proliferation signature" genes, including protein kinases and phosphatases, growth factors, growth factor receptors, and cyclin K. On the other hand, treatment of tumors with the decoy upregulated "reverse transformation" signature genes that are involved in the regulation of development, cell growth, and differentiation. Among the stimulated genes was that encoding transcription factor AP-2β, which, through binding to the AP-2 enhancer, up- or downregulates a number of genes involved in a broad range of biological functions.

In addition, other gene-specific *cis*-regulatory elements for transcription factors may be the targets for nucleic acid decoys to achieve downregulation of specific genes. These targets include AP-1, AP-2, SSRE, MEF-2, CarG box, VP16, GRE/HRE/MRE, heat shock RE, SRE (**s**terol **r**esponse **e**lement), TGF-β responsive element, HIF-1, and others.

2.2.5   Control of Gene Expression by Aptamers

The term aptamer was coined by Ellington and Szostak (from the Latin "*aptus*," meaning fitting) [29] as single-stranded nucleic acid molecules capable of specific binding of diverse molecular targets—amino acids, antibiotics, carbohydrates, lipids, peptides, proteins, nucleic acids, and even entire organisms. Aptamers may be based on either RNA or DNA, resulting in RNA aptamers or DNA aptamers. By virtue of their defined three-dimensional structures and multiple interactions with target molecules, aptamers are able to bind targets with excellent specificities and high affinities. In many aspects, aptamers may be viewed as the nucleic acid-based functional analogs of proteinaceous antibodies. The specificity and affinity of aptamer-target interaction can rival those of monoclonal antibody-antigen interaction [30].

By employing an iterative process of selection and amplification, called **s**ystematic **e**volution of **l**igands by **ex**ponential enrichment (SELEX) [31], aptamers against virtually any molecular target may be generated from large synthetic nucleic acid libraries containing single-stranded random sequences of RNA or DNA with typically 10^{14}–10^{15} unique sequences that can be easily generated and manipulated in the laboratory. Folding of the vast number of different RNA/DNA sequences results in three-dimensional conformations of immense diversity, which guaranties the functional (i.e., target-binding) diversity of different RNA/DNA sequences. For any given molecular target, it is likely that there exists at least one active RNA/DNA aptamer sequence that can fold into a complex three-dimensional conformation required for specific target binding. By applying a set of defined selection criteria, such as binding affinity/specificity and conditions, RNA/DNA sequences with desired functions (even at extremely low abundance, in principle a single copy) can be selectively isolated and amplified through multiple (typically, 6–20) rounds of selection, reverse transcription, PCR amplification, and transcription. In addition, sequence mutations with a defined mutation rate can be artificially introduced during the SELEX process. Although the manual SELEX procedure is highly repetitive, laborious, and time-consuming and often results in only a limited number of aptamers, the entire SELEX process has been automated [32] to allow for the high-throughput generation of large numbers of aptamers against a molecular target.

Anti-VEGF Aptamers Angiogenesis is a physiological process of growing new blood vessels from pre-existing ones. Angiogenesis plays important roles in both normal tissue growth/development (such as wound healing) and pathological development and maintenance of a variety of proliferative disorders such as tumor and ocular neovascularization. <u>V</u>ascular <u>e</u>ndothelial <u>g</u>rowth <u>f</u>actor (VEGF) is one of the best-characterized factors involved in angiogenesis. High levels of VEGF have been found to be associated with tumors and ocular neovascularization, including diabetic retinopathy and <u>a</u>ge-related <u>m</u>acular <u>d</u>egeneration (AMD).

Using SELEX, Ruckman et al. [33] isolated a number of 2′-F-pyrimidine RNA aptamers against human VEGF$_{165}$ (one of several VEGF isoforms). By sequence analysis, the aptamers were grouped into three major families, each representing a conserved primary sequence motif with binding affinities for VEGF$_{165}$ ranging from $Kd = 2$ pM to 9 nM. Truncation of the original aptamers yielded three minimal aptamers (one from each family, 23–29 nt): T22.23 (family 1, Kd = 90 nM) GCGGUAGGAAGAAUUG-GAAGCGC; T2.29 (family 2, Kd = 40 nM) GCGAACCGAUGGAAUU-UUUGGACGCUCGC; T44.27 (family 3, Kd = 10 nM) CGGAAUCAUG-GAAUGCUUAUACAUCCG. Further modification of all but two purines with 2′-OMe in each aptamer and addition of a 3′-inverted T resulted in aptamers named t22-OMe, t2-OMe, and t44-OMe with Kd = 72, 130, and

49 pM, respectively. No binding of $VEGF_{121}$, or $PlGF_{129}$ (placenta growth factor, a protein with 53% homology to VEGF) (at up to 100 nM) was observed for the aptamers, indicating their high binding specificity.

All three modified aptamers (t22-OMe, t2-OMe, and t44-OMe) were shown to potently inhibit the binding of VEGF to either one of the two VEGF receptors, Flt-1 (*fm*s-like tyrosine kinase) and KDR (kinase insert domain-containing receptor). The IC_{50} values (concentration at which 50% inhibition is achieved) for aptamer competition with Flt-1 and KDR are in the order of 100 pM and 1 pM, respectively. In addition, aptamer t44-OMe can act as an effective antagonist of intradermal VEGF-induced vascular permeability, inhibiting 48% of VEGF-induced vascular permeability at 0.1 mM. Conjugation of the aptamer with 40-kDa PEG (polyethylene glycol) led to PEG-t44-OMe with a slight reduction ($\sim$4-fold) in binding affinity to $VEGF_{165}$; however, the PEG-conjugation substantially enhanced the aptamer's biological activity, achieving 83% inhibition of VEGF-induced vascular permeability at 0.1 mM, while a similar scrambled control oligonucleotide-PEG conjugate showed no activity at the same concentration.

PEG-t44-OMe was renamed NX 1838 and later pegaptanib sodium and went through successful clinical trials for the treatment of AMD. Approved by the US FDA, the aptamer was marketed as Macugen by OSI Pharmaceuticals (Long Island, US) and is currently the only aptamer-based agent with clinical application.

Anti-HIV Reverse Transcriptase Aptamers The conversion of the HIV genetic information, stored in the form of RNA, into the DNA (cDNA) form is a critical step in the process of HIV infection. The RNA-to-cDNA conversion is catalyzed by the viral enzyme reverse transcriptase (HIV RT). High affinity binding of HIV RT by a chemical agent can in principle effectively sequester the enzyme, thereby disabling its reverse transcriptase activity. In an early viral targeting experiment with aptamers, Tuerk et al. [34] isolated RNA aptamers that were shown to specifically bind HIV RT and to reverse transcriptase activity. In cellular experiments, the aptamers were shown to strongly inhibit HIV-1 replication.

Several aptamers are currently in the preclinical or clinical testing stage. Aptamers have been validated as potential therapeutic agents for applications such as inhibition of infection, anticoagulation, anti-inflammation, antiangiogenesis, antiproliferation, and immunotherapy. Two aptamers have already entered clinical development: ARC1779 developed by Archemix (Cambridge, US) to selectively reduce platelet aggregation and thrombosis by inhibition of von Willebrand Factor, started human phase I clinical trials in December of 2006; an antithrombin DNA-based aptamer (ARC183, 15 nt) is in clinical trials as an anticoagulant for use in coronary artery bypass grafting.

Since the initial development of the SELEX method, numerous RNA/DNA aptamers against a variety of targets have been isolated. The Ellington Lab Aptamer Database (http://aptamer.icmb.utexas.edu/) contains information of these aptamers. Although artificial nucleic acid aptamers for a variety of targets (ligands) have been isolated from synthetic DNA/RNA libraries containing random sequences, the mechanism of specific aptamer–ligand interaction has also been exploited in nature. Riboswitches, discovered by the Breaker laboratory [35], are *cis*-active natural RNA aptamers that participate in regulating gene expression through conformation changes upon binding by specific metabolites.

2.2.6 Gene Expression Modulation by Ribozymes and DNAzymes

Ribozymes are RNA-based catalytic molecules or RNA enzymes that, like protein enzymes, are capable of catalyzing a wide variety of chemical reactions. First discovered in the process of *Tetrahymena* pre-rRNA splicing [36] and bacterial tRNA maturation [37], naturally occurring ribozymes include the hammerhead ribozyme (Figure 2.10), the hairpin ribozyme (Figure 2.10), the hepatitis delta virus (HDV) ribozyme, the Varkud satellite (VS) ribozyme, group I and group II introns, the RNA component of RNase P, and rRNA. In addition, increasing evidence strongly suggests that snRNAs in the

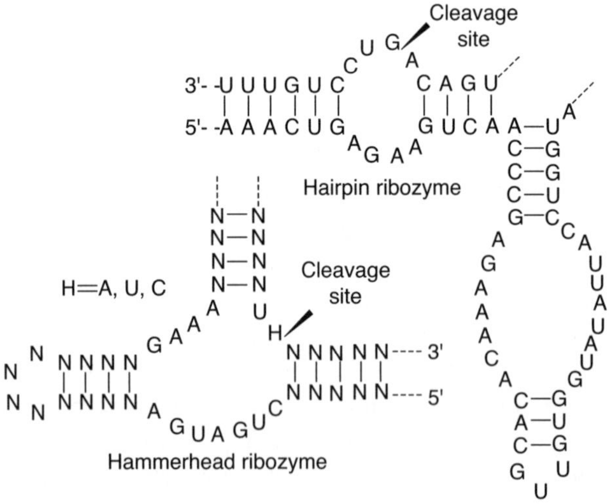

FIGURE 2.10 Secondary structures of hammerhead and hairpin ribozymes. Both ribozymes achieve specific cleavage of target RNA by complementary binding of the two arms of the ribozymes to target RNA sequences.

spliceosome may turn out to be the catalytic components. These hydrolytic ribozymes can be grouped according to their sizes into two classes—small ribozymes (hammerhead, hairpin, HDV, and VS ribozymes) and large ribozymes that include RNase P RNA and group I and II introns. Excluding rRNA, all naturally occurring ribozymes catalyze a single type of hydrolytic reaction—phosphodiester bond cleavage of the RNA backbone (Figure 2.10).

In addition to natural ribozymes, numerous artificial ribozymes have been isolated from large RNA libraries containing random sequences by *in vitro* selection techniques [29, 31, 38]. Compared with natural ribozymes, selected artificial ribozymes can catalyze a broader range of chemical reactions—from the hydrolytic cleavage of RNA backbone phosphodiester bonds to many biologically relevant metabolic reactions such as RNA capping, phosphorylation, carboxy group activation, thioester formation, peptide bond formation, and carbon–carbon bond formation. Taking the advantage of natural selection, degenerate random RNA libraries based on natural ribozymes such as the hammerhead and hairpin ribozymes have also been used to isolate derivatives of natural ribozymes with catalytic activities matching or exceeding those of natural ribozymes.

Although naturally occurring DNA-based enzymes have yet to be discovered, a variety of artificial DNAzymes (deoxyribozymes) have been created by *in vitro* selection from large random DNA libraries [39]. Comparable to ribozymes, DNAzymes can catalyze phosphorylation, DNA capping, and RNA backbone phosphodiester bond cleavage. The DNAzyme 10–23 has been widely used for RNA cleavage at a specific site (Figure 2.11).

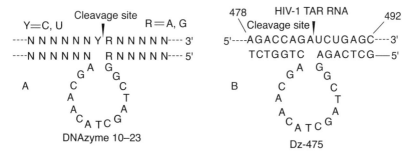

FIGURE 2.11 (a) Secondary structure of the general RNA-cleaving DNAzyme 10–23. (b) Structure of Dz-475, an HIV-1 TAR-cleaving DNAzyme, based on the structure of the 10–23 DNAzyme. In both (a) and (b), the top strand is a target RNA with a specific sequence, while the other strand is the sequence of a DNAzyme, with a catalytic core (15-nt loop) in the middle and two arms that recognize the target sequence by Watson–Crick base pairing.

For gene regulation purposes, only a special class of ribozymes and DNAzymes—the RNA hydrolases—are exploited to degrade defined target mRNAs. Since small nucleic acid molecules are easy to synthesize and economical to apply, small ribozymes and DNAzymes are commonly used for artificial gene regulation. These RNA hydrolases have in common a small catalytic core (made of either RNA or DNA) that is connected to two DNA/RNA arms (Figures 2.10 and 2.11). The catalytic core is usually highly conserved, while both the sequence and length of the two arms may change without affecting catalytic activity. A general principle for ribozymes and DNAzymes involves specific sequence recognition of the target mRNA by ribozymes or DNAzymes, followed by hydrolytic cleavage of an RNA backbone phosphodiester bond at a specific location. If the target mRNA sequence is unique, RNA cleavage rendered by ribozymes or DNAzymes should reduce the mRNA level of target gene, thereby leading to downregulation of its expression.

Recognition of a target RNA sequence is achieved through binding (Watson–Crick base pairing) of the two arms of the ribozyme or DNAzyme (catalytic core) to a specific mRNA sequence. After RNA hydrolysis at a defined site, the cleaved RNA pieces dissociate from the ribozyme/DNAzyme, and the enzyme can recruit a new mRNA molecule for hydrolytic destruction.

Anti-HIV Ribozymes   Numerous experiments have been reported in which ribozymes were designed to target various portions of HIV-1 RNA. Earlier experiments used a single ribozyme to target one specific site. Later on, different ribozymes were joined together as a single ribozyme-containing molecule that simultaneously target multiple sites. For example, Ramezani et al. [40] constructed a multiribozyme (Rz_{1-14}) containing 14 individual hammerhead ribozymes. The multiribozyme can simultaneously target the following genes or important RNA sequences in HIV-1 RNA: the 5′-UTR by cutting ACUCUG**UA**ACUAGAGA; *pro* (codes for protease) by cutting ACACC**UU**CAACAUAAU; *pol* (codes for integrase) by targeting U**U**UCGG**UU**UAUUACAG and GGGGCA**UA**GUAAUACA; *vif* (p23, encoding viral infectivity factor) by cutting AUUGGG**UC**UGCAUACA, and *env* (gene for envelope surface glycoprotein gp120) by targeting multiples cleavage sites—UAAUCAG**UU**UAUGGGAU, CCAUGUG**UA**AAAUUAAC, CG-GCUGG**UU**UUGCGAUU, AGCACAG**UA**CAAUGUAC, UACAAUG**UA** CACAUGGA, ACUGCUG**UU**AAAUGGCA, UUAAUUG**UA**CAAGACCC, ACAUUAG**UA**GAGCAAAA, and AGCAAUG**UA**UGCCCUC. Specific cleavage of HIV-1 RNA by ribozymes occurs between the two bold-faced nucleotides **UH (H = A, C, U)**. *In vitro* RNA cleavage experiments showed that Rz_{1-14} was able to cut target RNA sequences specifically at the defined sites. Nonspecific RNA cleavage was not observed. When challenged with

HIV-1, stable MT4 transductants expressing Rz_{1-14} exhibited and maintained significant inhibition against HIV-1 replication for the 60-day testing period.

Anti-HIV DNAzymes   A number of DNAzymes based on the 10–23 format have been designed to target HIV-1 RNA, including the conserved TAR region of the 5′ leader sequence (5′-LTR) of the HIV genome. In one experiment [41], a DNAzyme (Dz-475) (Figure 2.11b) was shown to cleave an *in vitro*-transcribed TAR fragment. Using HeLa cells, Dz-475 was able to inhibit HIV-1 gene expression by 40% over a mutated version of Dz-475 (M), and by 80% over an unrelated DNAzyme. Quantitation of isolated RNA showed a reduction of 10–12-fold relative to untreated samples or samples treated with an unrelated DNAzyme. The mutated DNAzyme Dz-475 (M) also showed a fourfold reduction in RNA. Therefore, Dz-475 appeared to achieve downregulation of HIV-1 gene expression by two different mechanisms, antisense inhibition and hydrolysis by DNAzyme, with similar efficiencies. Furthermore, when Dz-475 was introduced (at 2 μg dosage) into CXCR4- and CCR5-expressing HeLa-CD4 indicator (MAGI) cell lines, HeLa cells expressing an integrated copy of human CD4 and the HIV-1 long terminal repeat [LTR] fused to the beta galactosidase reporter gene, there was about 50% reduction of infectious virus production after either T-tropic (**T** cell-tropic) or M-tropic (**m**acrophage-tropic) virus challenge. In addition, Dz-475 was shown to inhibit HIV-1 replication in T cells, human PBMCs (**p**eripheral **b**lood **m**ononuclear **c**ells), and ACH2 cells (chronically infected T-cell line).

2.2.7 RNA Interference by siRNAs and miRNAs

In eukaryotic cells, innate posttranscriptional mechanisms exist for specific gene downregulation (gene silencing) at the mRNA level, mediated by small pieces (19– 26 nt) of RNA. The phenomenon of RNA-induced specific gene silencing is termed RNAi—RNA interference. RNAi can be induced by either siRNAs [42] or miRNAs [43–45]. siRNAs are double-stranded small RNAs, typically with a 2-nt overhang at the 3′ end of both strands. On the other hand, miRNAs are single-stranded small RNAs. *In vivo*, the RNase III-type enzyme Dicer is responsible for producing both siRNA and miRNA from double-stranded RNA (dsRNA) and hairpin RNA, respectively. A siRNA then forms a ribonucleoprotein complex termed **R**NA-**i**nduced **s**ilencing **c**omplex (RISC) that recognizes its target RNA sequence complementary to the siRNA and cleaves it in the middle. Natural siRNAs are formed from transposons, dsRNA viruses, and bidirectionally transcribed sequences. It is believed that the siRNA-based gene silencing mechanism plays a role in restricting transposon mobilization and as a defense mechanism against invading foreign RNA species. On the other hand, a miRNA forms a RISC-like complex that suppresses gene expression by either inhibiting translation (antisense-like mechanism) or inducing mRNA cleavage (siRNA-like mechanism), depending on the degree of its complementarity with a target mRNA sequence. Unlike siRNAs, miRNAs play important roles in the development of multicellular organisms.

On the basis of the innate RNAi mechanisms, specific gene silencing in eukaryotic cells may also be achieved by introducing artificially designed siRNAs [46] and miRNAs. The ability to silence virtually any gene in eukaryotes from nematodes to humans has dramatically changed the ways scientists conduct research in biological sciences. For example, siRNAs are, in many cases, replacing traditional gene-knockout methods to study functions of specific genes. Using siRNA arrays, mapping of global gene functions (functional genomics) can now be performed on a large scale. At the same time, the discovery of RNAi-based gene silencing approaches has generated unprecedented excitement and optimism in molecular biomedicine. With its great promise of becoming the next generation of nucleic acid-based pharmaceuticals with high potency and low toxicity, RNAi is being actively researched by in academia and the pharmaceutical industry. The rest of this book contains various chapters that deal with various aspects of RNAi technology, and is a manifestation of current intense research efforts focused on transforming RNAi principles into future clinical therapeutics.

2.3 COMPARISON OF DIFFERENT METHODS OF ARTIFICIAL GENE REGULATION

From the above introduction and description of different nucleic acid-based strategies for artificial modulation of gene expression, it is clear that each gene regulation mechanism has distinct advantages and disadvantages, which is summarized below.

The antigene approach by TFOs targets the source information (only one or two copies of DNA, in the nucleus) by forming triplex structures at Pu–Py tracts (~20 nt). Triplex DNA regions may either block transcription initiation or inhibit elongation. Therefore, effective TFOs can in principle completely shut down specific gene function by targeting the earliest stage in the gene expression pathway. The selectivity of TFOs is expected to be very high, due to the rare occurrence of Pu–Py tracts in the genome. However, TFOs have to be delivered to the nucleus and effective target Pu–Py tracts cannot be located within the regions of nucleosomes (DNA complexes with histones). In addition, G-rich TFOs may bind cellular proteins, resulting in both TFO depletion and undesired nonspecific activities.

Antisense strategy is based on the simple principle of Watson–Crick base pairing between mRNA and ASO. The resulting heteroduplex structure may either activate cellular RNase H to cleave the target mRNA and/or block translation through steric hindrance. Virtually, any mRNA can be targeted by ASO, and RNase H-activating ASO may be used multiple times for the destruction of target mRNA. However, exogenous ASOs have to be extensively modified to achieve their intended effects. A common modification by phosphorothioate may result in binding of cellular proteins and lead to nonspecific cytotoxicities. Other chemical modifications may inactivate the RNase H mechanism. Furthermore, large quantities of ASO would be needed to achieve and maintain a certain level of gene expression inhibition. Finally, low target specificity may arise from the formation of untargeted mRNA–ASO heteroduplexes that are not perfectly base paired.

DNA/RNA decoys achieve gene downregulation by sequestrating transcription factors through specific binding. The advantage of decoys is their easy design (typically the same sequence as that of the enhancer of a target gene) and synthesis (small oligonucleotides). However, since a transcription factor may be involved in more than one gene's expression, a decoy may affect more than one target gene. In addition, because transcription factors themselves are not targeted, continued expression of transcription factors would necessitate the use of large quantities of decoys to sustain the downregulation of target genes. Additional concerns may arise from the problems of disposing accumulated decoy-transcription factor complexes.

Downregulation of gene expression by DNA/RNA aptamers is achieved by a similar mechanism to that of decoys, but the binding targets can be either a transcription factor or any other functional cellular protein. While DNA/RNA aptamers may be more complex than decoys and require SELEX for isolation, specific aptamers with high binding affinities may be generated against almost any target protein. Aptamers may achieve high efficiency at low concentrations and with great target specificity. However, similar potential problems to those for decoys exist: continued use of aptamers in order to maintain low cellular levels of target protein and potential disposal problems of large quantities of aptamer–protein complexes.

Ribozymes/DNAzymes may be used to control gene expression by cleaving target mRNAs. The effect parallels that from ASOs, but ribozymes/DNAzymes do not rely on cellular machinery to achieve target inactivation. Similar chemistry may be used to modify ribozymes/DNAzymes to achieve higher cellular stability, although some restrictions apply to ribozymes/DNAzymes. For ribozyme/DNAzyme design, the two mRNA-binding arms may be fine-tuned to attain (a) desired binding affinity of target mRNA sequences, (b) discrimination of nontarget RNA sequences, and (c) fast dissociation of cleaved RNA fragments. In addition, the mispairing of RNA substrates with ribozymes/DNAzymes leads to lower catalytic activities. As a result, ribozymes/DNAzymes may exhibit higher target specificities than

ASOs. Because of intrinsic stability and easy synthesis of DNA over RNA, DNAzymes may be more desirable agents than ribozymes for gene regulation applications.

Finally, RNAi technology represents the latest addition to the nucleic acid-based weaponry for gene control. By enlisting the help of the innate eukaryotic cellular RNAi machinery, artificial small RNAs (siRNAs and miRNAs) can elicit powerful attacks on virtually any target mRNA. When recruited by RISC, siRNAs are protected from hydrolytic nucleases and the catalytic action of RISC can destroy multiple copies of a target mRNA. Therefore, siRNAs can exert lasting RNAi effects and display unrivaled high potency at low concentrations (nM). Experiments have shown that siRNAs can achieve gene downregulation at up to 100 times lower concentrations than required by antisense mechanism. While extensive chemical modifications are necessary for *in vivo* applications of other nucleic acid-based strategies (except for endogenously expressed RNA decoys, ribozymes and RNA aptamers), unmodified siRNAs and miRNAs are effective RNAi agents that can be directly applied to cells to achieve desired gene downregulation. Despite its short history, RNAi has emerged as the preferred tool for modulation of gene functions over other nucleic acid-based technologies, as demonstrated by the vast volume of and fast-growing publications on the subject. The name change of Ribozyme Pharmaceuticals to Sirna Therapeutics (San Francisco, US) and its recent purchase by Merck (Whitehouse Station, US) for 1.1 billion dollars probably reflect well the general belief on RNAi as the next generation of molecular therapeutics. Although problems associated with RNAi remain, such as inefficient intracellular delivery, off-target effects, and activation of interferon signaling pathways, the current unparalleled research efforts on RNAi will greatly enhance our understanding on RNAi mechanism and yield solutions to existing problems. In addition, the combination of RNAi with other nucleic acid-based technologies such as decoys and ribozymes [47] may achieve superior effects of gene control over using any one method alone. On the basis of the action mechanism and available data, RNAi-based strategy will undoubtedly evolve into a highly efficient and specific gene-control technology that holds great promise for transforming current small molecule-based medicine into future gene sequence-based molecular therapeutics.

REFERENCES

1. Mattick, J. S. and Makunin, I. V. (2006). Non-coding RNA. *Hum Mol Genet* **15**: R17–29.
2. Zamecnik, P. C. and Stephenson, M. L. (1978). Inhibition of Rous sarcoma virus replication and cell transformation by a specific oligodeoxynucleotide. *Proc Natl Acad Sci U S A* **75**: 280–4.

3. Stephenson, M. L. and Zamecnik, P. C. (1978). Inhibition of Rous sarcoma viral RNA translation by a specific oligodeoxyribonucleotide. *Proc Natl Acad Sci U S A* **75**: 285–8.

4. Crooke, S. T. (1998). Molecular mechanisms of antisense drugs: RNase H. *Antisense Nucleic Acid Drug Dev* **8**: 133–4.

5. Zamaratski, E., Pradeepkumar, P. I., and Chattopadhyaya, J. (2001). A critical survey of the structure-function of the antisense oligo/RNA heteroduplex as substrate for RNase H. *J Biochem Biophys Methods* **48**: 189–208.

6. Summerton, J., Stein, D., Huang, S. B., Matthews, P., Weller, D., and Partridge, M. (1997). Morpholino and phosphorothioate antisense oligomers compared in cell-free and in-cell systems. *Antisense Nucleic Acid Drug Dev* **7**: 63–70.

7. Iversen, P. L. (2001). Phosphorodiamidate morpholino oligomers: favorable properties for sequence-specific gene inactivation. *Curr Opin Mol Ther* **3**: 235–8.

8. Dominski, Z. and Kole, R. (1994). Identification and characterization by antisense oligonucleotides of exon and intron sequences required for splicing. *Mol Cell Biol* **14**: 7445–54.

9. Kole, R. and Sazani, P. (2001). Antisense effects in the cell nucleus: modification of splicing. *Curr Opin Mol Ther* **3**: 229–34.

10. Reed, J. C., Stein, C., Subasinghe, C., Haldar, S., Croce, C. M., Yum, S., and Cohen, J. (1990). Antisense-mediated inhibition of BCL2 protooncogene expression and leukemic cell growth and survival: comparisons of phosphodiester and phosphorothioate oligodeoxynucleotides. *Cancer Res* **50**: 6565–70.

11. Kitada, S., Miyashita, T., Tanaka, S., and Reed, J. C. (1993). Investigations of antisense oligonucleotides targeted against bcl-2 RNAs. *Anitsense Res Dev* **3**: 157–69.

12. Dean, N. M., McKay, R., Condon, T. P., and Bennett, C. F. (1994). Inhibition of protein kinase C-alpha expression in human A549 cells by antisense oligonucleotides inhibits induction of intercellular adhesion molecule 1 (ICAM-1) mRNA by phorbol esters. *J Biol Chem* **269**: 16416–24.

13. Krieg, A. M., Yi, A. K., Matson, S., Waldschmidt, T. J., Bishop, G. A., Teasdale, R., Koretzky, G. A., and Klinman, D. M. (1995). CpG motifs in bacterial DNA trigger direct B-cell activation. *Nature* **374**: 546–9.

14. Chan, J. H., Lim, S., and Wong, W. S. (2006). Antisense oligonucleotides: from design to therapeutic application. *Clin Exp Pharmacol Physiol* **33**: 533–40.

15. Zuker, M. (2003). Mfold web server for nucleic acid folding and hybridization prediction. *Nucleic Acids Res* **31**: 3406–15.

16. Ding, Y., Chan, C. Y., and Lawrence, C. E. (2004). Sfold web server for statistical folding and rational design of nucleic acids. *Nucleic Acids Res* **32**: W135–41.

17. Ho, S. P., Britton, D. H., Stone, B. A., Behrens, D. L., Leffet, L. M., Hobbs, F. W., Miller, J. A., and Trainor, G. L. (1996). Potent antisense oligonucleotides to the human multidrug resistance-1 mRNA are rationally selected by mapping RNA-accessible sites with oligonucleotide libraries. *Nucleic Acids Res* **24**: 1901–7.

18. Felsenfeld, G. and Rich, A. (1957). Studies on the formation of two- and three-stranded polyribonucleotides. *Biochim Biophys Acta* **26**: 457–68.

19. Felsenfeld, G., Davies, D. R., and Rich, A. (1957). Formation of a three-stranded polynucleotide molecule. *J Am Chem Soc* **79**: 2023–4.

20. Frank-Kamenetskii, M. D. and Mirkin, S. M. (1995). Triplex DNA structures. *Annu Rev Biochem* **64**: 65–95.

21. Ritchie, S., Boyd, F. M., Wong, J., and Bonham, K. (2000). Transcription of the human c-Src promoter is dependent on Sp1, a novel pyrimidine binding factor SPy, and can be inhibited by triplex-forming oligonucleotides. *J Biol Chem* **275**: 847–54.

22. Sullenger, B. A., Gallardo, H. F., Ungers, G. E., and Gilboa, E. (1990). Overexpression of TAR sequences renders cells resistant to human immunodeficiency virus replication. *Cell* **63**: 601–8.

23. Lee, T. C., Sullenger, B. A., Gallardo, H. F., Ungers, G. E., and Gilboa, E. (1992). Overexpression of RRE-derived sequences inhibits HIV-1 replication in CEM cells. *New Biol* **4**: 66–74.

24. Hiebert, S. W., Lipp, M., and Nevins, J. R. (1989). E1 A-dependent transactivation of the human MYC promoter is mediated by the E2F factor. *Proc Natl Acad Sci U S A* **86**: 3594–8.

25. Morishita, R., Gibbons, G. H., Horiuchi, M., Ellison, K. E., Nakama, M., Zhang, L., Kaneda, Y., Ogihara, T., and Dzau, V. J. (1995). A gene therapy strategy using a transcription factor decoy of the E2F binding site inhibits smooth muscle proliferation in vivo. *Proc Natl Acad Sci U S A* **92**: 5855–9.

26. Morishita, R., Sugimoto, T., Aoki, M., Kida, I., Tomita, N., Moriguchi, A., Maeda, K., Sawa, Y., Kaneda, Y., Higaki, J., and Ogihara, T. (1997). In vivo transfection of cis element "decoy" against nuclear factor-kappaB binding site prevents myocardial infarction. *Nat Med* **3**: 894–9.

27. Park, Y. G., Nesterova, M., Agrawal, S., and Cho-Chung, Y. S. (1999). Dual blockade of cyclic AMP response element- (CRE) and AP-1-directed transcription by CRE-transcription factor decoy oligonucleotide: gene-specific inhibition of tumor growth. *J Biol Chem* **274**: 1573–80.

28. Cho, Y. S., Kim, M. K., Cheadle, C., Neary, C., Park, Y. G., Becker, K. G., and Cho-Chung, Y. S. (2002). A genomic-scale view of the cAMP response element-enhancer decoy: a tumor target-based genetic tool. *Proc Natl Acad Sci U S A* **99**: 15626–31.

29. Ellington, A. D. and Szostak, J. W. (1990). In vitro selection of RNA molecules that bind specific ligands. *Nature* **346**: 818–22.

30. Gold, L. (1995). Oligonucleotides as research, diagnostic, and therapeutic agents. *J Biol Chem* **270**: 13581–4.

31. Tuerk, C. and Gold, L. (1990). Systematic evolution of ligands by exponential enrichment: RNA ligands to bacteriophage T4 DNA polymerase. *Science* **249**: 505–10.

32. Cox, J. C., Rudolph, P., and Ellington, A. D. (1998). Automated RNA selection. *Biotechnol Prog* **14**: 845–50.

33. Ruckman, J., Green, L. S., Beeson, J., Waugh, S., Gillette, W. L., Henninger, D. D., Claesson-Welsh, L., and Janjic, N. (1998). 2′-Fluoropyrimidine

RNA-based aptamers to the 165-amino acid form of vascular endothelial growth factor (VEGF165). Inhibition of receptor binding and VEGF-induced vascular permeability through interactions requiring the exon 7-encoded domain. *J Biol Chem* **273**: 20556–67.

34. Tuerk, C., MacDougal, S., and Gold, L. (1992). RNA pseudoknots that inhibit human immunodeficiency virus type 1 reverse transcriptase. *Proc Natl Acad Sci U S A* **89**: 6988–92.

35. Winkler, W., Nahvi, A., and Breaker, R. R. (2002). Thiamine derivatives bind messenger RNAs directly to regulate bacterial gene expression. *Nature* **419**: 952–6.

36. Kruger, K., Grabowski, P. J., Zaug, A. J., Sands, J., Gottschling, D. E., and Cech, T. R. (1982). Self-splicing RNA: autoexcision and autocyclization of the ribosomal RNA intervening sequence of Tetrahymena. *Cell* **31**: 147–57.

37. Guerrier-Takada, C., Gardiner, K., Marsh, T., Pace, N., and Altman, S. (1983). The RNA moiety of ribonuclease P is the catalytic subunit of the enzyme. *Cell* **35**: 849–57.

38. Robertson, D. L. and Joyce, G. F. (1990). Selection in vitro of an RNA enzyme that specifically cleaves single-stranded DNA. *Nature* **344**: 467–8.

39. Breaker, R. R. and Joyce, G. F. (1994). A DNA enzyme that cleaves RNA. *Chem Biol* **1**: 223–9.

40. Ramezani, A., Ma, X. Z., Nazari, R., and Joshi, S. (2002). Development and testing of retroviral vectors expressing multimeric hammerhead ribozymes targeted against all major clades of HIV-1. *Front Biosci* **7**: a29–36.

41. Chakraborti, S. and Banerjea, A. C. (2003). Inhibition of HIV-1 gene expression by novel DNA enzymes targeted to cleave HIV-1 TAR RNA: potential effectiveness against all HIV-1 isolates. *Mol Ther* **7**: 817–26.

42. Fire, A., Xu, S., Montgomery, M. K., Kostas, S. A., Driver, S. E., and Mello, C. C. (1998). Potent and specific genetic interference by double-stranded RNA in *Caenorhabditis elegans*. *Nature* **391**: 806–11.

43. Lagos-Quintana, M., Rauhut, R., Lendeckel, W., and Tuschl, T. (2001). Identification of novel genes coding for small expressed RNAs. *Science* **294**: 853–8.

44. Lau, N. C., Lim, L. P., Weinstein, E. G., and Bartel, D. P. (2001). An abundant class of tiny RNAs with probable regulatory roles in *Caenorhabditis elegans*. *Science* **294**: 858–62.

45. Lee, R. C. and Ambros, V. (2001). An extensive class of small RNAs in *Caenorhabditis elegans*. *Science* **294**: 862–4.

46. Elbashir, S. M., Harborth, J., Lendeckel, W., Yalcin, A., Weber, K., and Tuschl, T. (2001). Duplexes of 21-nucleotide RNAs mediate RNA interference in cultured mammalian cells. *Nature* **411**: 494–8.

47. Li, M., Li, H., and Rossi, J. J. (2006). RNAi in combination with a ribozyme and TAR decoy for treatment of HIV infection in hematopoietic cell gene therapy. *Ann N Y Acad Sci* **1082**: 172–9.

CHAPTER 3

USE OF siRNA OLIGONUCLEOTIDES TO STUDY GENE FUNCTION

KRISTIN A. WIEDERHOLT and ADAM N. HARRIS

3.1 INTRODUCTION

RNA interference (RNAi) describes the phenomenon in which double-stranded RNA (dsRNA) can inhibit gene expression via sequence-specific degradation of homologous mRNA sequences. This highly evolutionarily conserved process was first discovered in 1998 by Andrew Fire and Craig Mello in the nematode worm *Caenorhabditis elegans* and later found in a wide variety of organisms, including mammals. Although the molecular details are still being uncovered, an intricate model has emerged which establishes the processing of dsRNA into shorter 20–23 base pairs (bp) fragments by the enzyme Dicer. These shorter fragments are called small interfering RNAs (siRNAs). The antisense strand of the siRNA duplex is responsible for guiding the nucleotide recognition and cleavage of the target RNA by the <u>R</u>NA-<u>i</u>nduced <u>s</u>ilencing <u>c</u>omplex (RISC), an RNA-induced silencing multimeric protein complex, which subsequently functions in silencing the complementary messenger RNA (mRNA) targets (reviewed in Reference 1)

RNAi is a powerful gene-silencing technique, which has gained widespread acceptance for studying gene function and validating gene targets. There are a number of important factors that must be considered in order to achieve high-quality RNAi experimental results. Here, we provide a user's guide for newcomers as well as discuss complex issues involving the target sequence design process, methods to deliver siRNA, experimental design considerations, and methods to detect gene inhibition and resulting phenotypes.

RNA Interference: Application to Drug Discovery and Challenges to Pharmaceutical Development, Edited by Paul H. Johnson
Copyright © 2011 John Wiley & Sons, Inc.

3.2 SUCCESSFUL siRNA DESIGN STRATEGIES

The use of siRNA to inhibit gene expression is superior to other modes of gene inhibition, such as gene targeting by homologous recombination or small molecule inhibitors, because siRNA duplexes can be rationally designed to any gene based simply on knowledge of the target RNA sequence. However, it is imperative to understand the empirical guidelines and limitations for effective siRNA design. For example, the activity and specificity of RNAi duplexes are highly dependent on target site selection. Studies have shown shifting the target site by as few as 1–2 nucleotides (nt) can have a dramatic effect on activity [2].

The first siRNA design guidelines published by Elbashir et al. [3] recommended searching for the sequence motif $AA(N_{19})TT$ and using deoxythymidine dinucleotide (dTdT) overhangs at each 3′ end of the siRNA duplex. Since the initial design recommendations were published, several research groups have assessed the activity of a large number of duplexes and employed bioinformatic analyses to derive additional design criteria. These research efforts are intended to increase the "hit-rate"—the fraction of functionally active duplexes among those tested—and specificity of the siRNAs. An overview of these findings is described below as a guide for researchers new to the design process (see also Figure 3.1).

3.2.1 Obtain mRNA Sequence for Target Selection

Rational siRNA design begins with identification of the nucleotide sequence for the gene of interest. A number of publicly available databases provide searchable interfaces to find nucleotide sequences for target genes. These databases include the DNA Data Bank of Japan (DDBJ), European Molecular Biology Laboratory (EMBL), and the U.S. National Center for Biotechnology Information (NCBI). When obtaining sequence information for siRNA design, it is important to understand how the information is defined and its primary source. For illustration purposes, this section focuses on the information and nomenclature available in the NCBI database.

Entrez Gene is a searchable interface in NCBI for gene-specific information available from several databases including the Reference Sequence (RefSeq) database. The RefSeq database is manually curated to provide nonredundant, full-length sequence data accurately linked to gene names. Use of the RefSeq mRNA nucleotide information denoted by an NM (mRNA) or XM (predicted mRNA) accession number (see Figure 3.2) is recommended to ensure that the correct sequence is used and to avoid targeting functionally inactive regions such as introns [4].

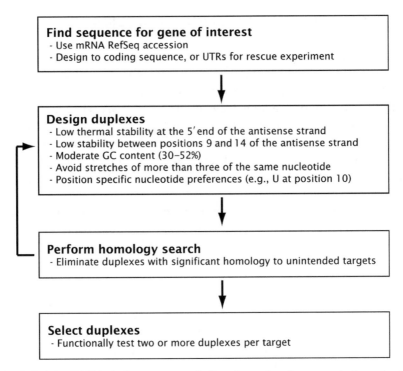

FIGURE 3.1   RNAi design process. A flowchart showing a typical method by which siRNA duplex designs are generated, from identifying the sequence for the gene of interest to selecting duplexes to be tested.

Once mRNA sequence information is located for the gene of interest, it is important to consider which region of the gene to target. Designing duplexes to target the coding sequence is the preferred approach although this is not a requisite. RNAi duplexes targeting the 5′ or 3′ untranslated regions (UTR) have been shown to successfully suppress gene expression [5, 6] and can be useful for gene rescue experiments (see Section 3.6). Depending on the research goals, a region that is unique or common to different splice variants can be selected for the design. Failure to target all splice variants may result in incomplete knockdown of gene function. However, in order to determine the functional importance of a specific protein isoform, variant-specific siRNA design may be successfully employed.

3.2.2 Optimal Length of siRNA Duplexes

In the endogenous RNAi pathway, Dicer, an RNase III enzyme, cleaves long dsRNA into duplexes about 20–23 nt in length. To exploit the mechanism of

AKT1 (NM_001014431.1)

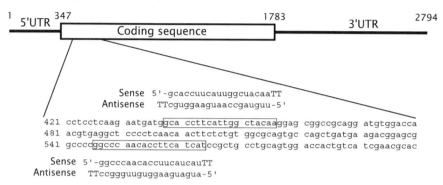

FIGURE 3.2   Design example. Schematic showing the UTRs (lines) and coding sequence (open box) of the human AKT1 gene, represented by RefSeq accession NM_001014431.1. Numbers along the top indicate sequence position within the accession. The gene sequence between nucleotides 421 and 600 is shown in detail below the diagram and two target sites picked by a design algorithm are shown (boxed text). The sequences of two siRNA duplexes corresponding to the target sites are shown above and below the gene sequence. The siRNAs consist of sense and antisense strands of 21 nt each which form 19 bp of duplex and have 3′ dTdT overhangs.

the endogenous pathway, the rational design of duplexes typically involves selecting complementary 21-nt RNAs that form a 19-bp duplex with two nucleotide 3′ overhangs [7]. While choosing duplexes of 21 mers is common practice, it is not an absolute requirement because longer duplexes have also been shown to effectively enter the RNAi pathway and efficiently inhibit target gene expression [8, 9]. For application in mammalian cells, it is not recommended to exceed 30 bp since longer duplexes are associated with induction of interferon and cell death [10, 11]. Researchers have reported that in some instances duplexes composed of strands longer than 21 nt can result in a higher level of activity [8]. Thus, selection of 21-mer siRNAs is commonly employed, but use of longer duplexes may provide additional benefits.

3.2.3   Thermodynamics and Nucleotide Composition

Target site selection is one of the key elements in producing highly functional duplexes. Duplex unwinding and loading of the guide strand is necessary for formation of the active RISC. Technically, either strand of an siRNA duplex can load into the RISC and act as the guide strand. Duplexes for which loading of the antisense strand, the strand capable of base pairing to and cleaving the target RNA, is favored over the sense strand tend to be more effective [12]. The orientation of strand loading is controlled in part by the relative thermal stability at the two ends of the duplex. Duplexes with low thermal stability at the 5′ end of the antisense strand, relative to the 5′ end of sense strand, correlate with functional activity [13]. To achieve favorable thermodynamic properties, duplexes are selected that are AU rich on the 5′ end of the antisense strand and GC rich on the 5′ end of the sense strand. Some duplexes with favorable thermodynamics result in only 50% inhibition [13], while some duplexes with unfavorable thermodynamics result in high level of inhibition, indicating that there are other factors that contribute to functional activity. For example, low thermal stability between nucleotides 9 and 14 of the antisense strand has been shown to be more common in active than in inactive duplexes [13].

In addition to thermodynamic parameters, the nucleotide composition of the duplex plays a role in dictating the level of activity. In general, duplexes with moderate to low GC content (30–52%) [14] that avoid homopolymeric stretches of more than three of the same nucleotide correlate with a higher functionality. Research studies have demonstrated a number of nucleotide preferences at specific positions. For example, duplexes with an A at position 3 and 19, U at position 10, A or U at position 19 of the sense or passenger strand [15] correlate with high activity. Other parameters such as the secondary structure of the duplex and target RNA may also affect activity. Avoiding sequences that contain internal repeats or palindromes is recommended to prevent the siRNA strands from folding back on themselves [15].

Taken together, these research studies demonstrate that there are a number of different parameters responsible for the effectiveness of siRNA duplexes. The most successful *in silico* prediction algorithms take into consideration weighted averages of the factors discussed and may include other criteria. There are a number of algorithms available freely on the World Wide Web that will generate designs on the basis of input of accession numbers or target gene sequences. While many of these algorithms design duplexes with a high rate of success, it is always important to test at least three duplex designs per target gene to increase the likelihood of finding at least one, and preferably two (see Section 3.6), functional duplexes.

3.3 siRNA TARGET SPECIFICITY

Although RNAi has gained widespread acceptance for inhibiting gene expression, there are growing concerns regarding siRNA specificity. Introduction of some siRNAs into cells can lead to changes in the phenotype that are unrelated to inhibition of the target gene. Some of these nonspecific effects can be attributed to "off-target effects"—inhibition of unintended target genes. Duplexes with partial homology to other targets can inhibit gene expression by cleaving the target [16, 17] or altering protein expression through an miRNA-like mechanism [18, 19], depending on the level of homology. Other nonspecific effects can be attributed to aptamer effects resulting from a particular sequence motif. Recent publications have demonstrated that the sequence motifs 5'-UGUGU-3' and 5'-GUCCUUCAA-3' can induce an interferon response [20, 21], and there may be other yet unidentified deleterious motifs. Understanding and controlling the specificity of RNAi is critical because nonspecific effects can complicate interpretation of RNAi experiments or lead to false positive results.

One approach to minimizing off-target effects is to eliminate duplexes with significant homology to other targets during the design process. The successful application of this approach requires an understanding of the factors responsible for the recognition and cleavage of the intended RNA by the active RISC. Early studies reported that a single mismatch in the middle of the antisense strand of an siRNA is sufficient to discriminate between target and nontarget RNAs [22], and initially researchers thought this could be universally applied for the design of highly specific duplexes. Subsequent microarray profiling studies [16, 23] and bioinformatic analyses of siRNAs resulting in false positives in high-throughput screening assays have shown the situation is far more complex than originally anticipated [24].

siRNAs with matches as short as 6–7 nt between nucleotides 2 and 8 from the 5' end of the antisense strand, known as the "seed" region, and nontargeted RNAs can mediate off-target gene regulation [23–25]. Systematic activity studies have shown that the introduction of single nucleotide mismatches to targets can reduce or abolish activity of duplexes to varying degrees; the extent of the effect depends on the position and composition of the mismatch [26, 27]. A common finding among these studies is that siRNA-guided destruction of the target RNA is mediated primarily by the seed recognition sequence from nucleotides 2 to 8 and the cleavage region comprising nucleotides 10 and 11. Selecting sequences containing mismatches in these regions with respect to unintended targets can reduce off-target effects. Avoiding full homology in these regions to potential off-target genes can reduce off-target effects but does not guarantee their complete elimination.

Comparative sequence analysis of the target sequence with other known transcripts during the design process is critical to maximizing RNAi specificity and reducing the potential for off-target effects. There are a number of publicly available tools that provide a quick and easy way to search for possible nucleotide matches to unintended targets. A commonly used tool is the Basic Local Alignment Search Tool (BLAST) available from NCBI. The output of a BLAST search displays pairwise alignments with targets found in the query database and can differ depending on the database and parameters or stringency criteria selected. The stringency can be increased or decreased by changing the word size—the minimum nucleotide length found to be considered a match—or the statistical significance threshold value (E value). Increasing the stringency can reduce the number of matches reported but might result in missing a significant match. The default word size match is 11 nt and can be used to eliminate duplexes with partial matches of this length to unintended targets during the design process. However, this process would not necessarily identify a six-nucleotide match in the seed region.

Advanced alignment programs such as SSearch use the Smith–Waterman algorithm to look for these smaller word size matches. While it can find these smaller matches, the Smith–Waterman algorithm is very processor-time intensive. Homology searches for s6 nt in a target genome will result in a long list of matches, many of which may have no biological consequences. Utilizing BLAST analyses during the initial design process is recommended in order to eliminate sequences with strong homology to other targets. Subsequently, use of a more stringent algorithm such as Smith–Waterman alignment should be applied to duplexes that pass the BLAST filter. Bioinformatics can reduce the potential for off-target effects but will not completely eliminate them. Good experimental design, in addition to bioinformatics, should be employed to ensure high-quality results.

3.4   CHEMICALLY MODIFIED siRNAs

Chemical synthesis of siRNA duplexes provides the opportunity to incorporate natural and unnatural chemical modifications during the synthesis process. In addition, a wide range of molecules such as dyes can be post-synthetically conjugated to duplexes modified with an appropriate functional group. Chemical modifications can be employed to enhance the specificity, activity, and stability toward nucleases of siRNA, the last of which can be an important consideration for researchers moving into *in vivo* model systems.

The first-generation siRNA duplexes were composed of unmodified ribonucleotides that typically have 3'dTdT overhangs. This reduces the synthesis cost but provides a comparable level of activity [3, 28]. Besides deoxythymidine substitution, virtually any position of the duplex can be modified including the phosphate backbone, the sugar, nucleotide bases, or the 5' and 3' hydroxyl groups (Figure 3.3). Incorporation of chemical modifications can impart beneficial properties; however, not all chemically modified duplexes maintain a high level of activity.

Loading of the guide strand into the RISC requires the ATP-dependent phosphorylation of the 5' hydroxyl group [29]. Researchers have

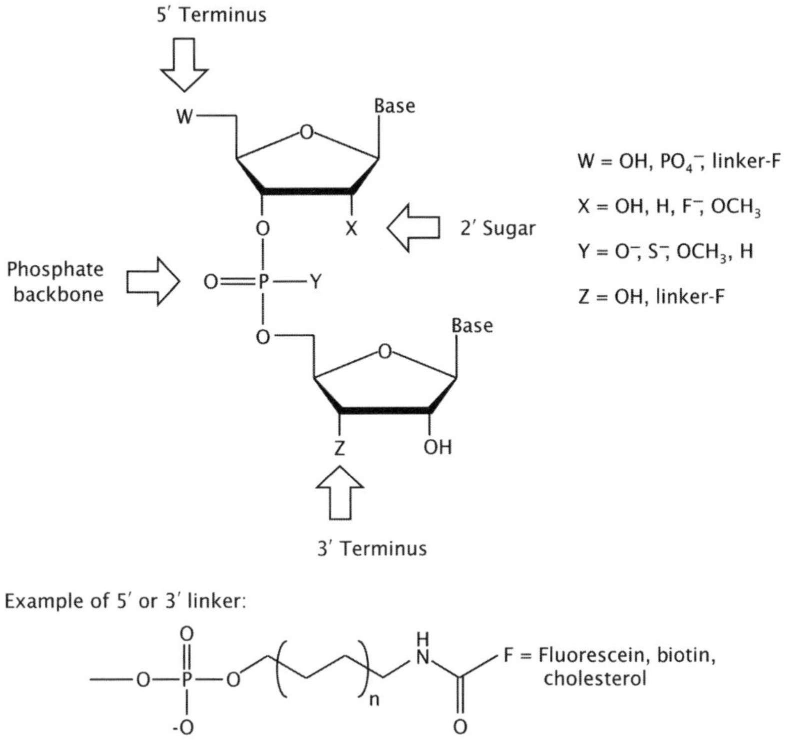

5′ Terminus

Base

W

2′ Sugar

Phosphate
backbone

$O=P-Y$

Base

W = OH, PO₄⁻, linker-F

X = OH, H, F⁻, OCH₃

Y = O⁻, S⁻, OCH₃, H

Z = OH, linker-F

3′ Terminus

Example of 5′ or 3′ linker:

F = Fluorescein, biotin,
cholesterol

FIGURE 3.3 Chemical modifications for siRNA Schematic indicating various positions that can be modified at the termini, phosphate, or sugar moieties in an RNA strand. Possible modifications are designated by W, X, Y, and Z. An example of a terminal linker used to conjugate additional macromolecules to the siRNA strand is shown at the bottom.

hypothesized that the addition of a 5′ phosphate during the chemical synthesis might increase loading efficiency of the antisense strand into the RISC [30]. However, functional activity comparisons of duplexes made with and without a 5′ phosphate group have revealed the same level of activity [28]. In addition, conjugating fluorescent dyes or molecules such as cholesterol to the 3′ or 5′ ends of siRNA duplexes can be useful for assessing uptake across the cell membrane (see Section 3.5) or enhancing biodistribution *in vivo* [31]. The 3′ end of either strand or the 5′ end of the sense strand can be modified without a loss in activity. However, modification of the 5′ end of the antisense strand or blocking phosphorylation of its hydroxyl group is not recommended, as it results in a loss of activity.

Replacing some of the phosphodiester linkages in the RNA backbone with alternatives such as phosphorothioate can enhance the nuclease stability of siRNAs without a loss in activity; however, phosphorothioate may also lead to increased toxicity when applied to cells. A less toxic method to enhance the nuclease stability of siRNA duplexes is by modifying the sugar residue, such as substitution of the 2′ hydroxyl with O-methyl or fluoro groups [32]. In addition to enhancing siRNA stability, use of 2′-O-methyl (2′OMe) nucleotides at specific positions, most notably position 2 on the antisense strand, has been shown to reduce off-target effects [33]. More extensive modification of the antisense strand with 2′OMe results in a loss of activity [34–36]. Applied to the sense strand, these modifications can enhance specificity by inactivating or preventing the sense strand from cleaving unintended targets. Modifications can impart beneficial properties to the duplexes, but not all chemically modified constructs are functionally active, and some may require screening of more target sites than unmodified siRNAs to find the requisite functional activity.

3.5 DELIVERING siRNA INTO CELL CULTURE

Use of synthetic siRNA requires a transfection protocol for delivery to the interior of the cell. Unmodified RNA duplexes are rapidly degraded in cell culture medium, and even those stabilized by chemical changes are unable to enter cells without the aid of a delivery vehicle. This section will primarily discuss the most common method for siRNA introduction—complexation with cationic lipids—but will conclude with a brief section on electroporation.

3.5.1 Cationic Lipid-Mediated Transfection of siRNA

The most common method by which siRNA is transfected is complexation with cationic lipids. Many different lipid formulations have been employed for this purpose, and their relative efficiencies vary by cell type. There is no universal lipid that gives optimal delivery to all cell types, but some have fairly broad ranges while others are narrow "specialty" reagents. By definition, all cationic lipids have a hydrophobic region and a positively charged head group, although many different variations on this chemical structure have been generated. The head group interacts with the negatively charged phosphate backbone of nucleic acids (such as plasmid DNAs or siRNAs), while the lipid regions allow the formation of lipoplexes that provide protection from the aqueous environment of the culture medium [37]. The lipoplexes can include an outside layer of positively charged head groups, which is thought to interact with negatively charged proteoglycans on the cell surface. When applied to cells, the lipoplexes are endocytosed as vesicles. If the nucleic acid payload is able to escape from these endosomes before it is degraded in lysosomes, it enters the cytoplasm. In the case of DNA-based plasmid vectors, subsequent entry into the nucleus for expression is required. However, siRNAs are active directly in the cytoplasm, which can result in their transfection being more efficient even if the same lipid and cell type are used.

3.5.2 Optimization of siRNA Transfection with Cationic Lipids

The goal of siRNA transfection is usually to maximize the transfection efficiency, which is calculated as the percentage of cells to which the specific duplex siRNAs are successfully delivered. Due to the high potency of RNAi, generally only low levels of siRNA need to be delivered to any given cell to achieve sufficient knockdown. However, untransfected cells will not exhibit gene silencing and will continue to express the target mRNA and protein. Thus, for downstream assays that assess the effect of knockdown on the cell population, the background expression from untransfected cells will reduce the overall percent knockdown, and optimizing the transfection efficiency is desirable.

The process of transfection can often be disruptive to cellular function, regardless of the payload. Perturbation of the cell cycle, decreased proliferation, and cell death can result from high concentrations of lipoplexes introduced into the medium. Thus, it is important to properly control for these effects of transfection (see Section 3.6). In addition, undesirable effects of transfection on the cells, including general toxicity, should be monitored, and any optimization of transfection should seek to balance these effects against the efficiency obtained. How much toxicity is tolerable depends in part on the nature of the downstream assays, which will be performed to monitor the outcome of target gene silencing.

There are four key variables that need to be optimized for transfection: the cationic lipid used, the cell density, the concentration of the lipid, and the concentration of the siRNA. These factors may be closely connected, and thus, a matrix of conditions (as shown by the hypothetical transfection conditions in Figure 3.4) should be tested.

As mentioned above, many cationic lipids, some commercially available, have been created and tested. There may already be optimized transfection protocols available for some of these reagents for a variety of cell types. When those data are limiting, a panel of lipids may need to be screened for best results. A limited optimization within the recommended parameters for each lipid can be attempted to quickly identify those with enough promise for further evaluation.

There are two factors to consider when determining the optimal cell density. First, different lipids work best at different densities; for example, some lipids exhibit toxicity at low cell densities but yield high transfection efficiencies at densities near confluence. Second, the experimental design may favor

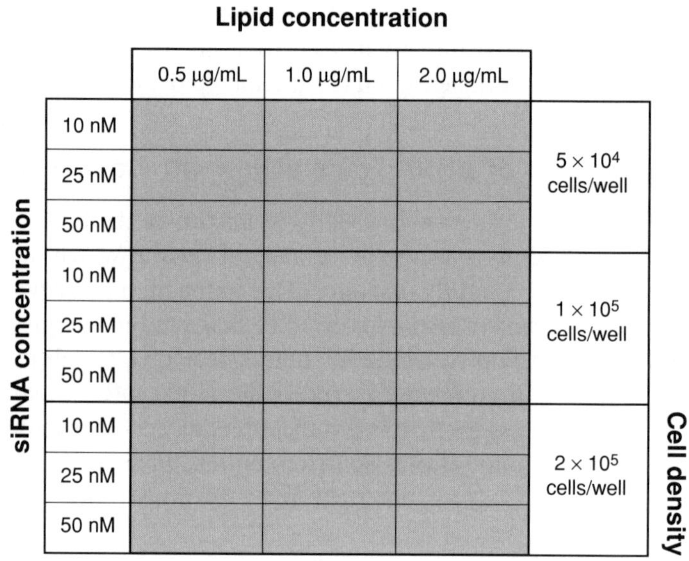

Lipid concentration

FIGURE 3.4   Example transfection optimization conditions. A matrix of test conditions is shown that vary three key parameters: lipid concentration (top), siRNA concentration (left), and cell density (right). Values are based on typical transfection protocol for 24-well dishes.

one density over another. If knockdown will be measured or the phenotype exhibited early (one to two days posttransfection), then a high plating density can be used without the cells overgrowing. This may provide more material for the downstream assay, enabling a smaller well size to be used to increase throughput. On the other hand, if the assay will not take place until three or four days after transfection, seeding at low density may enable the experiment to be performed without the need for transferring the cells.

Optimal lipid concentrations will vary with the lipid used and the plating density. Generally, the more dense the cells are, the more lipid that should be employed. Toxicity analysis using dead cell stains, detecting cellular enzymes released into the medium by lysis, or cell proliferation assays should be performed, and the toxicity associated with higher lipid concentrations should be counterbalanced with increased delivery rates. Transfecting a panel of negative controls (see Section 3.6.3) and comparing the toxicity to no treatment is recommended.

Finally, siRNA concentration has a dose-dependent effect on activity. Generally, the higher the duplex concentration used, the higher the transfection efficiency, and ultimately, the knockdown. However, as the concentration increases, the targeted gene silencing activity will begin to plateau while weaker off-target effects may continue to build. The best strategy is to start with a relatively high amount of siRNA, establish that knockdown can be achieved, and then reduce the siRNA concentration to the lowest effective dose. Measuring the siRNA level as its final concentration in the medium, 20–50 nM is a good starting point, although there are many siRNAs that are functional at significantly lower concentrations.

3.5.3 Fluorescently Labeled RNA Duplexes as Tools for Transfection Optimization

The final metric for determination of transfection success is knockdown of the target gene. However, transfection optimization requires the covariance of several parameters, and the various methods available for the measurement of target gene expression are not expedient for initial multivariable testing. For this reason, fluorescently labeled RNA duplexes—uptake controls—are often employed. Fluorescent duplexes enable rapid and simple readout of transfection success, reducing the turnaround time between rounds of optimization. They can be visualized under a fluorescent microscope or detected by flow cytometry within a day of transfection.

The uptake controls themselves can be active siRNA duplexes, commonly with a fluorescent tag linked to the 5′ end of the sense strand—a position in which the tag does not seem to interfere with gene silencing. However, in many cases it can be difficult to estimate overall efficiencies with these labeled siRNAs using microscopy because of the weak particulate fluorescence pattern observed. It is often unclear from visual inspection whether the duplexes have actually entered the cells or have merely attached to the outside of the plasma membrane. For this reason, stabilized fluorescent control duplexes using modified chemistries have been created, which produce brighter intracellular signals (see Figures 3.3 and 3.5). These may preferentially localize to nuclei, making data interpretation simple after co-staining with a nuclear dye.

To verify that an unlabeled siRNA behaves in the same manner as a fluorescently labeled duplex and because higher concentrations of fluorescent duplexes may be needed for detection than is required for siRNA-mediated knockdown, it is important to always include follow-up with transfection of a positive control siRNA (see Section 3.6) to confirm knockdown.

3.5.4 Delivery of siRNAs Using Electroporation

Some cells, especially primary and suspension cells, are refractory to transfection with cationic lipids. A commonly used alternative delivery method is electroporation. Electroporation uses short, high-voltage electric pulses to open transient pores in membranes of cells through which nucleic acids may enter (reviewed in Reference 38). Initially used for introduction of plasmids

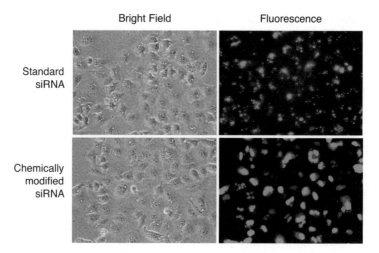

FIGURE 3.5   Fluorescent transfection indicators. A549 cells transfected with 6-FAM-labeled standard siRNA (upper panels) or chemically modified siRNA (lower panels) are shown in bright field (left) and fluorescent (right) images. Chemical modifications stabilize the duplex giving a clearer indication of cellular uptake. (For a color version of this figure, see plate 1.)

into bacteria, the technique was associated with high rates of cell death. However, subsequent optimization has enabled electroporation to become effective for delivery of siRNA with greater than 90% viability in some mammalian cell types.

Although some newer devices allow cells to be electroporated while attached to tissue culture plates, most require the cells to be moved to electrode-containing cuvettes. Current electroporators typically generate square wave pulses, and the key optimizing parameters are the length, strength, and number of pulses applied. In addition, a pulsing medium with low conductivity is usually recommended to decrease cell death. After electroporation, provided the cells are given a few minutes to reseal their membranes, they can be returned to plates and standard culturing conditions. The same controls during transfection and subsequent readout (see Sections 3.6 and 3.7.1) can be applied to both cationic lipid and electroporation techniques.

3.6   EXPERIMENTAL DESIGN

To achieve high-quality RNAi results, proper experimental design is critical [39, 40]. Key controls need to be employed, including screening of multiple RNA duplexes for each target, using appropriate negative and positive controls, confirming knockdown by more than one method, and in some cases,

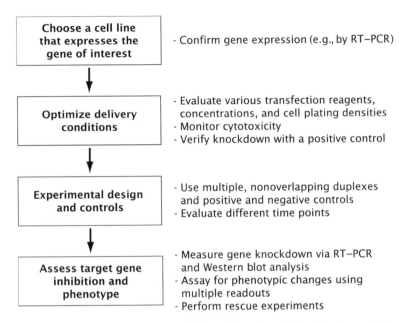

FIGURE 3.6   RNAi experiment workflow. Flowchart indicating the workflow for a typical RNAi experiment. A cell line is identified that expresses the target gene, then transfection conditions are optimized. Following transfection optimization, the siRNAs are transfected using proper controls and knockdown is determined by multiple methods.

performing a rescue experiment. This section describes these considerations and gives recommendations for when they should be applied (see Figure 3.6).

3.6.1 Using Duplexes in Pools or Individually

Although most siRNA duplexes created using the latest rational design algorithms will be functional, there remains a percentage that will fail. Even among the active duplexes, knockdown levels will vary. One approach to simplifying RNAi experiments is to pool together three or four different duplexes targeting the same gene and introduce them into a single cell population simultaneously.

The principal advantage of pooling is that it virtually eliminates knockdown failures, because it is rare for none of the members of the pool to be active. This can be especially useful in screening assays with many different target genes to reduce the size of the experiment because a single pool targeting each gene is transfected instead of individually transfecting the same three or four duplexes.

One perceived advantage of pooling is an amelioration of off-target effects by reducing the concentration of the individual duplexes. Researchers have shown that the off-target profile for some siRNAs can be titrated away by reducing the concentration of duplex delivered to the cell [17, 41]. Typically the sum of the concentrations of the duplexes in the pool is the same as the concentration at which a single duplex would be used in a similar experiment. The total knockdown activity of pooled duplexes on the target gene will relate to the sum of the concentrations of the active duplexes, but the off-target activities of those duplexes will in most cases relate to the now reduced concentrations of individual duplexes. This is because each duplex, by virtue of being designed to a different site in the target gene, is expected to have a unique off-target signature.

Some data have been interpreted to suggest that simple pools limited to three or four duplexes may not sufficiently reduce the dose of the individual duplexes to eliminate off-targeting [42]. On the other hand, pools of tens to hundreds of duplexes produced enzymatically by cleavage of long dsRNA by Dicer dramatically reduce off-target gene knockdown [42]. However, a critical disadvantage of pooling is that it eliminates the benefit of knockdown with redundant active duplexes discussed in the next section.

3.6.2 Knockdown with Two or More Active Duplexes

Whenever possible, at least two active duplexes derived from nonoverlapping sites in the target gene should be identified. Using these duplexes in each gene silencing experiment is a simple but very powerful control for off-target and sequence-motif-linked nonspecific effects. As discussed in the pooling section above, individual, nonoverlapping duplexes are expected to have different off-target gene signatures. In addition, it is unlikely for two duplexes linked only by inhibition of a common target to share sequence motifs leading to identical nonspecific effects such as stimulation of interferon-related genes. Thus, if the same phenotype is triggered by two or more independent duplexes, it increases the statistical probability of a correlation with target gene suppression. Conversely, if the duplexes have similar activity against the target gene but produce different phenotypes, this is an indicator of off-target or nonspecific activity. In these cases, additional active duplexes to the gene should be identified to delineate specific and nonspecific effects. While using duplexes separately rather than pooling during RNAi screens initially increases the number of wells needed to be transfected, the number of false positives can be decreased by allowing independent confirmation of bona fide phenotypes, thus reducing the number of target genes requiring validation in follow-up screens.

3.6.3 Negative Controls

Using multiple siRNAs that are active against the target gene can control for off-target and motif-induced nonspecific effects. However, it is important to include nontargeting or negative control duplexes in all RNAi experiments. These duplexes control for sequence-independent effects, which may occur from introducing small RNAs into cells. We recommend independently transfecting one or more negative control siRNAs rather than "lipid only" transfection or "buffer only" electroporation, as the presence of the duplexes complexed with lipid or in the pulsing medium may influence the final result on the cells. In addition, there may be effects related to the introduction of high levels of siRNA into cells. For example, RNAs transfected into the cell may out-compete endogenous small RNAs (such as miRNAs) for entry into RISC and disrupt normal gene regulation. Therefore, it is important that the negative control duplexes be designed in a sequence configuration capable of entering efficiently into the RNAi pathway (e.g., by having at least one end with low thermodynamic stability), yet not designed to target any specific gene. Two types of negative control duplexes have been applied in RNAi experiments: scrambled and universal.

A scrambled control has the same base composition as the target-specific duplex, but the order of the bases is rearranged, usually through several overlapping inversions. Both strands of the duplex are rearranged identically to maintain base pairing. If this option is chosen, it is important to keep two or three terminal base pairs on each end of the duplex unchanged, as this will allow for similar loading into the RISC. A separate scrambled control should be designed for each duplex siRNA target. It is important to subject the scrambled controls to homology searches such as BLAST in order to reduce their potential for unanticipated targeting.

Universal negative control siRNAs are similar in design to scrambled controls, but they are intended for use in conjunction with a broad number of target-specific duplexes. Universal controls do not match each target duplex in base composition, but may instead be classified into ranges of similar GC content. As with scrambled duplexes, they are designed to have no significant predicted silencing activity against the transcriptomes of the target species. While not mimicking the active duplexes as closely, a small number of universal controls can be designed (or purchased from commercial sources) and employed in all experiments. In addition, far fewer wells need to be reserved for universal versus scrambled controls when many target-specific siRNAs are being tested. Overall, given the potential for any given sequence to induce nonspecific or off-target effects, it is best to use a panel of negative controls to verify that they behave consistently and similar to no treatment in each experiment and enable the identification of outlying results.

3.6.4 Positive Controls

In addition to negative controls not expected to induce RNAi inhibition in the target cell, positive control siRNAs should be employed whenever practicable. These are previously validated duplexes targeting a gene known to be expressed in the cell line of interest. If chosen to target "housekeeping" genes which are ubiquitously expressed, only a small set of positive controls for each species whose cells will be tested may be needed.

Positive control duplexes serve several functions. First, they can be used to control for transfection (see Section 3.5), giving a positive indication that delivery has been successful. Second, positive control duplexes can confirm that the method used to measure knockdown (discussed in Section 3.7) is functioning properly. The relative success of novel duplexes being tested can be compared with standards indicating failure of knockdown (negative controls) and successful silencing (positive controls). A small window of measurement between failure and success may indicate that a low transfection efficiency has been achieved or that an inappropriate detection method is being used. Finally, positive controls can be used to test that phenotypic changes are detectable. Duplexes known to function against other members of the target gene's pathway or against genes in pathways involved in the same process (e.g., cell proliferation or apoptosis) can be used to determine the extent of the phenotype that can be expected from successful knockdown of the target.

3.6.5 Reversing the Knockdown

Perhaps the most powerful and convincing method for determining that a phenotype produced during an RNAi experiment is the consequence of suppression of the intended target is the gene rescue method (see Figure 3.7). Gene rescue is an attempt to reverse the knockdown phenotype by simultaneous introduction of both the siRNA and a vector expressing an RNAi-resistant version of the target gene. If the return of expression of the gene in the presence of the siRNA restores the normal phenotype to the cell, then the knockdown phenotype is not a result of off-target or nonspecific effects of siRNA introduction. Furthermore, this technique can also be used to express mutant, truncated, or chimeric forms of the target gene to determine which domains or residues are required for normal gene function and which mutations can induce abnormal function.

While powerful, the rescue technique can be difficult to employ. Creation of the RNAi-resistant gene expression construct is an extra step and potentially time-consuming. If the siRNAs are designed to the coding sequence of the target gene, two or more mutations can be introduced into the siRNA target sites in the rescue gene such that the amino acid sequence is left unchanged.

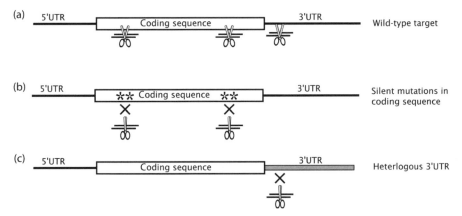

FIGURE 3.7 RNAi rescue constructs. Schematic showing two different approaches to using rescue constructs to confirm the specificity of phenotypes generated during an RNAi experiment. (a) Diagram of the endogenous target gene indicating the locations of the UTRs and coding sequence as in Figure 3.1. The positions of two siRNA target sites in the coding region and a site in the 3'UTR are indicated by double-lines and open scissors indicating cleavage. (b) Schematic of a rescue construct expression cassette, which will replace the activity of the wild-type gene during siRNA-mediated knockdown. Silent mutations (those not affecting the amino acid sequence) have been introduced into the siRNA target sites in the coding sequence (asterisks) to prevent cleavage by the duplexes specific for those sites (double-lines and closed scissors). (c) An alternative rescue construct approach wherein the entire wild-type 3'UTR is replaced by a heterologous 3'UTR in the expression vector. The duplex targeting the wild-type 3'UTR does not recognize a target site in the rescue gene.

Alternatively, if the siRNAs target the 3'UTR, the coding region of the target gene can be expressed from a vector with a heterologous 3'UTR sequence. Of the two approaches, using siRNA duplexes targeting the 3'UTR in combination with a vector containing a different 3'UTR is simplest and produces the most clear-cut results. In some cases, overexpression of the target gene can introduce its own phenotypic changes, so it may be necessary for the rescue construct to use the endogenous promoter or one of similar strength. A tunable, regulated promoter may provide an easier method for re-expression of the target gene at physiological levels.

Finally, the expression construct itself needs to be introduced into the cells, typically by transfection of plasmid DNA. This requires a separate optimization procedure, because conditions for delivery of plasmid DNAs often differ significantly from those for small RNAs, even if the same reagent is used. If the cells are difficult to transfect with plasmids, viral vectors (such as lentiviral, oncoretroviral, or adenoviral) may be needed. Because of the requirement for construction of specialized expression vectors and separate optimization of their delivery, the rescue gene control is usually not included in routine RNAi experiments. Instead, it may be used for final verification of an interesting knockdown phenotype, following careful confirmation of gene silencing using multiple duplexes and appropriate positive and negative controls.

3.7   DETECTION OF KNOCKDOWN

Once the siRNAs have been designed, the delivery method chosen, and the appropriate controls put in place, how can knockdown be measured? RNAi targets and destabilizes mRNA, leading to a decrease in steady-state protein levels and ultimately changes in the processes or structures in which the protein is involved. In this regard, there are various methods aimed to measure siRNA-induced gene silencing (see Figure 3.8). This section discusses these methods and the relative advantages of each. Importantly, it is often necessary to use more than one method to assess the success or failure of an RNAi experiment.

3.7.1   Detecting Knockdown at the mRNA Level by RT–PCR

The primary effect of RNAi is the degradation of target mRNAs, making RNA levels the most direct measure of silencing. The principal advantage of measuring knockdown at the level at which RNAi functions (transcript stability) rather than a downstream step (protein levels or cellular phenotype) is that it can give a clear answer as to the effectiveness of each siRNA without confounding influences such as protein stability, functional redundancy, and thresholds required for phenotypic effect.

The most common and simple method of measuring the level of a specific mRNA is by performing RT–PCR using either a one- or two-step protocol. The names of these protocols describe whether the reverse transcription (RT) and polymerase chain reaction (PCR) steps are performed in the same or separate reaction tubes. In the one-step protocol, gene specific primers are added and the RT and PCR reactions are performed in a single tube. In the two-step protocol, random hexamers and/or oligo dT are used to convert all mRNA present to cDNA using reverse transcriptase. A portion of this cDNA is then transferred to a separate tube to perform the PCR. While the one-step protocol may save time initially and require fewer tubes, the two-step protocol allows for multiple PCR reactions from a single cDNA reaction. The cDNA can be archived, which allows the researcher to return to the sample for analysis of additional genes at a later time. Another advantage of the two-step

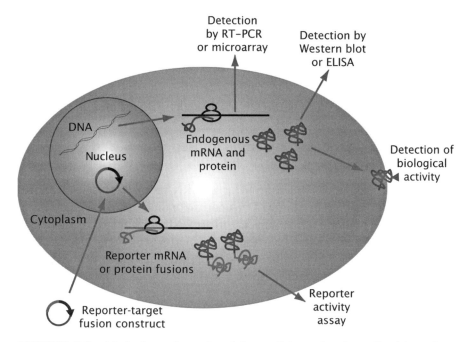

FIGURE 3.8   Methods to detect knockdown. Schematic of a cell with nuclear and cytoplasmic compartments indicated. The upper half shows endogenous mRNA (black line) levels can be determined by RT–PCR or microarray analysis, while endogenous protein (brown squiggle) levels can be measured by Western blot or ELISA. In addition, the normal biological activity of the protein, such as ligand binding (red triangle) may be assayed. The lower half shows a DNA construct that expresses a fusion of a reporter gene (blue) and the target gene (black) can be transfected into the cells. The levels of reporter-target fusion protein can then be measured in a standard activity assay.

protocol is that the RT and PCR steps can be optimized separately, which can facilitate the detection of low copy transcripts.

RT–PCR can be performed as an endpoint assay, whereby the amount of amplified DNA is assessed after a fixed number of cycles, typically by agarose gel electrophoresis. The conditions and cycle number must be chosen carefully to allow for proper quantitation. Alternatively, specialized methods and equipment can be used to assess amplification in "real time" with fluorescent readings taking place at least once per cycle.

One consideration when using RT–PCR to assess RNAi is the location of the primers with respect to the target site. After RISC-mediated cleavage of an mRNA, it is possible for the 5′ and 3′ cleavage products to persist, particularly if the target is very highly expressed. This may confound PCR analysis if the primers are distant from the cleavage site [43]. However, for many targets exonuclease-mediated degradation seems to occur with sufficient rapidity to eliminate cleavage products. Alternatively, if polyA+ RNA is isolated prior to RT–PCR and/or oligo dT primers are used in the RT reaction, the 5′ cleavage product will not be reverse transcribed. Therefore, it may be best to design PCR primers near or upstream of the siRNA target site(s) when possible.

3.7.2 Using Chimeric Transcripts for Reporter-Based Readout of RNAi

An alternative approach to measuring target mRNA transcript levels is to employ a reporter readout by cloning DNA corresponding to the complete target transcript or a portion thereof adjacent to the coding sequence of a reporter gene in a plasmid expression construct. The reporter can be a fluorescent protein such as a GFP or an enzyme with a fluorescent or luminescent substrate (e.g., beta-galactosidase, luciferase, or beta-lactamase). The target gene coding sequence can be cloned as a fusion with the reporter gene's open reading frame (usually C-terminally), or a short segment of the target gene can be cloned into the reporter's 3′UTR. When cotransfected into cells with siRNAs, the plasmid expresses a fusion transcript that can be cleaved by RISC. Live cells or lysates are assayed for reporter protein activity. The level of reporter activity detected with a target-specific siRNA compared with cotransfection with a negative control siRNA is used to quantitate knockdown.

There are several advantages to using the reporter-target gene fusion approach. First, it can be used to validate siRNA functionality in cells without requirement for the target gene to be expressed endogenously. Thus, an immortalized cell line can be substituted for difficult primary cells. The cell line can even be of a different species than the target gene as long as the promoter requirements for reporter gene expression are met. Second, the assay is largely insensitive to transfection efficiency, because the cells that take up the plasmid tend also to take up siRNA as well. Finally, the assays can generally be performed within 24 h of the transfection, are simple to apply to large numbers of samples and replicates, and can be highly quantitative. The principle drawback of this system is the requirement to create the fusion constructs.

3.7.3 Measuring Target Protein Levels

The cellular functions of protein-coding genes are carried out primarily by the encoded proteins themselves. While protein levels are integrally connected to mRNA levels, other factors, such as the rate of translation and protein turnover, influence this relationship. Thus, while mRNA levels are a more direct measure of RNAi, protein levels better connect the knockdown activity of siRNAs to a loss of gene function.

The most common methods to measure the levels of a target protein in the complex mixture of proteins present in cells use antibodies specific to the protein of interest. The protein is detected either by probing a Western blot containing proteins denatured by SDS-PAGE or performing an Enzyme Linked ImmunoSorbent Assay (ELISA), a quantitative measure of specific protein levels in solution.

When assessing inhibition of the protein, the half-life of the protein is an important consideration. By degrading mRNA, RNAi can prevent new protein from being produced, but existing protein will persist until it has been naturally degraded by proteases or diluted by cell division. If the half-life of the protein is long or unknown, it may be important to have an independent means (such as RT–PCR or a reporter fusion) by which to confirm siRNA function. Performing a time course experiment measuring the protein levels is recommended in order to identify the optimal conditions for inhibition. Very persistent proteins may require multiple rounds of transfection to maintain inhibition of the target gene while the protein level is in decline.

3.7.4 Assaying for Knockdown-Associated Phenotypes

Even protein levels are not direct measurements of protein activity in the cell, because some proteins need posttranslational modifications (such as phosphorylation) or cofactors to perform their function. A reduction in the overall amount of a protein in the cell may not reduce the active amount of protein. Furthermore, if the protein is in excess, then even a considerable reduction in its levels may have no effect. Therefore, it may be desirable to confirm knockdown by assaying for a particular cellular phenotype.

The choice of an appropriate phenotypic assay depends upon the expected functionality of the target gene. These may include cell cycle, proliferation, and apoptosis assays. As with any RNAi experiment, all critical controls should be used, including positive control duplexes affecting the same process, if available. It is also important to consider that failure to detect a phenotype associated with knockdown of a gene may be due to functional redundancy with other genes in the cell. If independent means have been tested to show the duplex is functional at the mRNA and/or protein levels, a result of no phenotypic effect is more easily interpreted.

3.8 CONCLUSION

Although the molecular mechanisms of the RNAi pathway are continuing to be elucidated, it is clear that RNAi-induced gene silencing is a powerful tool that enables researchers to study the function of genes in cell culture and *in vivo* model organisms. There are various experimental parameters that are critical for successful gene silencing by siRNAs. In this regard, we have highlighted the criteria for selection of RNAi sequences, efficient delivery methods, required controls, and assays for detection of RNAi-mediated gene silencing. Overall, careful optimization of these parameters will enhance reproducibility, minimize off-target effects and false positives, and contribute to successful RNAi screening of specified target genes.

ACKNOWLEDGMENTS

We thank Dr. Vasiliki Anest, Dr. Cheryl Denault, and Charles Adams for their critical reading of the manuscript.

REFERENCES

1. Dorsett, Y. and Tuschl, T. (2004). siRNAs: applications in functional genomics and potential as therapeutics. *Nat Rev Drug Discov* **3**: 318–29.
2. Holen, T., Amarzguioui, M., Wiiger, M. T., Babaie, E., and Prydz, H. (2002). Positional effects of short interfering RNAs targeting the human coagulation trigger tissue factor. *Nucleic Acids Res* **30**: 1757–66.
3. Elbashir, S. M., Harborth, J., Weber, K., and Tuschl, T. (2002). Analysis of gene function in somatic mammalian cells using small interfering RNAs. *Methods* **26**: 199–213.
4. Zeng, Y. and Cullen, B. R. (2002). RNA interference in human cells is restricted to the cytoplasm. *RNA* **8**: 855–60.
5. Hsieh, A. C., Bo, R., Manola, J., Vazquez, F., Bare, O., Khvorova, A., Scaringe, S. and Sellers, W. R. (2004). A library of siRNA duplexes targeting the phospho-inositide 3-kinase pathway: determinants of gene silencing for use in cell-based screens. *Nucleic Acids Res* **32**: 893–901.
6. McManus, M. T., Haines, B. B., Dillon, C. P., Whitehurst, C. E., Van Parijs, L., Chen, J. and Sharp, P. A. (2002). Small interfering RNA-mediated gene silencing in T lymphocytes. *J Immunol* **169**: 5754–60.
7. Elbashir, S. M., Harborth, J., Lendeckel, W., Yalcin, A., Weber, K., and Tuschl, T. (2001). Duplexes of 21-nucleotide RNAs mediate RNA interference in cultured mammalian cells. *Nature* **411**: 494–8.
8. Kim, D. H., Behlke, M. A., Rose, S. D., Chang, M. S., Choi, S., and Rossi, J. J. (2005). Synthetic dsRNA Dicer substrates enhance RNAi potency and efficacy. *Nat Biotechnol* **23**: 222–26.
9. Rose, S. D., Kim, D. H., Amarzguioui, M., Heidel, J. D., Collingwood, M. A., Davis, M. E., Rossi, J. J. and Behlke, M. A. (2005). Functional polarity is introduced by Dicer processing of short substrate RNAs. *Nucleic Acids Res* **33**: 4140–56.

10. Minks, M. A., West, D. K., Benvin, S., Greene, J. J., Ts'o, P. O., and Baglioni, C. (1980). Activation of 2',5'-oligo(A) polymerase and protein kinase of interferon-treated HeLa cells by 2'-O-methylated poly (inosinic acid) . poly(cytidylic acid), Correlations with interferon-inducing activity. *J Biol Chem* **255**: 6403–7.

11. Stark, G. R., Kerr, I. M., Williams, B. R., Silverman, R. H., and Schreiber, R. D. (1998). How cells respond to interferons. *Annu Rev Biochem* **67**: 227–64.

12. Schwarz, D. S., Hutvagner, G., Du, T., Xu, Z., Aronin, N., and Zamore, P. D. (2003). Asymmetry in the assembly of the RNAi enzyme complex. *Cell* **115**: 199–208.

13. Khvorova, A., Reynolds, A., and Jayasena, S. D. (2003). Functional siRNAs and miRNAs exhibit strand bias. *Cell* **115**: 209–16.

14. Chalk, A. M., Wahlestedt, C., and Sonnhammer, E. L. (2004). Improved and automated prediction of effective siRNA. *Biochem Biophys Res Commun* **319**: 264–74.

15. Reynolds, A., Leake, D., Boese, Q., Scaringe, S., Marshall, W. S., and Khvorova, A. (2004). Rational siRNA design for RNA interference. *Nat Biotechnol* **22**: 326–30.

16. Jackson, A. L., Bartz, S. R., Schelter, J., Kobayashi, S. V., Burchard, J., Mao, M., Li, B., Cavet, G. and Linsley, P.S. (2003). Expression profiling reveals off-target gene regulation by RNAi. *Nat Biotechnol* **21**: 635–7.

17. Semizarov, D., Frost, L., Sarthy, A., Kroeger, P., Halbert, D. N., and Fesik, S. W. (2003). Specificity of short interfering RNA determined through gene expression signatures. *Proc Natl Acad Sci USA* **100**: 6347–52.

18. Saxena, S., Jonsson, Z. O., and Dutta, A. (2003). Small RNAs with imperfect match to endogenous mRNA repress translation: implications for off-target activity of siRNA in mammalian cells. *J Biol Chem.*

19. Scacheri, P. C., Rozenblatt-Rosen, O., Caplen, N. J., Wolfsberg, T. G., Umayam, L., Lee, J. C., Hughes, C. M., Shanmugam, K. S., Bhattacharjee, A., Meyerson, M., and Collins, F. S. (2004). Short interfering RNAs can induce unexpected and divergent changes in the levels of untargeted proteins in mammalian cells. *Proc Natl Acad Sci USA* **101**: 1892–7.

20. Hornung, V., Guenthner-Biller, M., Bourquin, C., Ablasser, A., Schlee, M., Uematsu, S., Noronha, A., Manoharan, M., Akira, S., de Fougerolles, A., Endres, S., and Hartmann, G. (2005). Sequence-specific potent induction of IFN-alpha by short interfering RNA in plasmacytoid dendritic cells through TLR7. *Nat Med* **11**: 263–70.

21. Judge, A. D., Sood, V., Shaw, J. R., Fang, D., McClintock, K., and Maclachlan, I. (2005). Sequence-dependent stimulation of the mammalian innate immune response by synthetic siRNA. *Nat Biotechnol* **23**: 457–62.

22. Elbashir, S. M., Lendeckel, W., and Tuschl, T. (2001). RNA interference is mediated by 21- and 22-nucleotide RNAs. *Genes Dev* **15**: 188–200.

23. Jackson, A. L., Burchard, J., Schelter, J., Chau, B. N., Cleary, M., Lim, L., and Linsley, P. S. (2006). Widespread siRNA "off-target" transcript silencing mediated by seed region sequence complementarity. *RNA* **12**: 1179–87.

24. Lin, X., Ruan, X., Anderson, M. G., McDowell, J. A., Kroeger, P. E., Fesik, S. W., and Shen, Y. (2005). siRNA-mediated off-target gene silencing triggered by a 7 nt complementation. *Nucleic Acids Res* **33**: 4527–35.

25. Birmingham, A., Anderson, E. M., Reynolds, A., Ilsley-Tyree, D., Leake, D., Fedorov, Y., Baskerville, S., Maksimova, E., Robinson, K., Karpilow, J., Marshall, W. S., and Khvorova, A. (2006). 3′ UTR seed matches, but not overall identity, are associated with RNAi off-targets. *Nat Methods* **3**: 199–204.

26. Du, Q., Thonberg, H., Wang, J., Wahlestedt, C., and Liang, Z. (2005). A systematic analysis of the silencing effects of an active siRNA at all single-nucleotide mismatched target sites. *Nucleic Acids Res* **33**: 1671–7.

27. Schwarz, D. S., Ding, H., Kennington, L., Moore, J. T., Schelter, J., Burchard, J., Linsley, P. S., Aronin, N., Xu, Z., and Zamore, P. D. (2006). Designing siRNA that distinguish between genes that differ by a single nucleotide. *PLoS Genet* **2**: e140.

28. Elbashir, S. M., Martinez, J., Patkaniowska, A., Lendeckel, W., and Tuschl, T. (2001). Functional anatomy of siRNAs for mediating efficient RNAi in *Drosophila melanogaster* embryo lysate. *Embryol J* **20**: 6877–88.

29. Nykanen, A., Haley, B., and Zamore, P. D. (2001). ATP requirements and small interfering RNA structure in the RNA interference pathway. *Cell* **107**: 309–21.

30. Rivas, F. V., Tolia, N. H., Song, J. J., Aragon, J. P., Liu, J., Hannon, G. J., and Joshua-Tor, L. (2005). Purified Argonaute2 and an siRNA form recombinant human RISC. *Nat Struct Mol Biol* **12**: 340–9.

31. Soutschek, J., Akinc, A., Bramlage, B., Charisse, K., Constien, R., Donoghue, M., Elbashir, S., Geick, A., Hadwiger, P., Harborth, J., John, M., Kesavan, V., Lavine, G., Pandey, R. K., Racie, T., Rajeev, K. G., Rohl, I., Toudjarska, I., Wang, G., Wuschko, S., Bumcrot, D., Koteliansky, V., Limmer, S., Manoharan, M., and Vornlocher, H. P. (2004). Therapeutic silencing of an endogenous gene by systemic administration of modified siRNAs. *Nature* **432**: 173–8.

32. Monia, B. P., Johnston, J. F., Sasmor, H., and Cummins, L. L. (1996). Nuclease resistance and antisense activity of modified oligonucleotides targeted to Ha-ras. *J Biol Chem* **271**: 14533–40.

33. Jackson, A. L., Burchard, J., Leake, D., Reynolds, A., Schelter, J., Guo, J., Johnson, J. M., Lim, L., Karpilow, J., Nichols, K., Marshall, W., Khvorova, A., and Linsley, P. S. (2006). Position-specific chemical modification of siRNAs reduces "off-target" transcript silencing. *RNA* **12**: 1197–205.

34. Amarzguioui, M., Holen, T., Babaie, E., and Prydz, H. (2003). Tolerance for mutations and chemical modifications in a siRNA. *Nucleic Acids Res* **31**: 589–95.

35. Braasch, D. A., Jensen, S., Liu, Y., Kaur, K., Arar, K., White, M. A., and Corey, D. R. (2003). RNA interference in mammalian cells by chemically-modified RNA. *Biochemistry* **42**: 7967–75.

36. Czauderna, F., Fechtner, M., Dames, S., Aygun, H., Klippel, A., Pronk, G. J., Giese, K., and Kaufmann, J. (2003). Structural variations and stabilising modifications of synthetic siRNAs in mammalian cells. *Nucleic Acids Res* **31**: 2705–16.

37. Martin, B., Sainlos, M., Aissaoui, A., Oudrhiri, N., Hauchecorne, M., Vigneron, J. P., Lehn, J. M., and Lehn, P. (2005). The design of cationic lipids for gene delivery. *Curr Pharm Discov* **11**: 375–94.

38. Gehl, J. (2003). Electroporation: theory and methods, perspectives for drug delivery, gene therapy and research. *Acta Physiol Scand* **177**: 437–47.

39. (2003). Whither RNAi? *Nat Cell Biol* **5**: 489–90.

40. Echeverri, C. J., Beachy, P. A., Baum, B., Boutros, M., Buchholz, F., Chanda, S. K., Downward, J., Ellenberg, J., Fraser, A. G., Hacohen, N., Hahn, W. C., Jackson, A. L., Kiger, A., Linsley, P. S., Lum, L., Ma, Y., Mathey-Prevot, B., Root, D. E., Sabatini, D. M., Taipale, J., Perrimon, N., and Bernards, R. (2006). Minimizing the risk of reporting false positives in large-scale RNAi screens. *Nat Methods* **3**: 777–9.

41. Persengiev, S. P., Zhu, X., and Green, M. R. (2004). Nonspecific, concentration-dependent stimulation and repression of mammalian gene expression by small interfering RNAs (siRNAs). *RNA* **10**: 12–8.

42. Myers, J. W., Jones, J. T., Meyer, T., and Ferrell, J. E. (2003). Recombinant Dicer efficiently converts large dsRNAs into siRNAs suitable for gene silencing. *Nat Biotechnol* **21**: 324–8.

43. Javorschi, S., Harris, A., Castro, K., Madden, K., Kusser, W., and Gleeson, M. (2004). Kinetics of RNA interference studied by real-time PCR with LUX fluorogenic primers. *PharmaGenomics* **4**: 44–8.

CHAPTER 4

GENOME SCANNING BY RNA INTERFERENCE

RODERICK L. BEIJERSBERGEN and OLIVER C. STEINBACH

4.1 INTRODUCTION

RNA interference (RNAi) on a genome-wide scale can be used for deciphering complex biological and pathological processes as well as the identification of potential new targets for drug intervention. High-throughput RNAi screening combined with high-content readouts allows for the identification of genes, pathways, and targets associated with increasingly complex phenotypes. This chapter discusses the different technologies and their application in functional genomic screening.

RNA is one of the most versatile biomolecules for the fundamental function of living systems: storage (messenger RNA: mRNA), control (small interfering RNA: siRNA and microRNA: miRNA) and decoding (transfer RNA:tRNA and ribosomal RNA: rRNA) of genetic information, enzymatic activity (rRNA), scaffolding-defined three-dimensional structures (rRNA), and signaling (immunostimulating RNA: isRNA). These natural activities have been developed into powerful research tools and drugs. The newly discovered RNA inhibitory activity mediated by short double-stranded RNA (dsRNA) (siRNA and miRNA) has further boosted the utilization of RNA for deciphering genetic pathways, regulatory mechanisms, and in drug development.

Molecular biology has entered into a new era when these noncoding RNAs (ncRNA) were found to play a role in aspects of cellular regulation (gene expression, development, chromatin remodeling, and possible rebuilding of chromosomal DNA). Diverse phenomena originally named "quelling" (fungi), "RNAi" (animals), and "cosuppression" or "posttranscriptional gene silencing" (plants) are all following essentially the same fundamental

RNA Interference: Application to Drug Discovery and Challenges to Pharmaceutical Development, Edited by Paul H. Johnson
Copyright © 2011 John Wiley & Sons, Inc.

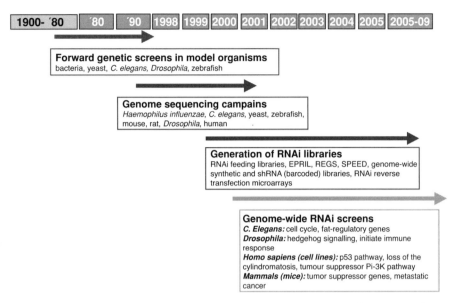

FIGURE 4.1   History and landmark events in the development of RNAi as a functional screening tool.

mechanism involving ncRNAs now collectively called "RNAi." Here, non-coding dsRNA (dsRNA) eventually degrades or inhibits the translation of the target RNA, thereby causing a knockdown of gene expression, as opposed to the permanent mutational alteration of the gene, traditionally known as "knockout." In 1998, the Andrew Fire and Craig Mello teams first realized that they could inactivate expression of specific genes in *Caenorhabditis elegans* by injecting the worms with dsRNAs complimentary in sequence to the gene they wanted to inactivate [1]. In a series of elegant experiments, it was demonstrated that dsRNA induces posttranscriptional degradation of homologue transcripts entering a cellular pathway that is commonly referred to as RNAi, and has been observed in a variety of organisms including plant, fungi, insects, worms, protozoans, and mammals [2–13].

The discovery of RNAi coincided with the explosion of genomic sequencing projects such as the sequencing campaigns in *Haemophilus influenzae*, bacteria, yeasts, *C. elegans*, zebrafish, mouse, rat, *Drosophila*, and human (Figure 4.1) [14–17]. The fact that RNAi applications can be scaled up for use in high-throughput techniques led to the creation of genome-wide RNAi reagents and applications. This without doubt accelerated the identification of critical pathways involved in disease manifestation and eventually its application in the drug discovery process.

Another reason for the rapid adoption of siRNA is that research aimed at optimizing traditional antisense oligonucleotides (ODNs) had already solved many important problems. For example, cellular uptake of ODNs is a major obstacle for efficient gene inhibition inside cells. By the time siRNA appeared, a wide variety of efficient delivery systems for nucleic acids had been developed and were commercially available. In addition, researchers using traditional antisense ODNs had already described potential pitfalls and developed criteria for the essential control experiments needed to produce convincing results. Although successful in some applications, antisense ODN and ribozyme-based gene-silencing technologies have been difficult to apply universally (Table 4.1) [18, 19].

Since the discovery that dsRNA can specifically inhibit expression of homologous genes, RNAi has become one of the most widely used methods for studying loss-of-function phenotypes in model organisms as well as mammalian cells, and therefore represents the latest addition to the family of antisense technologies. Not surprisingly, RNAi is also increasingly used across the whole pharmaceutical research process.

4.2   DISSECTION OF PHYSIOLOGICAL AND PATHOLOGICAL PROCESSES WITH GENETIC SCREENS

Thanks to progress in genomics and proteomics, mutational analysis, gene massive parallel expression profiling, cDNA-based functional screens and a plethora of public-domain genomics and proteomics data collections such as the human genome project and the cancer genome atlas, biological processes and diseases are increasingly deciphered at the cellular and molecular level. The scientific challenge is to achieve an accurate understanding of pathways at these levels, which is the focus of an emerging area of research known as functional genomics and systems biology. Further, those modern technologies and resources deliver a plethora of possible candidate targets for future drugs. Target validation and particularly target invalidation has become a crucial step in the drug discovery process. However, the availability of overwhelming amounts of genomic, transcriptomic, and proteomic data has, paradoxically, made it difficult to select a promising molecular target for a full-scale drug development effort. The field of target validation aims to uncover the few "real" drug targets among myriads of "omics"-candidates, and thus, reduce costly attrition later in development [20].

The traditional approach of deciphering biological networks using forward genetics starts with a phenotype and then identifies the gene(s) or mutation that control or cause that trait. There have been many prominent examples for this approach in model organisms such as bacteria, yeast, *C. elegans*, *Drosophila*, and zebrafish [21–24]. In contrast stands reverse genetics, in which one goes from a gene/sequence, often discovered via high-throughput

TABLE 4.1 Properties of Different Gene-Silencing Strategies for Screening

Strategy	Advantage	Disadvantage
Low-molecular weight agents	• Easy to administer • Often inexpensive	• Often nonspecific • Not available • Off-target effects
Antisense ODN	• Easy to synthesize • Inexpensive • Modifications for selectivity and efficacy	• Exogenous delivery only protein binding • Off-target effects e.g. interferon induction
Ribozymes	• Simple catalytic domain • Delivery as free molecules or vector expression • Tissue-specific delivery • Administration to subcellular compartments	• Specific cleavage triplets • Protein binding
DNAzymes	• Inexpensive • Good catalytic properties • Modifications for systemic delivery	• Exogenous delivery only • Off-target effects
siRNA Libraries of pooled siRNAs Libraries of multiple, individual siRNAs per gene	• Highly effective at low concentrations • Delivery as free siRNA molecules • No library maintenance required • Quick screening • Ease of use • Pooled siRNAs: lower number of plates and automation needed in primary screen • Available from commercial vendors	• Expensive • Finite resource • Off-target effects interferon-response induction • High transfection efficacy required • Assays of short duration • Short kinetic of gene/protein knockdown • Reconfirmation of each hit with individual siRNA (in case pools are used) • Higher automation need • Issues with *in vivo* delivery and stability
shRNA single-well or pooled libraries, expression shRNAs or miRNA embedded shRNAs	• Delivery by short hairpin expression vector • Low cost • Tissue specific expression if vector established • Unlimited resource • Long-term assays • Larger repertoires of target cells • *In vivo* delivery and stability less challenging for certain organ systems	• Viral vectors require special expertise and containment • Significant library maintenance (DNA/virus preparation) • Requirement of easy DNA/Plasmid transfection • Challenges in vector and virus construction

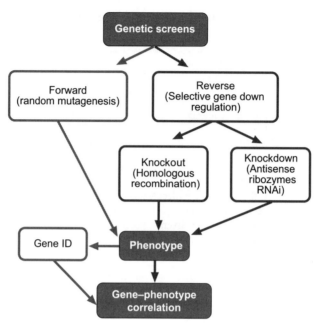

FIGURE 4.2   Schematic workflow of forward- and reverse genetic screens. While in the forward genetic approach the process starts with a phenotypic observation and the underlying gene, (mal-)function needs then to be identified. In reverse genetic screens, the starting point is a known gene(sequence) and its biological function and phenotypic manifestation is deciphered through the use of knockout and knockdown methodology.

sequencing and bioinformatics technologies, to its biological function (Figure 4.2) [25].

Reverse genetic methods are more amenable to whole genome high-throughput analysis than is forward genetics. There is functional information for only ~15% of human genes at present. Loss-of-function genetic screens aim to identify gene function through inactivation of a gene (or its corresponding mRNA). Various technologies have been developed to study the effects of gene suppression in mammalian cells, including genetic suppressor elements [26–29], antisense vectors [30], ribozymes [31], aptamer libraries [32], and more recently, RNAi [33–40]. Through its use in large-scale screens and selection experiments, RNAi is expected to provide great impact on cell biology.

In addition to its reverse genetic approaches, double-strand-mediated gene silencing has been adapted to move genetics forward in both model organisms (e.g., *C. elegans*, *Drosophila melanogaster*, and *Arabidopsis thaliana*) and mammalian cell systems to discover genes responsible for complex cellular phenotypes by the use of large-scale collections of RNAi molecules or constructs targeting all predicted genes. This, combined with functional genomics applications such as transcriptional profiling and sophisticated high-content cell-based assays, provides a unique opportunity to perform high-throughput genetics in these complex cell systems.

Both approaches, forward and reverse genetic screens, have moved into higher organisms in the recent past mainly because of the applicability of RNAi in mammalian systems. RNAi provides a "loss-of-function" approach, which has been widely used in the last couple of years first for general interest in the analysis of gene function, eventually expanded into more complex pathway analysis including disease pathway association and consequently in drug discovery, for identification and validation of potential drug target candidates. The focus of such screens is lately evolving more toward drugable gene families rather than genome-wide approaches as the latter is expensive, complex and sometimes confusing [41–46].

Many of the methodologies that are used in RNAi screening—such as how to establish phenotypic assays, perform large-scale screens and select candidate hits—are similar to those used in "classical" genetic screening approaches. The phenotypes to be scored might differ, for example, cell-based screens might require automation and new analysis methods. However, when applied across the genome, an RNAi screen is essentially a forward genetics screen using a reverse genetics technique, and thus, has similar promises and constraints. Past successes of classical genetic screens have been in large part due to clearly defined and easy to score phenotypes that were then traced to mutations in relevant genes. Prime examples include screens for vulval development defects in *C. elegans* and eye development phenotypes in *Drosophila*, which together identified most of the major components of the Ras signaling pathways [47–50]. However, a genetic screen generates a set of mutants for which the molecular lesion is not known, and identifying the mutated gene is often cumbersome and time consuming. In addition, some genetic screening methods such as transposon-mediated mutagenesis suffer from target bias.

Two major advantages of RNAi screens over classical genetic screens are that the sequences of all identified genes are immediately known and lethal mutations are easier to identify because it is not necessary to recover mutants. These features affect postscreening analyses, allowing more sophisticated data analyses on identified (and missed) genes. RNAi screens of functional subgroups based on sequence or other criteria are also possible, and sequence can be taken into account when choosing genes to study in detail. However, RNAi also has disadvantages, such as the variability and incompleteness of knockdowns and the potential nonspecificity of reagents. In addition, whereas classical genetic screens can identify alleles that uncover regulatory mechanisms, RNAi is purely a loss-of-function technique targeting the mature message (Table 4.2).

TABLE 4.2   Features of Classical Genetic and RNAi-Screens

Classical Genetic Screen	RNAi Screen
• Gain-of-function alleles can be isolated, which can uncover regulatory mechanisms • Tissue-specific alleles can be recovered • Insights into structure–function relationships can be obtained from point mutations	• RNAi-mediated knockdown results in a reduced level of wild-type product
• Every gene should be mutable using this approach	• Not every gene is susceptible to RNAi— some tissues are resistant and genes encoding proteins with long half-lives are hard to knock down effectively
• The cloning stage is laborious	• The gene sequence is known immediately
• Maternal-effect genes with zygotic requirement are hard to identify	• Can introduce double-stranded RNA at different developmental stages, bypassing earlier requirements
• Mutations usually affect single genes	• Multiple genes with shared sequence can be knocked down, thereby uncovering redundancy
• Mutant alleles are heritable	• Knockdown is usually not heritable, except when the silencing construct is expressed as a transgene(s)

Most researchers use RNAi as a simple reverse genetics tool to understand the function of one or a few genes essentially using RNAi for gene-by-gene analysis method for a confounding phenotype. On the other hand, RNAi represents an ideal strategy to decipher the role of hundreds or thousands of genes simultaneously in screens for specific phenotypic changes. These forward genetic approaches may help to gain insight into complex physiological and pathological processes.

Large-scale RNAi screens have already reproduced many previously hard-won genetic discoveries, and have identified new genes that appear to function in well-studied biological processes such as in *C. elegans* (cell cycle, fat-regulatory genes) [33, 51–54], *Drosophila* (*Imd, Wnt* and hedgehog signaling, initiate immune response) [53, 55], and *Homo sapiens* (p53 pathway, loss of the cylindromatosis tumor suppressor, PI3-K pathway) [56–58]. Boutros and colleagues targeted almost all of the predicted *Drosophila* mRNAs to analyze their possible roles in cell growth and viability. Importantly, these and other

RNAi-based screens have identified the role of genes that have conserved orthologs in mice and humans (see Table 4.3 and following sections).

Multiple large-scale RNAi-based genetic screens in mammalian cells using vector-based short hairpin RNA (shRNA) expression have been reported [51, 71]. These large-scale genetic screens have successfully identified a number of novel genetic elements of the interrogated signaling or metabolic pathways. On the other hand, certain known components of these pathways were not identified even if the respective targeting constructs were present in the applied RNAi libraries. This discrepancy may be explained by the fact that sometimes not all pathway components can be assessed by the same phenotypic screen. Moreover, despite careful design and use of multiple targeting sequences, some genes may not be effectively silenced to a level to produce the assayed phenotype. Furthermore, some genes previously implicated in a pathway are merely modifiers that only display a phenotype in a particular setting and are not recaptured in these readouts. On the other hand, many unexpected genes are identified as well but it has become clear that the functional validation of each si/shRNA molecule represents an even bigger challenge than the construction of the library (see following sections).

Many of these screens have also provided evidence that RNAi pathways are under genetic control in these organisms, a discovery that may have significant impact on the use of RNAi both in basic research and in clinical applications. The challenge in pharmaceutical target validation is to provide the usefulness of a specific target *in vitro* and ideally *in vivo* (animal model) as well. Correlation of a target's presence with disease relevant parameter or analytes (e.g., through expression profiling) or *in vivo* phenotype is not good enough—it is also essential to demonstrate that the target has a causal role in producing that phenotype. Although there is no one universal solution for every target, there is a clear consensus among pharmaceutical companies that tools such as RNAi can be used to invalidate the vast majority of candidates identified through correlative target validation work [72, 73]. RNAi-based technologies can be used to study the effects of inhibition in the original disease phenotype. A significant effect on the disease phenotype indicates that the target in question could well play an important role in the disease itself.

4.3 LARGE-SCALE RNAi-BASED SCREENS IN MAMMALIAN CELLS

4.3.1 Exogenous Delivery Versus Endogenous Expression RNAi Screening

Soon after the basic requirements to create successful RNAi reagents for mammalian systems were established, multiple groups started to assemble

TABLE 4.3 Genetic RNAi-Screens in Different Model Organisms

Model Organism	RNAi Reagent/Delivery Method	Library, Number of Targeted Genes	Assay	References
Viruses and bacteria (HCV, WNV, Trypanosoma)	Synthetic siRNA	<100 pathogen genes, ≤22.000 human genes	Virus/bacteria replication, infectivity	[59–61]
Worms (*C. elegans*)	Long dsRNA Bacterial feeding libraries dsRNAi library Soaking Injection	17.000 -> 90% of known genes	Viability, embryonic lethality sterility, embryogenesis, fat metabolism/accumulation, genomic stability, mitochondrial function, life span, transposon silencing	[54, 62, 63]
Flies (*Drosophila*)	Cell-bathing in long dsRNA containing medium Cell transfection Embryo injection	20.000 -> 90% of known genes	Viability, growth, cell morphology, cell signaling, initiate immune response Hedgehog signaling Cardiogenesis	[39, 64, 65]
Cultured mammalian cells (human and mouse cells)	Transfected chemically synthesized siRNA libraries Transfected plasmid shRNA library Infected retroviral shRNA libraries	50–8.000 genes 1–3 siRNAs per gene 2–9 shRNAs per gene	TRAIL-induced apoptosis NF-kB signaling P53-dependent proliferation arrest 26S proteasome function	[51, 66, 67]
Mammals *in vivo*	Lipids, nanoparticles Electroporation Adeno- and lentivirus Hydrodynamic intravascular injection Normal intravascular injection Sonoporation	400 genes, pools of siRNAs, shRNAs (48 each)	Ocular neovascularization, age related macular degeneration, viral infection, tumor suppressor genes, metastatic cancer, respiratory inflammation	[51, 68–70]

si/shRNA libraries that targeted increasingly larger numbers of genes. These have been successfully applied to study a variety of cellular processes. Initial studies examined the function of a relatively small set of genes in specific signaling or metabolic pathways. Very recently, much larger RNAi libraries attempting genome-wide coverage have been created [74, 75]. Generating such libraries and delivering them into mammalian cells has presented real challenges that have been solved in part by using strategies borrowed from technical breakthroughs in the fields of gene sequencing and chemical genetics.

In (mammalian) RNAi experiments, two parameters primarily determine the choice of targeting molecule and delivery method: the cell type and the desired duration of the silencing effect. For example, if one is interested in the short-term consequences of knocking down a particular gene in an easy-to-transfect cell line, probably the most effective approach is to use synthetic siRNAs. When the goal is long-lasting gene silencing, it is more appropriate to use shRNAs expressed from plasmids or, in the case of hard-to-transfect cells, from lenti- or retrovirus-based vectors [76a] (Figure 4.3).

This chapter is focused on the two most widely used approaches: (a) exogenous delivery of siRNA molecules and (b) endogenous expression of shRNAs. These two RNAi reagents each come in several flavors. For example, apart from the chemically synthesized siRNAs, siRNAs have been made by nuclease cleavage of long *in vitro* transcribed dsRNAs: esiRNAs [76b]. The improvements in design algorithms to select the most efficient target sequences has led to a high frequency of functional siRNAs that result in very efficient knockdown of the desired target. Further improvements in siRNA stability, structure and improved transfection methods have resulted in robust homogenous inactivation of target gene expression in a plethora of cell lines as well as primary cells. A disadvantage of the application of siRNAs is the transient gene expression-inhibition effect restricting the use of siRNAs to short-term assays. This limitation is overcome with the development of vector-based systems driving the expression of short hairpins that can be processed into both siRNAs and miRNAs. The shRNAs can be expressed as pol III transcripts or embedded in a miRNA structure driven by Pol II promoters. The expression cassettes for both shRNA and miRNAs can be introduced by transfection of plasmids or viral infection. Upon integration, these vectors cause a stable and effective gene silencing. For plasmid-derived shRNAs different viral delivery systems are available (e.g., Moloney virus-based vectors, lentiviral vectors, adenoviral vectors allowing the introduction in a wide variety of cell types [76a, 76c–79]. The application of regulatory elements in the promoters driving the expression of these shRNA or miRNAs can be used for inducible long-term gene silencing even *in vivo* in animal models (Table 4.3).

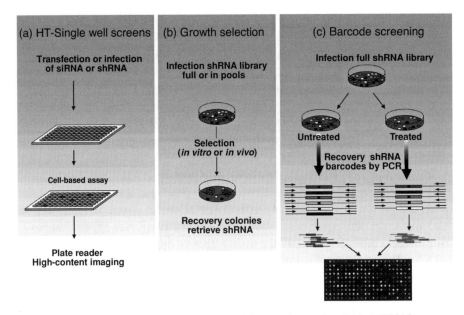

FIGURE 4.3 Large-scale cell-based RNAi screening technologies. RNAi screens in human cells usually require multiple independent (a) siRNAs, either in individual wells or delivered as pools. Other methods include (a, b) transfection or viral transduction of hairpin expression constructs, small hairpin (sh)RNAs that are intracellular transcribed and processed into small interfering RNAs (siRNAs). (c) In siRNA barcode screens, a large population of cells is infected with the shRNA library and divided into two populations. One is treated (or selected), whereas the other population serves as a reference for the hybridization. From each population, genomic DNA is isolated and shRNA cassettes are recovered by PCR. The PCR products are used as templates for an *in vitro* linear amplification reaction to generate RNA probes that are subsequently labeled with fluorescent dyes. The probes from the selected cells and reference population are hybridized to a DNA microarray containing the complementary sequences from the complete shRNA library. (For a color version of this figure, see plate 2.)

Today, several large shRNA or shRNA mircollections are available and mostly constructed from designed ODNs but can also be generated from cDNA fragments. The latter approach includes EPRIL [80], REGS [81], or SPEED [82] technologies. In addition, multiple technologies have been developed to produce siRNAs *in vitro* through RNase III/Dicer digestion of *in vitro* produced long dsRNAs [79, 83, 84]. Multiple companies and academic resource centers in Europe and in the United States are involved in the development and distribution of such RNAi tools [85–87].

Both synthetic and DNA-mediated RNAi methods are compatible with high-throughput screening (HTS) methodologies. However, the relatively high cost of synthetic siRNA has biased most public efforts toward vector-encoded shRNA libraries. Although the initial cost of acquiring whole genome synthetic libraries is large, the screening cost thereafter is fairly low depending on the type of readout (cost per screening point can be around 0.2 cents per data point [88, 89]). Because synthetic siRNA libraries are available as lyophilized, deprotected, arrayed reagents of constant quality, they can be directly used for screening. This relative ease of use has resulted in the broad application of siRNA libraries and reagents for both screening efforts and validation experiments.

In principle gene silencing by RNAi has two major aspects, one concerning the effectiveness of knockdown and a second associated with off-target effects. The improvements in design algorithms for siRNAs have led to a high frequency of efficient knockdown. However, at this moment, shRNA design is not optimal and a significant fraction of designed shRNAs will not lead to efficient gene silencing. As a consequence, multiple shRNAs are used per gene to increase the chance of sufficient knockdown required for the phenotype of interest. The use of multiple independent si or shRNAs also addresses the issue of off-target effects. To establish a clear link between the gene of interest and the cellular phenotype studied, one needs at minimum two independent siRNA sequences that produce the phenotype. The largest gene knockdown experiments performed to date have used large collections of shRNA vectors containing multiple short interfering/short hairpin (si/sh)RNAs per gene [51, 59, 90]. It is clear that increased numbers of si/sh RNAs per gene contribute to a more reliable screening tool with less false positives or negatives. The increased number of siRNA sequences present in such a pool increases knockdown efficiency, while reducing the frequency of off-target effects as measured by gene expression [91, 92]. Although the siRNA sequence can significantly influence its potency (level of knockdown achieved) and specificity (stimulating phenotype through knockdown of the target gene only), it is strongly associated with the chance of off-target effects. Reconfirmation of gene annotation sequence analysis of gene family homologues and splice variants, etc. is strongly recommended before designing siRNAs by using one of many public or proprietary algorithms. In addition, rules have to be put in place to prevent miRNA seed complementarity or sequence similarity with $5'$ or $3'$ UTRs.

The availability of many different technology platforms as the basis for large collections of RNAi reagents has greatly expanded the number of screening models. In addition to single-well screens with single-well readouts, several examples have been described where pooled shRNA libraries are used. In these screens, the identity of the shRNA is determined by DNA microarray hybridization or sequencing. Although the approach of pooled library screening is powerful and cost-effective, it is difficult to combine with more complex cellular (or subcellular) readouts. An interesting alternative for large-scale single-well screens with complex readouts is the use of glass slides on which siRNA, shRNA, or esiRNA reagents are spotted [41, 45, 93, 94]. These spots can contain siRNAs together with lipid transfection reagents or infectious virus. The siRNAs or shRNAs are then introduced into the cells that are grown on these slides by reverse transfection or infection, respectively. The phenotypic effects of this "reverse" transfection or infection of hundreds or thousands of gene products can be detected using specific cell-based bioassays including staining with antibodies or dyes for specific organelles. Most approaches to mammalian RNAi that are discussed above are compatible with the cell microarray format: siRNA, shRNAs, esiRNAs, or virus shRNAs can be printed onto microscope slides, and these printed microarrays can be stored or used directly. As this technology matures, RNAi cell microarrays will provide an economical way to systematically screen the genome [66, 95].

4.3.2   Genome-Wide Versus Focused RNAi Screens

Whole-genome RNAi libraries are most commonly used in the academic research communities. Because many researchers in the pharmaceutical industry are focused on finding targets that can be progressed toward drug development multiple focused siRNA— or arrayed adenoviral shRNA—libraries are directed against the small-molecule drugable genome. The drugable genome consists of ~4700 transcripts corresponding to ~3700 gene loci. Therefore, every transcript is represented in the library by three or more RNAi constructs directed against it to increase the chances for target suppression and to allow for multiple, independent siRNA constructs to confirm the observed, specific phenotype thereby eliminating off-target effects.

Therefore, the RNAi community is increasingly focused on the tractable target classes of the genome, usually those classes that are drugable through small molecule agonists or antagonists. Several academic and industrial research groups are following on the heels of this work to carry out more specialized focused RNAi screens. There are a number of examples for gene-family focused screens especially in the field of kinases as attractive potential pharmaceutical targets in cancer [38, 51]; [96, 97]; [98–101].

4.3.3   *In Vivo* RNAi Screens

The use of RNAi screening technologies *in vivo*, has been extensively used in the model organisms *C. elegans* and *Drosphila* [102, 103]. These screens have resulted in the identification of many components of cellular pathways implicated in disease. However, these animal models often cannot reflect the complex physiological of pathological disease processes present in mammals and particular humans. Although RNAi screens in mammalian cell lines performed *in vitro* have identified a number of physiologically or pathologically relevant genes, these models can often be biased by the use of cell lines *in vitro* and where many complex physiological or disease processes have no simple *in vitro* correlates, such as organ development or metastasis.

In the past decades, the generation of knockout mouse models has been instrumental in the identification and validation of genes in normal and pathological situations. Apart from the "classical" knockout models, more sophisticated models, including inducible and tissue specific knockouts, have further strengthened this technology [104, 105].

RNAi technologies now also provide an efficient approach to systematically investigate the genetic basis of normal and disease physiology in animal models. The feasibility of RNAi screens *in vivo* was first demonstrated in a study where a series of shRNA vectors was analyzed for their ability to promote liver tumorigenesis in a mosaic mouse model [87]. The recovery of tumor cells from these animals allowed for the identification of specific shRNAs affecting the disease process. Although at this moment such screens are with limited numbers of genes, the further development of new technologies for readout and recovery will expand the use of *in vivo* RNAi screens.

4.4 DESIGN AND PRACTICAL IMPLEMENTATION OF A HIGH-THROUGHPUT RNAi SCREENS

4.4.1 Choosing Components for RNAi Screening—Library, Cellular System and Delivery Method

Like classical genetic screens in the past, the success of large-scale RNAi surveys depends on a careful development of phenotypic assays in a relevant biological context. The development of an effective functional siRNA screen represents a multi-pass approach. Several factors in the RNAi workflow and experimental design need to be optimized to ensure the success of a high-throughput experiment, such as RNAi reagent selection, delivery methods, functional readouts, and collection, analysis and interpretation of data. The assay used for screening ultimately reflects the aim of the experiment, be it the study of genes in a particular pathway or the identification of genes involved in a disease process. The key practical issues when performing RNAi screens in mammalian cells are assay development, library selection, on-target validation, and performing follow-up experiments [41]. An outline for building an RNAi screen is shown in Figure 4.4.

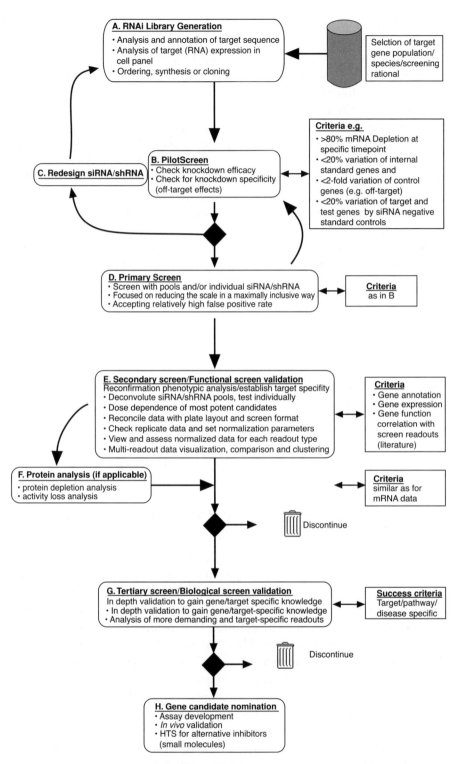

FIGURE 4.4 Schematic workflow of an RNAi screen. For details refer to chapter.

The first step, component discovery, involves developing and performing the biological screen of interest. In a poorly understood system, a small set of targets (e.g. kinases) can be examined to look for genes in a specific functional class or pathway that might affect the system of interest. This was, for instance, done to identify the long sought-after gene encoding vitamin K epoxide reductase, an important drug target, by an RNAi screen in human cells that was focused on a set of genes in a particular chromosomal region [106]. For more developed pathway analysis, a genome-wide screen can be performed to gain comprehensive view of the system, network, or signaling cascade, as was done in a *C. elegans* genome-wide screen for genes involved in endocytosis [107]. Library selection will depend on the target cell type and whether long-term or transient inactivation of gene products is required.

The choice of cell type should also be carefully considered being suitable for efficient, high-throughput siRNA transfection. In addition, some cell types may be more biologically responsive than others to the particular RNAi effect under study. The cell type chosen for RNAi experiments should be easy to transfect at high efficiencies and compatible with the downstream screening assay. It is advisable to perform initial RNAi experiments with more than one cell type, as there are numerous publications that show that there can be highly significant differences between the levels of responsiveness of different cell lines to knock down of genes involved in the cell cycle [38, 108].

The use of siRNAs relies on efficient delivery into cells, but there are several cell types that are partially or completely refractory to transfection. In addition, because siRNAs are quickly diluted in dividing cells, the silencing effect usually lasts for a few days at most, and it can be maintained for a week or more in nondividing cells or when chemically stabilized molecules are used. Both of these limitations can be overcome by using shRNAs and viral-transduction methods.

In the large number of RNAi studies reported to date, siRNAs have been shown to be effective in a broad range of different cell types, from commonly used cell lines to primary cultured cell (see Tables 4.3 and 4.4) Since viral-based vectors can transduce many cell types with approximately equal efficiency, the difference in target suppression and phenotype can be attributed to shRNA expression levels and critical factors in determining the effectiveness of the shRNA. This could possibly be the expression of, for example, Argonaut proteins [130] or the IFN response (IFR) elicited by adenoviral shRNA constructs [131, 132]. The cellular environment can affect both the efficiency and specificity of si/shRNAs. Therefore, careful optimization is needed to achieve the desired balance between these two factors, and at the same time, to eliminate potential toxic effects caused by increased concentration of the siRNA in the cell.

4.4.2 Choosing Components for RNAi Screening—Assay

A robust and specific assay is the most important element of a successful RNAi screen. Its development is usually the most time-consuming aspect, requiring repetitive work and careful attention to detail while minor changes in parameters are tested and optimized, but the time spent in assay development is rewarded in the results of the final screen.

Cell culture-based screens open up new avenues for HTS and are particularly suitable for dissecting basic cellular processes. In contrast to whole-animal assays, cell-based phenotypes are comparatively reductionist and particular care has to be taken to choose the appropriate biological context. The simplest cell-based assay is a homogeneous or bulk-cell assay, in which the phenotypes of many cells are averaged across each well in a microtiter-plate. At the other extreme are imaging screens, in which an image of each well (or spot) is taken and then individual cells are scored, potentially with many phenotypic descriptors. An example of such an assay is the combination of determining cell number, DNA content, an apoptotic marker and a mitotic marker such as histone H3 phosphorylation. Also a more in depth analysis of the expression and subcellular distribution of a protein is one of the advantages of high-content automated confocal microscopes. Time-lapse imaging has recently been adapted to RNAi screens, allowing dynamic processes such as mitosis to be investigated [133, 134]. One of the great advantages of this type of research is that the assays do not have to be highly complex to yield valuable information about cellular pathways and responses [41].

In the increasingly image-based RNAi screening, there is a strong need to improve ways to capture such readouts in space and time. Cell biologists traditionally depict these events by confining themselves to the level of a single cell, or to many population-averaged cells. Applying such relatively complex assays to a high-throughput setup, in which a quantitative statement about each single cell is generated, needs sophisticated computational infrastructure and image analysis algorithms, and a high degree of method standardization. Currently, the methodology of "high-throughput and high-content imaging" is at an early stage but rapidly developing. These screens generate a large amount of data, easily exceeding a terabyte per screen. Open-source software packages have been developed for image databases and automated image analysis [135, 136].

Like any good genetic screen, an RNAi screen needs an assay that is specific for the biological process being investigated. Unfortunately, often the ease of the assay is inversely proportional to its specificity. Cell lethality is probably the easiest phenotype to score, but it does not give much information about a gene's function. By contrast, an assay in which the function of synapses is directly measured using electrophysiological techniques is specific, but also laborious or not feasible on a genome-wide scale. Often, large-scale RNAi screens have to find a compromise between specificity and practicality. Even the range of (whole-animal) assays that can be used is vast. These can be simple visual assays of morphological defects, changes in the expression of green fluorescent protein (GFP) reporters, synthetic phenotypes, sensitivity or resistance to drugs or small molecules, or any other assay that gives a reproducible output. Biological processes that are difficult or impossible to access in cell culture, such as organ function or organ formation and behavior, can be probed using whole-animal RNAi screening. Processes that occur at the level of single cells are also amenable to RNAi screening.

Signaling pathways can be easily investigated by good reporter assays, for example, luciferase-based transcriptional reporters, protein modification reporters, protein-interaction reporters such as Y2H and fluorescence resonance energy transfer (FRET) protein localization reporters, reporters for cell size, cellular morphology, cellular internalization, secretion, and many others [41]. Reporter assays require a specific methodology of detection such as fluorescence readers or high-content screening systems.

After development of the initial assay and thorough quality control of its robustness, certain parts of the screen can be subject to automation. Automated steps at every stage of the screening process increase the robustness and reproducibility of the actual screen. It is important that the automated process of screening is supported by an integrated laboratory information management system to ensure seamless project management, from project concept to target output. Using such a platform, it is possible to screen and rescreen an arrayed siRNA library in complex cellular assays in just a few weeks or month [137].

4.4.3 Pilot Screen

Once the screening assay is developed, a small-scale "pilot" screen of a few (hundred) random genes plus the positive and negative controls is usually done before undertaking a whole-genome screen. This will ensure that the hit rate is not too high and that the screen can be feasibly carried out on a large scale. For example, if 10% of random genes score as positive in the pilot screen, the assay is probably not very specific and should be redesigned. Likewise, if the positive controls are not reproducibly detected, the assay might not be sensitive enough. Bottlenecks in screening can also be identified during the pilot screen. In addition, scoring parameters can be finalized or sometimes altered if unexpected phenotypes are seen. At the conclusion of the pilot screen, the assay should be running under the exact conditions that will be used during the genome-wide screen.

4.4.4 Primary Screen

The scope of the primary screen is to reduce the scale of the library. The initial gene candidate selection should be as comprehensive as possible, even at the expense of detecting false positive hits. Different statistical methods have been developed and are used for data normalization and hit prioritization [138]. An initial hit rate, depending on the screen, can vary between 2% and 5%. Although top-down ranking of hits can be valuable, one has to bear in mind that off-target effects can be as strong as real biologically significant hits [139].

The second step, or validation round, is to confirm whether hits are real and reproducible and "on target" by an examination of the target transcript and protein levels. Obtaining multiple distinct targeting constructs per gene provides evidence that the hits are on target. Subsequently, target transcript and protein levels are examined to establish a strong knockdown versus phenotype correlation. After this step, a high confidence hit list can be generated for further analysis and follow-up. Components are classified into organized subgroups by probing the literature and doing comparative analysis with homologous genes in other organisms. An integrative genomics approach can yield insights into the function of the genes identified and place them in cellular networks or signaling pathways. In a confirmation step, further validation experiments of putative targets are done in a panel of different cellular models, assessing dose to exclude context dependence and specificity tests, for example, the exclusion of off-target effects ("clean-up step"). These experiments will increase the confidence of target specific effects versus the off-target siRNA effects. In the final step that is contextual or systems analysis, hypothesis generation takes over and additional experiments help define gene relationships and provide mechanistic insight. For example, systematic genetic epistasis experiments can help to define the order of components that function in a signaling pathway. On the basis of their functional characteristics and their known and/or predicted and experimentally validated biochemical functions (in-depth validation step), the newly identified candidate targets are prioritized for in-depth biological characterization or nomination for the drug discovery process (Figure 4.5).

4.5 RNAi SCREEN VALIDATION

4.5.1 Technical RNAi Screen Validation and Data Normalization

Primary screens are usually conducted in duplicate, triplicate, or more to increase the confidence of positives and to avoid the false negatives that arise in large-scale screening. All candidate hits are normally retested in the original

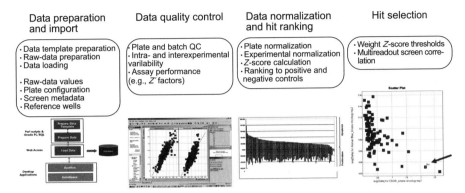

Data preparation and import	Data quality control	Data normalization and hit ranking	Hit selection
· Data template preparation · Raw-data preparation · Data loading · Raw-data values · Plate configuration · Screen metadata · Reference wells	· Plate and batch QC · Intra- and interexperimental variability · Assay performance (e.g., Z' factors)	· Plate normalization · Experimental normalization · Z-score calculation · Ranking to positive and negative controls	· Weight Z-score thresholds · Multireadout screen correlation

FIGURE 4.5   Data analysis workflow for high-throughput RNAi screens. After preparation and import of data (which can be significant for high-content screens), data are analyzed to calculate certain quality control parameters, for example, outliers between replicate measurements, intra- and interplate effects and artifacts; such measurements are flagged for downstream analysis. Quantitative phenotypic data are then normalized to a standard and scored according to predefined criteria such as the significance of the phenotypes compared with positive or negative controls, or the rank of hits. The overall quality of the screen and potential background signal in comprehensive data sets can be quantified, for example, with Z' factors, as a measure of the statistical power of the assay to discriminate between positive and negative hits before candidates for further workup are selected on the basis of predefined thresholds. (For a color version of this figure, see plate 3.)

assay to confirm that they are positive (hit validation). The end result of the primary screen will be a list of reagents that reproducibly score as positive in the primary assay. In experimental systems in which false positives caused by off-target effects are common, such as when using siRNAs in mammalian cells or long dsRNAs in *Drosophila* cell culture, it is advisable to retest hits using independent, nonoverlapping RNAi reagents.

The gene knockdown itself can be validated by various methods. The most widely used are quantitative real-time RT–PCR analysis at the mRNA level [140] and Western blot analysis at the protein level. The latter is restricted to a small number of proteins because antibodies for the protein of interest are not always available. Alternatively a sense clone could be tagged to a GFP protein, cotransfected, and subsequently, the change of fluorescence measured by FACS analysis or other means [141, 142]. Finally, rescue experiments can further strengthen the identified gene in a biological process. Where possible, mutant cDNAs can be generated that are no longer subject to the siRNA or shRNA-mediated degradation. Alternatively, cDNAs from different species can be used preferably at expression levels identical to endogenous gene expression. The use of P1 clones containing a large genomic region has also been very useful.

Although the aim is to be able to clearly say whether each gene tested scores as positive, there is usually a range in the strength of the phenotypes observed. Therefore, a scoring strategy needs to be developed, which can be qualitative—such as yes, maybe, no or not scorable—or quantitative; the latter is common in homogeneous and imaging assays. The positive controls of different strengths will help to determine the range of signals that can be detected. Typically, the cutoff point at which a gene is scored as positive is determined by analyzing the data from the whole screen.

4.5.2 Control Experiments

When setting up the experiment, it is vital to include adequate positive and negative controls to ensure that the high volume of data can be correctly interpreted and to account for variation in the different parameters of the procedure. Positive and negative controls should be selected to develop the primary screen assay in order to achieve high signals with the positive controls and low noise with the negative ones; where possible, positive controls should encompass a range of strengths to develop an assay that can identify both weak and strong hits. Selecting only strong positive controls will give a biased assessment of the assay quality. The positive and negative controls will give important information on the reproducibility, robustness, and ease of the assay—an assay that is successful when used on a small number of genes might not be amenable to being scaled up. Further optimization, by altering parameters such as time, procedures and equipment is important for improving signal-to-noise ratio.

Positive and negative (nonsilencing) control siRNAs should be used in each experiment. Positive control siRNAs are molecules that are known to provide high knockdown of a target gene that produces the desired phenotype. Routine transfection of positive control siRNAs shows that transfection and assay conditions remain optimal. Small molecules or bioactive compounds that produce the phenotype under study can also be used as positive controls for assay conditions. For example, an apoptosis-inducing drug could be used as a positive control for an apoptosis-screening assay. Alternatively, an inhibitory compound could be used to inhibit upstream components of the pathway under study. However for a quality statement of the screening paradigm itself the use of si/shRNA as weak or strong positive controls is essential. Nonsilencing control siRNAs can be siRNAs with no homology to any known mammalian gene or siRNAs that are homologous to a gene that is not present in the cells under study (e.g., GFP). Data from transfection of nonsilencing siRNAs can be used to analyze the extent of nonspecific effects that may have occurred as a result of siRNA transfection. Phenotypic effects observed after knockdown must always be confirmed by one or more additional siRNAs targeted to different regions of the same mRNA.

4.5.3 Management and Mitigation of Off-Target Effects in RNAi Screens

While siRNA mediated gene knockdown was originally reported to be highly specific, recent studies have demonstrated RNAi-mediated "off-target" gene modulation resulting from mRNA cleavage or translational repression of genes with partial homology to either strand of the duplex siRNA and other toxic effects that can generate measurable phenotypes [143]. Off-target effects can generate measurable phenotypes. siRNAs have been identified that induce cell death in a target-independent, sequence-dependent manner [66, 144].

siRNA signatures are a sum of on- and off-target gene regulation [145–150]. The different gene-silencing mechanisms of short interfering (si)RNAs and miRNAs present a challenge for siRNA design. On the one hand, mismatches between the mRNA target and the 3′ and central regions of the siRNA are usually detrimental for gene silencing; hence, an optimal siRNA should contain mismatches with other transcripts in these regions to avoid off-target effects. On the other hand, translational repression by miRNAs requires a near-perfect matching in the 5′ region, whereas a central bulge and partial binding in the 3′ region seem to be preferential for translational repression [118,151–154].

Combining high specificity with high potency is the most important challenge facing traditional antisense ODNs and siRNA. Both can affect unintended targets that are partially complementary. Furthermore, as with any exogenous compound, cells can respond by activating an array of biological pathways. For example, cytosine–guanine motifs are known to stimulate immune function. Cells respond to duplex RNA by signaling interferon viral defense mechanisms. Moreover, ODNs can exert effects by interacting with cellular components other than their intended targets. The primary strategy for minimizing the effects of such misleading interactions is sound experimental design including multiple target ODNs, functional control ODNs, dose–response and rescue experiments, assaying target and nontarget message and protein levels.

Possible solutions to mitigate these artifacts are improved bioinformatics (through improving annotation of target sequence) and siRNA design to generate more efficient siRNAs. Chemical modifications, for example, to inactivate sense strand or increase stability (longer half-life) and high-purity siRNA tools can add significant specificity. From an experimental point of view by using the lowest possible siRNA concentration, siRNA pooling and siRNA redundancy, that is, more than one siRNA/target, as well as careful monitoring of global cellular effects by, for example, expression analysis add further confidence to the phenotypic results. Finally, rescue experiments (mutated target sequence, complementation by sense sequence) are the best biological proofs of specificity, however, technically very demanding [143, 155, 118].

4.5.4   Biological RNAi Screen Validation

Internal and external cues create a highly variable population of cells, with the full range of possible cellular states. It is important to realize that this is the situation in an unperturbed population of cells. Therefore, a genetic perturbation in a population of individual cells will create a different distribution of cellular states with additional dimensions. This observation raises important questions as to how RNAi phenotypes arise in human tissue culture cells.

4.5.5   Penetrance and Expressivity of Phenotype

In classical genetics, a gene loss-of-function phenotype is penetrant when it is manifest in a proportion of individuals within a genetically homogenous population. Depending on the frequency of the particular cellular state in which the phenotype is apparent, the phenotype might have a very low penetrance. There are numerous examples from classical genetics where a low penetrance of a particular loss-of-function phenotype is still significant [136]. Moreover, in mutants that are genetically null (complete lack of gene product), it can occur that the penetrance is less than 100% [156].

A related phenomenon known from classical genetics is the expressivity or severity of a phenotype, which is the variability in the degree with which a phenotype becomes apparent in an individual organism, and by analogy, an individual cell. As with penetrance, expressivity can also be modified by genetic and environmental influences. Both parameters need to be taken into account when either qualitative or quantitative statements are made. In fact, expressivity can be used to define a phenotypic threshold [136].

4.5.6   Genetic Redundancy and Pleiotropic Effects

In several cases, silencing of a gene via RNAi leads to no obvious phenotype, even though the gene is known to have an important role (usually concluded from overexpression of dominant, active or negative forms). The lack of a phenotype by RNAi can be explained by genetic or functional redundancy, where the activity of a gene is lost, yet compensated by the function of a different gene or a different pathway. In model organisms, redundant genes are discovered by conducting synthetic screens and studied by performing double mutant analyses. Genetic techniques in human cell lines are limited, but similar studies could be undertaken by combinatorial RNAi screens, or by combining RNAi with dominant-negative mutants or small molecule inhibitors [157, 158].

Unlike genetic redundancy, gene loss-of-function can also result in multiple phenotypes. What classical geneticists refer to as pleiotropy can also be observed in a population of cultured cells, with different cells showing different phenotypes, and/or the same cells sharing more than one phenotype. While different cells showing different phenotypes could be explained by the perturbation acting on different cellular states, different phenotypes within one cell could be the result of the gene product participating in more than one biological process, or has signaling functions on multiple target molecules.

Indirect effects determining an RNAi phenotype will also be complicated by a potential indirect, although "on-target," effect of gene silencing. A phenotype can be the result of affecting a general, essential cellular process, or affecting a process that "feeds" into the one perturbed by the knockdown. An obvious example of the first case is that genes regulating the translational capacity or the metabolic status of a cell are expected to have widespread influences on various biological activities. Examples of the latter might be imagined as effects that act through changing the distribution of cellular states. Even though such phenotypes are interesting and important for the understanding of a cellular process, they will not inform us about the components of the core machinery of the studied process [159].

4.5.7 Pathway Analysis and Decision Support

Candidate and target selection for follow-up experiments require the collection and analysis of a wealth of diverse information beyond DNA sequence and protein structure and role. Whereas initial target information is quite structured, it consists of a name and alternate names, DNA and protein sequences, protein structure, related genes, and so forth, a target selection decision must be based on a wide range of largely unstructured information, which is often derived from the published literature. Questions that must be considered in selecting a target include physiological and pathological role of the protein, diseases that the target could intervene, alternative approaches to achieving the same therapeutic aim, potential for side effects, patent and competitive landscape, and resources required.

The differences between structured and unstructured information present information management challenges, because it is usually not possible to rely on formal databases to manage all aspects of target selection. Summary annotation of candidate genes does not provide the necessary depth and context to support full assessment. They require powerful indexing and retrieval methods to ensure that collected information is accessible. Collecting and assessing the information needed to make a target-selection decision ideally require the input of a wide range of experts from different scientific and functional areas. Target selection should not be the exclusive province of bioinformaticians, but ideally it ought to include input from chemistry, pathology, clinical development and even marketing, the legal department, and so forth. In drug target discovery criteria such as disease relevance, drugablility, amenability to HTS, feasibility of secondary test cascades, availability of reference compound, situation of intellectual property, freedom to operate, defined competition should provide a balanced target portfolio.

How the primary and secondary screen results are analyzed depends on the type of assay and screening mode (Figure 4.5). Qualitative data, which are more common in whole-animal screens, will be analyzed differently from quantitative cell-based data. But there are some general properties that distinguish the results of RNAi screens from classical screens. Because weak mutants are often discarded, a classical genetic screen usually yields a set of mutants that each displays a strongly penetrant phenotype. An RNAi screen will yield a set of genes with a large range of scores. Weak but genuine phenotypes can be caused either by partial knockdown of a gene with a strong effect (similar to a hypomorphic mutation) or a strong knockdown of a gene with a weak effect. For quantitative assays in particular, a rigorous procedure that includes statistical analyses of the genome-wide data is important for assessing the significance of hits. If the genome-wide screen used a qualitative primary assay, then secondary assay results are often used for most of the analyses and for defining the final gene list. It is common for the secondary assays to provide some simple quantitative data, such as percentage of animals that show a given phenotype. In this case, a simple statistical test could be applied to define the cutoff point for positives. In cases in which quantitative data are not available, the investigator's expert knowledge of the biological system can be used to make an informed decision, sometimes incorporating information from several assays. Further it is useful to define both high- and low-confidence lists. The false-positive and false-negative rates can be used to evaluate the success of an RNAi screen. The false-negative rate is usually estimated by measuring the hit rate for known positive genes. If the positive-control genes are strong hits, this only estimates the rate of identifying strongly positive genes. Comparing reproducibility between duplicate or triplicate wells can also provide information on false-negative rates. The false-positive rate of the primary screen can be estimated using the results of the secondary assays. In a well-designed and well-controlled screen, the final false-positive rate should be negligible.

Large-scale quantitative data sets require more sophisticated analyses, including the design of analysis workflows and their integration into all parts of the screening procedures (Figure 4.5). Other key requirements are assessing the reproducibility between technical replicates, identifying the outliers that often occur in high-throughput experiments, and integrating different measurements such as multiplex reporter-gene assays. Several (semi-) automated analytical approaches have been developed for the analysis of high-throughput screens [160–162].

An additional complexity arises in siRNA experiments when analyzing phenotypes of different strengths that are induced by independent siRNAs. Statistical tools that build scores based on multiple independent measurements might ultimately help to discriminate true from false hits [163]. The application of standardized (and automated) analysis routines is particularly important when comparing large-scale RNAi data sets to find different and common phenotypes.

4.5.8 *In Vivo* validation

Mammalian tissue culture and animal models are indispensable tools to study the genetic basis of human physiology and disease. Systematic manipulation of the genetic background by overexpression, deletion, or mutation of genes is the principal method for understanding complex biological processes. Indeed, transgenic, knockout, and knock-in mice are often the best available *in vivo* models for human disorders. However, generating these genetically engineered animals requires a significant amount of time, money, and effort. Furthermore, creating a more complex genetic environment with simultaneous gain- and loss-of-function mutations of multiple genes, as is often seen in human diseases, is frequently beyond the reach of these technologies and model systems.

The remarkable success of siRNA as a laboratory tool and for target validation has led to high expectations for siRNA as an *in vivo* platform. However, there have been few reports of the use of siRNA in animal models and the usefulness of synthetic siRNA in animal experimentation and preclinical drug development remains to be established. Little is known about biodistribution and pharmacokinetic properties. Using various intravenous and intraperitoneal injection strategies the sequence-specific inhibition of reporter and endogenous gene activity in liver, kidney, spleen, lung and pancreas could be demonstrated. Chemical modifications have been developed to improve thermal stability, resistance to nuclease digestion and pharmacokinetic properties as well as to reduce nonspecific effects and to regulate distribution to target tissues. Ultimately, optimizing various routes of delivery, including oral bioavailability, will be necessary to maximize the potential of siRNA in animal models as well as for pharmaceuticals [164–166]. A number of groups have also used plasmid-based shRNAs, instead of siRNAs, to obtain relatively long-lived gene silencing *in vivo* [167, 168]. A number of approaches have also been shown to improve cell and tissue delivery of siRNAs and shRNAs, including conjugating RNAs to membrane-permeable peptides and by incorporating specific binding reagents such as monoclonal antibodies into liposomes used to encapsulate siRNAs.

4.6 RNAi SCREENS—EXAMPLES

4.6.1 Cancer

Inhibition of growth, proliferation and metastasis of cancer cells is a challenge with major scientific and therapeutic impact. So not surprisingly targeting neoplastic cell structures with small molecules and lately RNAi is an extensively investigated field and various *in vitro* and *in vivo* studies using siRNA and shRNA have demonstrated the potential of the RNAi phenomenon to decipher and treat cancer (see Table 4.4). Malignant cells generally show dysregulation of cell cycle mechanisms, resulting in uncontrolled growth and resistance to death as a result of altered apoptotic pathways. These features are mediated by mutated or nonmutated, physiological regulated or dysregulated oncogenes, tumor suppressor genes or alternative genes involved in the pathways leading to such cancer-associated phenotypes. Consequently, many of those genes are part of a list of drugable genes of potential cancer targets being increasingly addressed with RNAi technology [18, 88, 169, 170].

Initial *in vitro* RNAi studies with cancer-associated genes silenced well-known and common oncogenes such as K-ras [171], mutated p53 [129] and BCR-Abl [172] followed by a number of investigations targeting other genes implying an important role in cancer including next to "classical cellular oncological targets" viral oncogenes, genes involved in therapy resistance among others, such as angiogenesis targets, the latter being a hallmark of cancer and many other serious diseases that are characterized by the uncontrolled growth of new blood vessels [173]. Here, to investigate HIF-1 regulation by the kinome a kinase-specific small interference RNA library using a hypoxia-response element luciferase reporter assay under hypoxic conditions was screened. This screen determined that depletion of cellular SMG-1 kinase, the newest and least studied member of the phosphoinositide 3-kinase-related kinase family, most significantly modified cellular HIF-1 activity in hypoxia.

RNAi has proven to be a powerful tool for the identification of genes involved in tumorigenesis, however, "positive" screens in which cells are

TABLE 4.4 Examples of Successful Cancer-Associated Screens and Identified Targets

Phenotype	Screening Method	Cancer Type (Cell Line)	Genes Screened	Hits Identified	Result	References
Apoptosis sensitization	siRNA single well	Cervix (HeLa)	Kinases (650) and phosphatases (222)	21 kinases and 12 phosphatases	Determinants of apoptosis induced by chemotherapy	[38]
B-Raf senescence	shRNA polyclonal screen sequencing	Normal tissue (fibroblast)	Genome	17 genes	IGFBP7 can block proliferation B-Raf mutant cells	[109]
Bypass p53 induced cell cycle arrest	shRNA polyclonal screen sequencing	Normal tissue (fibroblast)	8000 genes (mostly drugable)	5 genes	Novel genes that are essential for p53 function	[51]
Cell cycle	siRNA single-well microscopy	Osteosarcoma (U2OS)	Genome	1152 genes after cell cycle progression	130 genes found are increased in tumor expression	[110]
Cell cycle	esiRNA single-well microscopy	Cervix (HeLa)	17000 genes	1351 genes causing cell cycle arrest/cell division	One of the largest efforts to find genes involved in cell cycle	[92, 111]
Cell cycle and mitosis	siRNA single-well microscopy	Cervix (HeLa)	Genome	8 genes were validated in 2 cell lines		[112]
Cell cycle in presence of Taxol	shRNA single-well microscopy	Cervix (HeLa)	Ubiquitin associated genes (800)	14 new candidate spindle checkpoint regulators	USP44 in DUB for CDC20	[113]

(Continued)

TABLE 4.4 (*Continued*)

Phenotype	Screening Method	Cancer Type (Cell Line)	Genes Screened	Hits Identified	Result	References
Cisplatin/ Gemcitabine/ Paclitaxel	siRNA single-well viability	Cervix (HeLa)	Genome	53 genes that sensitize cell to cisplatin	Cells with mutant BRCA pathway are more sensitive to cisplatin treatment	[114]
Essential genes	shRNA polyclonal barcode screen	Diffuse large B-cell lymphoma	2500 genes	15 genes are essential for proliferation	CARD11, MALT1 ad BCL 10 are essential for DLBCL proliferation	[115]
Essential genes	shRNA barcode	Colon/breast cancer and normal tissue	3000 genes; kinases, phophatases	19 genes are essential for proliferation	First large approach to find essential genes in human cells	[116]
Essential genes	shRNA polyclonal barcode	12 cancer cell lines	Genome	268 genes that are essential in all 12 cell lines	Identification of imatinib and FAS-mediated cell death regulators	[117]
Gemcitabine sensitization	siRNA single-well apoptosis LEISA	Pancreas	645 kinases	10 kinases sensitized 2 pancreatic cancer cell lines to gemcitabine	Some identified kinases are potential targets for gemcitabine combination therapy	[118]
In vivo hepatocellular carcinoma	shRNA *in vivo* liver cancer	Normal hepatoblast	300 genes	13 new liver tumor suppressor genes	XPO4 suppresses tumor growth through EIF5A	[70]
Invasion in 3D cell culture	shRNA clinogenic assay sequencing	Melanoma (mouse)	Genome	22 genes	GAS 1 is metastasis suppressor that is deleted in human melanoma	[119]

104

K-Ras synthetic lethality	siRNA single-well viability	Colon (DLD-1 isogenic mutant RAS cell lines)	4000 genes		Survivin inhibition is more toxic to mutant RAS cells	[120]
K-Ras synthetic lethality	siRNA single-well viability	Monocytic leukemia, normal tissue	1000 kinases and phosphatases	1 kinase found in cell line panel with and without mutant RAS	Identification of STK33 kinase, inhibition is selectively toxic in mutant RAS cells	[121]
Mitotic index	shRNA single-well microscopy	Lung /A549, HT-29	1000 genes	87 genes (higher mitotic index); 15 genes (lower mitotic index)	On of the first single-well shRNA screens	[41]
NF-κB signaling	shRNA single-well NF-κB reporter	Osteosarcoma (U2OS)	Deubiquitinating enzymes	1 DUB that activates NF-κB signaling	Tumor suppressor CYLD functions through NF-κB activation	[56]
Pacitaxel sensitization	siRNA single-well viability	Lung (NCI-H1 155)	Genome	87 pacitaxel sensitizer loci	Inhibition of proteasome and genes involved in spindle checkpoint integrity sensitize to pacitaxel	[122]
Pacitaxel sensitization	shRNA single-well viability	Lung (A549)	74 tumor suppressor genes	shRNA for proteins with long half-life	Inhibition of MDR1 drug transporter sensitizes cells to pacitaxel	[123]
Resistance to HDAC inhibitors	shRNA polyclonal screen sequencing	Osteosarcoma (U2OS)	8000 mostly drugable genes	Suppression of Rad 23B causes cell resistance to HDAC inhibition	Possibility to combine HDAC inhibitors with proteasome inhibitors	[124]

(Continued)

TABLE 4.4 (*Continued*)

Phenotype	Screening Method	Cancer Type (Cell Line)	Genes Screened	Hits Identified	Result	References
Resistance to necroptosis	siRNA single well	Normal tissue (L929, mouse)	Genome	432 genes	Identification of genes involved in cancer and human diseases	[125]
Resistance to trastuzumab	shRNA polyclonal barcode	Breast	8000 mostly drugable genes	Knockdown of PTEN causes resistance to trastuzumab	Activation status of PI2k kinase pathway determines response to trastuzumab treatment	[126]
Soft agar Ras complementation	shRNA polyclonal screen barcode & sequencing	Normal tissue (HMEC)	8000 genes	18 genes allow growth in soft agar	Identification of REST as tumor suppressor	[36]
Tamoxifen	siRNA single-well viability	Breast (MCF-7)	779 kinases and related proteins	3 kinases that cause tamoxifen resistance	CDK10 is potential biomarker of tamoxifen response	[127]
Wnt signaling	shRNA single-well reporter and cell viability	Colon (HCT116)	1000 genes mostly kinases	9 genes affect viability and Wnt signaling	CDK8 is oncogene in colorectal cancer	[128]
Resistance to MDM2 inhibitors	shRNA barcode screen	Breast (MCF-7)	8000 mostly drugable genes	2 on target hits	Knockdown of the tumor suppressor 53BP1 causes resistance to MDM2 inhibition	[129]

rescued from cytotoxic conditions do not lead to the identification of potential therapeutic targets.

A study using a library of retroviral vectors that allows the inducible expression of shRNAs targeting 2500 human genes described a loss of function, or so-called Achilles heel screen, that enables the isolation of genes required for the proliferation and survival of cancer cells and thus the identification of putative anticancer drug targets. Each shRNA carried a unique identifier barcode, allowing the abundance of individual shRNAs to be monitored in a population of cells after shRNA expression has been induced. This showed that CARD11, an NF-κB pathway component, is required for proliferation of a subgroup of diffuse large B-cell lymphomas [115].

Synthetic screens for modifiers of a particular cancer chemical compound or knockdowns of other genes hold great promise for identifying genes, in particular, cancer pathways. A genome-wide RNAi library for enhancers of paclitaxel, a compound that inhibits the growth of microtubules and that is used as a cancer therapeutic was screened and 87 genes found that, when knocked down, sensitized a human lung-cancer cell line to paclitaxel-induced cytotoxity [122]. In a recent shRNA library-based barcode screen for resistance genes against Herceptin, an antagonistic epidermal growth factor receptor antibody now commonly used as a breast-cancer therapeutic, identified components of the phosphatase and tensin homologue (PTEN) pathway [126].

4.6.2 Neurology

Given the number of genes in mammalian genomes, methods that accelerate gene function analyses are urgently needed to speed up discoveries in neuroscience. Recent studies have shown that the potential of RNAi extends to applications in the mammalian nervous system. RNAi technique was successfully applied to neuroscience studies performed with mammalian cells *in vitro* and mammals *in vivo* to study gene function in fundamental neurobiological processes such as intracellular signaling, embryonic development, formation of cellular junctions, cell cycle, programmed cell death, neural plasticity, axon guidance, and membrane trafficking. Effective gene silencing using RNAi screening has been demonstrated in neuronal cell lines [174], neural stem cells [175], primary mammalian neurons [176], astrocytes [177], and Schwann cells [178]. Moreover, gene silencing by adenovirus vector shRNA expression has also been demonstrated in mouse brain *in vivo* [179]. Synthetic siRNA can be readily introduced into neurons and effectively inhibit the expression of endogenous and transfected genes, suggesting RNAi might be developed into a highly efficacious tool to study the roles of specific genes in neuronal development and functioning [176, 174].

The RNAi screening technique has also been extensively used to explore the functions of genes in the nervous system of invertebrates such as *C. elegans* and *Drosophila*, which have been the premier genetic model systems for a long time. Ion channel function [180], neuromuscular function [181], and synaptic vesicle endocytosis [182] are processes that were evaluated with RNAi in *C. elegans*. The function of human neurological disease genes, such as ataxin, was explored using RNAi in invertebrate models. The ortholog of human spinocerebellar ataxia type 2 gene was found to be essential for early embryonic patterning in *C. elegans*.

Recent studies using RNAi screening techniques in *Drosophila* have explored neural plasticity [183], control of photoreceptor axon and cortical axon topography in the developing visual system [184], axon guidance [185], sensory axon guidance and synaptic target recognition [186], neurodegeneration [187] and excitability [188].

These results show that RNAi is a powerful tool in the study of genes functioning in learning and memory in Aplysia by specifically inhibiting both the constitutive and induced expression of the genes. It is possible that RNAi is one of the physiologic mechanisms that regulate long-term gene expression in the brain [189–192].

4.6.3 Immunology and Infectious Diseases

Hepatitis C virus (HCV) isolates that are infectious in cell culture provide a genetic system to evaluate the significance of virus–host interactions for HCV replication. A systematic, focused RNAi screen was carried out wherein siRNAs were designed that target 62 host genes encoding proteins previously identified in protein–protein interaction screens, that physically interact with HCV RNA or proteins or belong to cellular pathways thought to modulate HCV infection. The silencing of 26 genes modulated virus production more than threefold [59].

Likewise the human immunodeficiency virus (HIV)-1 depends on the host cell machinery to support its replication. To discover cellular factors associated with HIV-1 replication, a genome-scale siRNA screen, revealing more than 311 host factors, including 267 that were not previously linked to HIV, was conducted. Surprisingly, there was little overlap between these genes and the HIV dependency factors described recently. This study highlights both the power and shortcomings of large-scale loss-of-function screens in discovering host–pathogen interactions [193].

RNAi screens were performed targeting 37 of the 72 RRM-domain proteins of *Trypanosoma brucei*. In eukaryotes, proteins containing RNA recognition motifs (RRMs) are involved in many different RNA processing reactions,

RNA transport, and mRNA decay. Kinetoplastids rely extensively on post-transcriptional mechanisms to control gene expression, so RRM-domain proteins are expected to play a prominent role. RNAi targeting eight of the genes caused clear growth inhibition in bloodstream trypanosomes, and milder effects were seen for 9 more genes. The small, single-RRM protein *Tb*RBP3 specifically associated with 10 mRNAs in trypanosome lysates, but RBP3 depletion did not affect the [60, 61].

4.7 LIMITATIONS OF RNAi SCREENING

The efficacy of siRNA-mediated suppression of gene expression depends on a number of factors, including not only the chosen siRNA sequence but also the structure of the siRNA, and the receptiveness of the cell type to siRNA uptake [194, 195]. In addition, the half-life of the target message and/or protein needs to be considered in order to achieve optimal silencing. The initial limitation of RNAi technology is designing an effective siRNA sequence [196]. Advancements in siRNA delivery (such as the enzymatic synthesis of siRNAs from T7 promoters) have placed constraints on which sequences of the target genes can even be considered for use. Many of these constraints depend on the type of polymerase ultimately used to recognize and amplify the siRNA sequence [197]. However, even following the recommended rules for siRNA design does not ensure effective silencing of the target gene [194, 195, 198].

Care should be taken not to overinterpret the negative data obtained with RNAi. To avoid off-target effects, proper controls, such as a second independent RNAi or complementation with a nontargeted cDNA, should be included. But most of all, the speed at which one can knock down expression of a single protein should not be taken as evidence that this procedure will circumvent any secondary effects. Even when studying mammalian cell division, one should realize that 2 days is twice a lifetime for most of the cells that we study [199].

Not all diseases can be captured into an *in vitro* cellular assay model. For example, good cellular assays that provide a direct link to the disease are difficult to design for certain central nervous system disorders, such as schizophrenia, and could make a program difficult or impossible to set up, unless one settles for the second best choice of phenotypes. This increases the risk of identifying targets that are not relevant. In addition, including an *in vivo* validation model early in the target validation process might be needed, resulting in a bias as the throughput of *in vivo* target validation is limited and researchers are not able to select genes based on disease-specific *in vitro* selection criteria [137].

4.8 SUMMARY AND OUTLOOK

Since its initial discovery in 1998 by Fire et al. [1], RNAi has become a fascinating area with enormous potential. Small noncoding RNAs such as siRNA, shRNA, and miRNA can interfere with gene expression in several ways: by cleaving the mRNA in a sequence-specific manner, by preventing translation of mRNA or by transcriptional silencing. RNAi and related phenomena began to be studied as a part of the biology of mainly lower organisms (such as *Neurospora* or *C. elegans*) or plants. Subsequently, however, it was discovered that equivalent cellular pathways exist in mammalian cells. As the study of these pathways progressed, it was soon evident that RNAi, more specifically, siRNA could be utilized as a tool to study mammalian gene function as it allowed down-regulation of gene expression, hence providing a simple alternative to creating cell lines or transgenic animals with knockout phenotypes. To facilitate these studies of gene function, a number of techniques aimed at easing the synthesis and screening of synthetic siRNA have been developed. Examples include the *in vitro* transcription of siRNAs and the development of prescreened siRNA libraries. With the advent of vector-based systems for the expression of shRNA, many of the problems associated with siRNA delivery, for example, low transfection efficiency and inappropriate subcellular localization, have begun to be solved. In parallel, viral vector-based systems allow the silencing effect of the shRNA to be prolonged and used in animal *in vivo* models [200].

An additional value of RNAi screens is that they can be combined with other functional genomics assays, such as, transcriptional profiling and protein interaction experiments, resulting in more "-ome" terminologies like "phenome," "transcriptome," "interactome" [201, 202]. The future of genetic screening will require increasingly sophisticated assays both for conventional genetics and for RNAi-based approaches. Stained fat bodies [54], fluorescent reporter protein for genome instability [203], longevity, and DNA repair [203, 204] are only a few examples for such specialized genetic screens.

RNAi is a powerful tool for pharmaceutical target discovery facilitating the expedited mining of genomic information. RNAi-based screening requires a highly defined workflow including automation, bioinformatics, multiple layers of control and a panel of robust assays. As with every technology that interferes with biological systems, there is the risk of artifacts (false positives and false negatives). With reasonable efforts, these can be managed and mitigated to a certain extent. Several selection criteria can play an important role in determining reliable target priority, for example, target tissue expression profiles, degree and quality of available intellectual property, druggablility and access to necessary molecular validation tools, all of which can help focus research efforts on the most promising gene candidates.

RNAi screening is becoming part of the standard experimental repertoire. Through the distribution of public-domain libraries and the establishment of screening centers that can provide automation for cell-based screens, performing genome-wide RNAi screens is within the reach of most laboratories. Similar to genetic screens, the RNAi screen is only the first step in the comprehensive analysis of biological phenomena—the end of the screen is the beginning of the experiment.

REFERENCES

1. Fire, A., et al. (1998). Potent and specific genetic interference by double-stranded RNA in *Caenorhabditis elegans*. *Nature* **391**(6669): 806–11.
2. Van Der Krol, A. R., et al. (1990). Flavonoid genes in petunia: addition of a limited number of gene copies may lead to a suppression of gene expression. *Plant Cell* **2**(4): 291–9.
3. Mol, J. N., et al. (1990). Regulation of plant gene expression by antisense RNA. *FEBS Lett* **268**(2): 427–30.
4. Napoli, C., Lemieux, C., and Jorgensen, R. (1990). Introduction of a chimeric chalcone synthase gene into petunia results in reversible co-suppression of homologous genes in trans. *Plant Cell* **2**(4): 279–89.
5. Romano, N., et al. (1992). Quelling: transient inactivation of gene expression in *Neurospora crassa* by transformation with homologous sequences. *Mol Microbiol*, **6**(22): 3343–53.
6. Silva, J., et al. (2004). RNA-interference-based functional genomics in mammalian cells: reverse genetics coming of age. *Oncogene* **23**(51): 8401–9.
7. Paddison, P. J., et al. (2002). Short hairpin RNAs (shRNAs) induce sequence-specific silencing in mammalian cells. *Genes Dev* **16**(8): 948–58.
8. Ketting, R. F., et al. (2001). Dicer functions in RNA interference and in synthesis of small RNA involved in developmental timing in *C. elegans*. *Genes Dev* **15**(20): 2654–9.
9. Bernstein, E., Denli, A. M., and Hannon, G. J. (2001). The rest is silence. *RNA* **7**(11): 1509–21.
10. Elbashir, S. M., et al. (2001). Duplexes of 21-nucleotide RNAs mediate RNA interference in cultured mammalian cells. *Nature* **411**(6836): 494–8.
11. Elbashir, S. M., et al. (2002). Analysis of gene function in somatic mammalian cells using small interfering RNAs. *Methods* **26**(2): 199–213.
12. Sijen, T., et al. (2001). On the role of RNA amplification in dsRNA-triggered gene silencing. *Cell* **107**(4): 465–76.
13. Andres, A. J. (2004). Flying through the genome: a comprehensive study of functional genomics using RNAi in Drosophila [review]. *Trends Endocrinol Metab* **15**(6): 243–7.

14. Adams, M. D., et al. (2000). The genome sequence of *Drosophila melanogaster*. *Science* **287**(5461): 2185–95.

15. Carninci, P., et al. (2005). The transcriptional landscape of the mammalian genome. *Science* **309**(5740): 1559–63.

16. Gibbs, R. A., et al. (2004). Genome sequence of the Brown Norway rat yields insights into mammalian evolution. *Nature* **428**(6982): 493–521.

17. Venter, J. C., et al. (2001). The sequence of the human genome. *Science* **291**(5507): 1304–51.

18. Lage, H. (2005). Potential applications of RNA interference technology in the treatment of cancer [review]. *Future Oncol* **1**(1): 103–13.

19. Sullenger, B. A. and Gilboa, E. (2002). Emerging clinical applications of RNA. *Nature* **418**(6894): 252–8.

20. Szymkowski, D. E. (2003). Target validation joins the pharma fold. *Targets* **2**: 8–10.

21. Stark, G. R. and Gudkov, A. V. (1999). Forward genetics in mammalian cells: functional approaches to gene discovery. *Hum Mol Genet* **8**(10): 1925–38.

22. . St. Johnston, D. (2002). The art and design of genetic screens: *Drosophila melanogaster*. *Nat Rev Genet* **3**(3): 176–88.

23. King, D. P. and Takahashi, J. S. (1996). Forward genetic approaches to circadian clocks in mice. *Cold Spring Harb Symp Quant Biol* **61**: 295–302.

24. Pickart, M. A., et al. (2004). Functional genomics tools for the analysis of zebrafish pigment. *Pigment Cell Res* **17**(5): 461–70.

25. Adams, M. D. and Sekelsky, J. J. (2002). From sequence to phenotype: reverse genetics in Drosophila melanogaster. *Nat Rev Genet* **3**(3): 189–98.

26. Gudkov, A. V., et al. (1993). Isolation of gentic suppressor elements, inducing resistance to topoisomerase II-interactive cytotoxic drugs, from human topoisomerase II cDNA. *Proc Natl Acad Sci U S A* **90**: 3231–5.

27. Gudkov, A. V., et al. (1994). Cloning mammalian genes by expression selction of gentic suppressor elements: association of kinesin with drug resistance and cell immortalization. *Proc Natl Acad Sci U S A* **91**: 3722–48.

28. Gudkov, A. V. and Ronnison, I. B. (1998). Isolation of genetic suppressor elements (gseS) from random fragmented cDNA libraries in retorviral vectors. In: G. Cowell and I. B. Ronisson (eds), *Protocols for cDNA Libraries*. Humana Press, Totowa, New Jersey.

29. Roninson, I. B., et al. (1995). Genetic suppressor elements: new tools for molecular oncology-thirteenth Cornelius P. Rhoads memorial award lecture. *Cancer Res* **55**: 4023–8.

30. Kimchi, A. (2003). Antisense libraries to isolate tumor suppressor genes. *Methods Mol Biol* **222**: 399–412.

31. Beger, C., et al. (2001). Identification of Id4 as a regulator of BRCA1 expression by using a ribozyme-library-based inverse genomics approach. *Proc Natl Acad Sci U S A* **98**(1): 130–5.

32. Colas, P., et al. (1996). Genetic selection of peptide aptamers that recognize and inhibit cyclin-dependent kinase 2. *Nature* **380**(6574): 548–50.

33. Kleino, A., et al. (2005). Inhibitor of apoptosis 2 and TAK1-binding protein are components of the Drosophila Imd pathway. *EMBO J* **15**: 15.

34. Muller, P., et al. (2005). Identification of JAK/STAT signalling components by genome-wide RNA interference. *Nature* **436**(7052): 871–5.

35. Baeg, G. H., Zhou, R., and Perrimon, N. (2005). Genome-wide RNAi analysis of JAK/STAT signaling components in Drosophila. *Genes Dev* **19**(16): 1861–70.

36. Westbrook, T. F., et al. (2005). A genetic screen for candidate tumor suppressors identifies REST. *Cell* **121**(6): 837–48.

37. Bernards, R. (2005). A functional approach to questions about life, death, and phosphorylation. *Cancer Cell* **7**(6): 503–4.

38. MacKeigan, J. P., Murphy, L. O., and Blenis, J. (2005). Sensitized RNAi screen of human kinases and phosphatases identifies new regulators of apoptosis and chemoresistance. *Nat Cell Biol* **7**(6): 591–600.

39. Boutros, M., et al. (2004). Genome-wide RNAi analysis of growth and viability in Drosophila cells. *Science* **303**(5659): 832–5.

40. Tewari, M. and Vidal, M. (2003). RNAi on the apoptosis TRAIL: the mammalian cell genetic screen comes of age. *Dev Cell* **5**(4): 534–5.

41. Moffat, J. and Sabatini, D. M. (2006). Building mammalian signalling pathways with RNAi screens [review]. *Nat Rev Mol Cell Biol* **7**(3): 177–87.

42. Cullen, L. M. and Arndt, G. M. (2005). Genome-wide screening for gene function using RNAi in mammalian cells [review]. *Immunol Cell Biol* **83**(3): 217–23.

43. Campbell, T. N. and Choy, F. Y. (2005). RNA interference: past, present and future [review]. *Curr Issues Mol. Biol* **7**(1): 1–6.

44. Sandy, P., Ventura, A., and Jacks, T. (2005). Mammalian RNAi: a practical guide [review]. *Biotechniques* **39**(2): 215–24.

45. Vanhecke, D. and Janitz, M. (2005). Functional genomics using high-throughput RNA interference [review]. *Drug Discov Today* **10**(3): 205–12.

46. Shi, Y. (2003). Mammalian RNAi for the masses [review]. *Trends Genet* **19**(1): 9–12.

47. Walhout, A. J. M., et al. (2000). Protein interaction mapping in *C. elegans* using proteins involved in vulval development. *Science* **287**: 116–22.

48. Brown, N. L., et al. (1991). Hairy gene function in the Drosophila eye: normal expression is dispensable but ectopic expression alters cell fates. *Development* **113**: 1245–56.

49. Carroll, S. B. and Whyte, J. S. (1989). The role of the hairy gene during Drosophila morphogenesis: stripes in imaginal discs. *Genes Dev* **3**: 905–16.

50. Fischer-Vize, J. A., Vize, P. D., and Rubin, G. M. (1992). A unique mutation in the Enhancer of split gene complex affects the fates of the mystery cells in the developing Drosophila eye. *Development* **115**: 89–101.

51. Berns, K., et al. (2004). A large-scale RNAi screen in human cells identifies new components of the p53 pathway. *Nature* **428**(6981): 431–7.

52. DasGupta, R., et al. (2005). Functional genomic analysis of the Wnt-wingless signaling pathway. *Science* **308**(5723): 826–33.

53. Foley, E. and P. H. (2004). O'Farrell, Functional dissection of an innate immune response by a genome-wide RNAi screen. *PLoS Biol* **2**(8): E203.

54. Ashrafi, K., et al. (2003). Genome-wide RNAi analysis of *Caenorhabditis elegans* fat regulatory genes. *Nature* **421**(6920): 268–72.

55. Panakova, D., et al. (2005). Lipoprotein particles are required for Hedgehog and Wingless signalling. *Nature* **435**(7038): 58–65.

56. Brummelkamp, T. R., et al. (2003). Loss of the cylindromatosis tumour suppressor inhibits apoptosis by activating NF-kappaB. *Nature* **424**(6950): 797–801.

57. Hudson, J. D., et al. (1999). A proinflammatory cytokine inhibits p53 tumor suppressor activity. *J Exp Med* **190**(10): 1375–82.

58. Carnero, A., et al. (2000). Loss-of-function genetics in mammalian cells: the p53 tumor suppressor model. *Nucleic Acids Res* **28**(11): 2234–41.

59. Lupberger, J., Brino, L., and Baumert, T.F. (2008). RNAi: a powerful tool to unravel hepatitis C virus-host interactions within the infectious life cycle. *J Hepatol* **48**(3):523–5.

60. Mack, K. D., et al. (2005). Functional identification of kinases essential for T-cell activation through a genetic suppression screen. *Immunol Lett* **96**(1): 129–45.

61. Krishnan, M. N., et al. (2008). RNA interference screen for human genes associated with West Nile virus infection. *Nature* **455**(7210): 242–5.

62. Vastenhouw, N. L., et al. (2003). A genome-wide screen identifies 27 genes involved in transposon silencing in *C. elegans. Curr Biol* **13**(15): 1311–6.

63. Nollen, E. A., et al. (2004). Genome-wide RNA interference screen identifies previously undescribed regulators of polyglutamine aggregation. *Proc Natl Acad Sci U S A* **101**(17): 6403–8.

64. Ramet, M., et al. (2002). Functional genomic analysis of phagocytosis and identification of a Drosophila receptor for *E. coli. Nature* **416**(6881): 644–8.

65. Hsieh, A. C., et al. (2004). A library of siRNA duplexes targeting the phosphoinositide 3-kinase pathway: determinants of gene silencing for use in cell-based screens. *Nucleic Acids Res* **32**(3): 893–901.

66. Jackson, A. L., et al. (2003). Expression profiling reveals off-target gene regulation by RNAi. *Nat Biotechnol* **21**(6): 635–7.

67. Bridge, A. J., et al. (2003). Induction of an interferon response by RNAi vectors in mammalian cells. *Nat Genet* **34**(3): 263–4.

68. Ventura, B. (2004). Is siRNA the tool of the future for in vivo mammalian gene research? The experts speak out. *Physiol Genomics* **18**(3): 252–4.

69. Bernards, R. (2008). RNAi Delivers insights into liver cancer. *Cell* **135**(5): 793–5.

70. Zender, L., et al. (2008). An oncogenomics-based in vivo RNAi screen identifies tumor suppressors in liver cancer. *Cell* **135**(5): 852–64.

71. Paddison, P. J., et al. (2004). A resource for large-scale RNA-interference-based screens in mammals. *Nature* **428**(6981): 427–31.

72. Chopra, M., et al. (2003). Using RNA interference to modulate gene expression. *Targets* **1**(3): 102–8.

73. Constans, A. (2002). RNAi for the Masses. *Scientist* **16**(9): 36.

74. Chatterjee-Kishore, M. (2006). From genome to phenome–RNAi library screening and hit characterization using signaling pathway analysis [review]. *Curr Opin Drug Discov Dev* **9**(2): 231–9.

75. Chatterjee-Kishore, M. and Miller, C. P. (2005). Exploring the sounds of silence: RNAi-mediated gene silencing for target identification and validation [review]. *Drug Discovery Today* **10**(22): 1559–65.

76a. Brummelkamp, T. R., Bernards, R., and Agami, R. (2002). A system for stable expression of short interfering RNAs in mammalian cells. *Science* **296**(5567): 550–3.

76b. Buchholz, F., et al. (2006). Enzymatically prepared RNAi libraries. *Nat Methods* **3**(9): 696–700.

76c. Abbas-Terki, T., et al. (2002). Lentiviral-mediated RNA interference. *Hum Gene Ther.* **13**(18): 2197–201.

77. Brummelkamp, T. R. and Bernards, R. (2003). New tools for functional mammalian cancer genetics. *Nat Rev Cancer* **3**(10): 781–9.

78. Banan, M. and Puri, N. (2004). The ins and outs of RNAi in mammalian cells [review]. *Curr Pharm Biotechnol* **5**(5): 441–50.

79. Michiels, F., et al. (2002). Arrayed adenoviral expression libraries for functional screening. *Nat Biotechnol* **20**(11): 1154–7.

80. Shirane, D., et al. (2004). Enzymatic production of RNAi libraries from cDNAs. *Nat Genet* **36**(2): 190–6.

81. Sen, G., et al. (2004). Restriction enzyme-generated siRNA (REGS) vectors and libraries. *Nat Genet* **36**(2): 183–9.

82. Luo, B., Heard, A. D., and Lodish, H. F. (2004). Small interfering RNA production by enzymatic engineering of DNA (SPEED). *Proc Natl Acad Sci U S A* **101**(15): 5494–9.

83. Arts, G.J., et al. (2003). Adenoviral vectors expressing siRNAs for discovery and validation of gene function. *Genome Res* **13**(10): 2325–32.

84. Williams, N.S., et al. (2003). Identification and validation of genes involved in the pathogenesis of colorectal cancer using cDNA microarrays and RNA interference. *Clin Cancer Res* **9**(3): 931–46.

85. Bernards, R., Brummelkamp, T. R., and Beijersbergen, R. L. (2006). shRNA libraries and their use in cancer genetics. *Nat Methods* **3**(9): 701–6.

86. Fewell, G. D. and Schmitt, K. (2006). Vector-based RNAi approaches for stable, inducible and genome-wide screens. *Drug Discov Today* **11**(21–22), 975–82.

87. Chang, K., Elledge, S. J., and Hannon, G.J. (2006). Lessons from nature: microRNA-based shRNA libraries. *Nat Methods* **3**(9): 707–14.

88. Willingham, A. T., et al. (2004) RNAi and HTS: exploring cancer by systematic loss-of-function [review]. *Oncogene* **23**(51): 8392–400.

89. Aza-Blanc, P., et al. (2003). Identification of modulators of TRAIL-induced apoptosis via RNAi-based phenotypic screening. *Mol Cell* **12**(3): 627–37.

90. Luo, J., et al. (2009). A genome-wide RNAi screen identifies multiple synthetic lethal interactions with the Ras oncogene. *Cell* **137**(5): 835–48.

91. Kittler, R., et al. (2007). Genome-scale RNAi profiling of cell division in human tissue culture cells. *Nat Cell Biol* **9**(12): 1401–12.

92. Kittler, R., et al. (2007). Genome-wide resources of endoribonuclease-prepared short interfering RNAs for specific loss-of-function studies. *Nat Methods* **4**(4): 337–44.

93. Ziauddin, J. and Sabatini, D. M. (2001). Microarrays of cells expressing defined cDNAs. *Nature* **411**(6833): 107–10.

94. Chang, F. H., et al. (2004). Surfection: a new platform for transfected cell arrays. *Nucleic Acids Res* **32**(3): e33.

95. Wheeler, D. B., Carpenter, A. E., and Sabatini, D. M. (2005). Cell microarrays and RNA interference chip away at gene function. *Nat Genet* **37**(30), Suppl: S25–30.

96. Shelton, J. G., et al. (2005). The epidermal growth factor receptor gene family as a target for therapeutic intervention in numerous cancers: what's genetics got to do with it? *Expert Opin Ther Targets* **9**(5): 1009–30.

97. Rabindran, S. K. (2005). Antitumor activity of HER-2 inhibitors. *Cancer Lett* **227**(1): 9–23.

98. Dietrich, S., et al. (2005). Role of c-MET in upper aerodigestive malignancies—from biology to novel therapies. *J Environ Pathol Toxicol Oncol* **24**(3): 149–62.

99. Corso, S., Comoglio, P. M., and Giordano, S. (2005). Cancer therapy: can the challenge be MET? *Trends Mol Med* **11**(6): 284–92.

100. Silva, C. M. (2004). Role of STATs as downstream signal transducers in Src family kinase-mediated tumorigenesis. *Oncogene* **23**(48): 8017–23.

101. Ward, J. P., et al. (2004). Protein kinases in vascular smooth muscle tone—role in the pulmonary vasculature and hypoxic pulmonary vasoconstriction. *Pharmacol Ther* **104**(3): 207–31.

102. Fraser, A. (2004). Towards full employment: using RNAi to find roles for the redundant. *Oncogene* **23**(51): 8346–52.

103. Perrimon, N. and Mathey-Prevot, B. (2007). Applications of high-throughput RNA interference screens to problems in cell and developmental biology. *Genetics* **175**(1): 7–16.

104. Jonkers, J. and Berns, A. (2002). Conditional mouse models of sporadic cancer. *Nat Rev Cancer* **2**(4): 251–65.

105. Jonkers, J. and Derksen, P. W. (2007). Modeling metastatic breast cancer in mice. *J Mammary Gland Biol Neoplasia* **12**(2-3): 191–203.

106. Li, T., et al. (2004). Identification of the gene for vitamin K epoxide reductase. *Nature* **427**(6974): 541–4.

107. Balklava, Z., et al. (2007). Genome-wide analysis identifies a general requirement for polarity proteins in endocytic traffic. *Nat Cell Biol* **9**(9): 1066–73.

108. Hahn, P., et al. (2005). A genomewide perspective of gene expression—integration of QIAGEN RNAi technologies and Affymetrix GeneChip Arrays. *QIAGEN News* **e8.**

109. Wajapeyee, N., et al. (2008). Oncogenic BRAF induces senescence and apoptosis through pathways mediated by the secreted protein IGFBP7. *Cell* **132**(3): 363–74.

110. Mukherji, M., et al. (2006). Genome-wide functional analysis of human cell-cycle regulators. *Proc Natl Acad Sci U S A* **103**(40): 14819–24.

111. Kittler, R., et al. (2004). An endoribonuclease-prepared siRNA screen in human cells identifies genes essential for cell division. *Nature* **432**(7020): 1036–40.

112. Rines, D. R., et al. (2008). Whole genome functional analysis identifies novel components required for mitotic spindle integrity in human cells. *Genome Biol* **9**(2): R44.

113. Stegmeier, F., et al. (2007). Anaphase initiation is regulated by antagonistic ubiquitination and deubiquitination activities. *Nature* **446**(7138): 876–81.

114. Bartz, S. R., et al. (2006). Small interfering RNA screens reveal enhanced cisplatin cytotoxity in tumor cells having both BRCA network and TP53 disruptions. *Mol Cell Biol* **26**(24): 9377–86.

115. Ngo, V. N., et al. (2006). A loss-of-function RNA interference screen for molecular targets in cancer. *Nature* **441**(7089): 106–10.

116. Schlabach, M. R., et al. (2008). Cancer proliferation gene discovery through functional genomics. *Science* **319**(5863): 620–4.

117. Luo, K., Harding, S. A., and Tsai, C. J. (2008). A modified T-vector for simplified assembly of hairpin RNAi constructs. *Biotechnol Lett* **30**(7): 1271–4.

118. Giroux, V., Iovanna, J., and Dagorn, J. C. (2006). Probing the human kinome for kinases involved in pancreatic cancer cell survival and gemcitabine resistance. *FASEB J* **20**(12): 1982–91.

119. Gobeil, S., et al. (2008). A genome-wide shRNA screen identifies GAS1 as a novel melanoma metastasis suppressor gene. *Genes Dev* **22**(21): 2932–40.

120. Sarthy, A. V., et al. (2007). Survivin depletion preferentially reduces the survival of activated K-Ras-transformed cells. *Mol Cancer Ther* **6**(1): 269–76.

121. Scholl, C., et al. (2009). Synthetic lethal interaction between oncogenic KRAS dependency and STK33 suppression in human cancer cells. *Cell* **137**(5): 821–34.

122. Whitehurst, A. W., et al. (2007). Synthetic lethal screen identification of chemosensitizer loci in cancer cells. *Nature* **446**(7137): 815–9.

123. Ji, D., Deeds, S. L., and Weinstein, E. J. (2007). A screen of shRNAs targeting tumor suppressor genes to identify factors involved in A549 paclitaxel sensitivity. *Oncol Rep* **18**(6): 1499–505.

124. Fotheringham, S., et al. (2009). Genome-wide loss-of-function screen reveals an important role for the proteasome in HDAC inhibitor-induced apoptosis. *Cancer Cell* **15**(1): 57–66.

125. Hitomi, J., et al. (2008). Identification of a molecular signaling network that regulates a cellular necrotic cell death pathway. *Cell* **135**(7): 1311–23.

126. Berns, K., et al. (2007). A functional genetic approach identifies the PI3 K pathway as a major determinant of trastuzumab resistance in breast cancer. *Cancer Cell* . **12**(4): 395–402.

127. Iorns, E., et al. (2008). Identification of CDK10 as an important determinant of resistance to endocrine therapy for breast cancer. *Cancer Cell* **13**(2): 91–104.

128. Firestein, R., et al. (2008). CDK8 is a colorectal cancer oncogene that regulates beta-catenin activity. *Nature* **455**(7212): 547–51.

129. Brummelkamp, T. R., et al. (2006). An shRNA barcode screen provides insight into cancer cell vulnerability to MDM2 inhibitors. *Nat Chem Biol* **2**(4): 202–6.

130. Diederichs, S., et al. (2008). Coexpression of Argonaute-2 enhances RNA interference toward perfect match binding sites. *Proc Natl Acad Sci U S A* **105**(27): 9284–9.

131. Semizarov, D., et al. (2003). Specificity of short interfering RNA determined through gene expression signatures. *Proc Natl Acad Sci U S A* **100**(11): 6347–52.

132. Persengiev, S. P., Zhu, X., and Green, M. R. (2004). Nonspecific, concentration-dependent stimulation and repression of mammalian gene expression by small interfering RNAs (siRNAs). *RNA* **10**(1): 12–8.

133. Neumann, B., et al. (2006). High-throughput RNAi screening by time-lapse imaging of live human cells. *Nat Methods* **3**(5): 385–90.

134. Bertelsen, M. and Sanfridson, A. (2005). Inflammatory pathway analysis using a high content screening platform. *Assay Drug Dev Technol* **3**(3): 261–71.

135. Carpenter, A. E., et al. (2006). CellProfiler: image analysis software for identifying and quantifying cell phenotypes. *Genome Biol* **7**(10): R100.

136. Sacher, R., Stergiou, L., and Pelkmans, L. (2008). Lessons from genetics: interpreting complex phenotypes in RNAi screens. *Curr Opin Cell Biol* **20**(4): 483–9.

137. van Es, H. H. and Arts, G. J. (2005). Biology calls the targets: combining RNAi and disease biology [review]. *Drug Discov Today* **10**(20): 1385–91.

138. Birmingham, A., et al. (2009). Statistical methods for analysis of high-throughput RNA interference screens. *Nat Methods* **6**(8): 569–75.

139. Scacheri, P.C., et al. (2004). Short interfering RNAs can induce unexpected and divergent changes in the levels of untargeted proteins in mammalian cells. *Proc Natl Acad Sci U S A* **101**(7): 1892–7.

140. Scherer, L., et al. (2004). RNAi applications in mammalian cells. *Biotechniques* **36**(4): 557–61.

141. Sui, G. and Shi, Y. (2005). Gene silencing by a DNA vector-based RNAi technology. *Methods Mol Biol* **309**: 205–18.

142. Harper, S. Q. and Davidson, B. L. (2005). Plasmid-based RNA interference: construction of small-hairpin RNA expression vectors. *Methods Mol Biol* **309**: 219–35.

143. Sarov, M. and Stewart, A. F. (2005). The best control for the specificity of RNAi. *Trends Biotechnol* **23**(9): 446–8.

144. Chi, J. T., et al. (2003). Genomewide view of gene silencing by small interfering RNAs. *Proc Natl Acad Sci U S A* **2**: 2.

145. Achenbach, T. V., Brunner, B., and Heermeier, K. (2003). Oligonucleotide-based knockdown technologies: antisense versus RNA interference. *Chembiochem* **4**(10): 928–35.

146. Scherer, L. J. and Rossi, J. J. (2003). Approaches for the sequence-specific knockdown of mRNA. *Nat Biotechnol* **21**(12): 1457–65.

147. Miyagishi, M., et al. (2004). Optimization of an siRNA-expression system with an improved hairpin and its significant suppressive effects in mammalian cells. *J Gene Med* **6**(7): 715–23.

148. Duxbury, M. S. and Whang, E. E. (2004). RNA interference: a practical approach. *J Surg Res* **117**(2): 339–44.

149. Sledz, C. A. and Williams, B. R. (2004). RNA interference and double-stranded-RNA-activated pathways. *Biochem Soc Trans* **32**(Pt 6): 952–6.

150. Scherr, M. and Eder, M. (2004). RNAi in functional genomics. *Curr Opin Mol Ther* **6**(2): 129–35.

151. Silva, J. M., et al. (2004). RNA interference microarrays: high-throughput loss-of-function genetics in mammalian cells. *Proc Natl Acad Sci U S A* **101**(17): 6548–52.

152. Snove, O., Jr., and Holen, T. (2004). Many commonly used siRNAs risk off-target activity. *Biochem Biophys Res Commun* **319**(1): 256–63.

153. Amarzguioui, M., et al. (2003). Tolerance for mutations and chemical modifications in a siRNA. *Nucleic Acids Res* **31**(2): 589–95.

154. Marques, J. T. and Williams, B. R. (2005). Activation of the mammalian immune system by siRNAs [review]. *Nat Biotechnol* **23**(11): 1399–405.

155. Du, Q., et al. (2005). A systematic analysis of the silencing effects of an active siRNA at all single-nucleotide mismatched target sites. *Nucleic Acids Res* **33**(5): 1671–7.

156. Lackner, M. R. and Kim, S. K. (1998). Genetic analysis of the *Caenorhabditis elegans* MAP kinase gene mpk-1. *Genetics* **150**(1): 103–17.

157. Castanotto, D., et al. (2007). Combinatorial delivery of small interfering RNAs reduces RNAi efficacy by selective incorporation into RISC. *Nucleic Acids Res* **35**(15): 5154–64.

158. Sahin, O., et al. (2007). Combinatorial RNAi for quantitative protein network analysis. *Proc Natl Acad Sci U S A* **104**(16): 6579–84.

159. Griffiths A. J. F., M. J., Suzuki, D. T., Lewontin, R. C., and Gelbart, W. M. (1997). *An Introduction to Genetic Analysis*. WH Freeman and Company, New York.

160. Malo, N., et al. (2006). Statistical practice in high-throughput screening data analysis. *Nat Biotechnol* **24**(2): 167–75.

161. Zhang, J. H., Chung, T. D., and Oldenburg, K. R. (1999). A simple statistical parameter for use in evaluation and validation of high throughput screening assays. *J Biomol Screen* **4**(2): 67–73.

162. Boutros, M. and Ahringer, J. (2008). The art and design of genetic screens: RNA interference. *Nat Rev Genet* **9**(7): 554–66.

163. Konig, R., et al. (2007). A probability-based approach for the analysis of large-scale RNAi screens. *Nat Methods* **4**(10): 847–9.

164. Dillon, C. P., et al. (2005). RNAi as an experimental and therapeutic tool to study and regulate physiological and disease processes [review]. *Ann Rev Physiol* **67**: 147–73.

165. McManus, M. T., et al. (2002). Small interfering RNA-mediated gene silencing in T lymphocytes. *J Immunol* **169**(10): 5754–60.

166. Rubinson, D. A., et al. (2003). A lentivirus-based system to functionally silence genes in primary mammalian cells, stem cells and transgenic mice by RNA interference. *Nat Genet* **33**(3): 401–6.

167. Paroo, Z. and Corey, D. R. (2004). Challenges for RNAi in vivo [review]. *Trends Biotechnol* **22**(8): 390–4.

168. Xie, F. Y., Woodle, M. C., and Lu, P. Y. (2006). Harnessing in vivo siRNA delivery for drug discovery and therapeutic development [review]. *Drug Discovery Today* **11**(1–2): 67–73.

169. Lu, P. Y., Xie, F. Y., and Woodle, M. C. (2005). Modulation of angiogenesis with siRNA inhibitors for novel therapeutics [review]. *Trends Mol Med* **11**(3): 104–13.

170. Hannon, G. J. and Rossi, J. J. (2004). Unlocking the potential of the human genome with RNA interference [review]. *Nature* **431**(7006): 371–8.

171. Martinez, L. A., et al. (2002). Synthetic small inhibiting RNAs: efficient tools to inactivate oncogenic mutations and restore p53 pathways. *Proc Natl Acad Sci U S A* **99**(23): 14849–54.

172. Scherr, M., et al. (2003). Specific inhibition of bcr-abl gene expression by small interfering RNA. *Blood* **101**(4): 1566–9.

173. Chen, R. Q., et al. (2009). Kinome sirna screen identifies SMG-1 as a negative regulator of hypoxia-inducible factor-1alpha in hypoxia. *J Biol Chem* **284**(25): 16752–8.

174. Gan, L., et al. (2002). Specific interference with gene expression and gene function mediated by long dsRNA in neural cells. *J Neurosci Methods* **121**(2): 151–7.

175. Wood, M. J., et al. (2003). Therapeutic gene silencing in the nervous system. *Hum Mol Genet* **12** 2: R279–R84.

176. Krichevsky, A. M. and Kosik, K. S. (2002). RNAi functions in cultured mammalian neurons. *Proc Natl Acad Sci U S A* **99**(18): 11926–9.

177. Oh, W. J., et al. (2002). Nuclear proteins that bind to metal response element a (MREa) in the Wilson disease gene promoter are Ku autoantigens and the Ku-80 subunit is necessary for basal transcription of the WD gene. *Eur J Biochem* **269**(8): 2151–61.

178. Higuchi, H., et al. (2003). Functional inhibition of the p75 receptor using a small interfering RNA. *Biochem Biophys Res Commun* **301**(3): 804–9.

179. Xia, H., et al. (2002). siRNA-mediated gene silencing in vitro and in vivo. *Nat Biotechnol* **20**(10): 1006–10.

180. Bianchi, L., et al. (2003). A potassium channel-MiRP complex controls neurosensory function in *Caenorhabditis elegans*. *J Biol Chem* **278**(14): 12415–24.

181. Schulze, E., et al. (2003). The maintenance of neuromuscular function requires UBC-25 in *Caenorhabditis elegans*. *Biochem Biophys Res Commun* **305**(3): 691–9.

182. Harris, T. W., Schuske, K., and Jorgensen, E. M. (2001). Studies of synaptic vesicle endocytosis in the nematode *C. elegans*. *Traffic* **2**(9): 597–605.

183. Billuart, P., et al. (2001). Regulating axon branch stability: the role of p190 RhoGAP in repressing a retraction signaling pathway. *Cell* **107**(2): 195–207.

184. Dearborn, R. Jr., et al. (2002). Eph receptor tyrosine kinase-mediated formation of a topographic map in the Drosophila visual system. *J Neurosci* **22**(4): 1338–49.

185. Georgiou, M. and Tear, G. (2002). Commissureless is required both in commissural neurones and midline cells for axon guidance across the midline. *Development* **129**(12): 2947–56.

186. Marie, B. and Blagburn, J.M. (2003). Differential roles of engrailed paralogs in determining sensory axon guidance and synaptic target recognition. *J Neurosci* **23**(21): 7854–62.

187. Syntichaki, P., et al. (2002). Specific aspartyl and calpain proteases are required for neurodegeneration in *C. elegans*. *Nature* **419**(6910): 939–44.

188. Zhang, H., et al. (2002). The Drosophila slamdance gene: a mutation in an aminopeptidase can cause seizure, paralysis and neuronal failure. *Genetics* **162**(3): 1283–99.

189. Smalheiser, N. R., Manev, H., and Costa, E. (2001). RNAi and brain function: was McConnell on the right track? *Trends Neurosci* **24**(4): 216–8.

190. Genc, S., Koroglu, T. F., and Genc, K. (2004). RNA interference in neuroscience [review]. *Brain Research*. Mol Brain Res **132**(2): 260–70.

191. Miller, V. M., Paulson, H. L., and Gonzalez-Alegre, P. (2005). RNA interference in neuroscience: progress and challenges [review]. *Cell Mol Neurobiol* **25**(8): 1195–207.

192. Yamada, S., et al. (2007). Identification of twinfilin-2 as a factor involved in neurite outgrowth by RNAi-based screen. *Biochem Biophys Res Commun* **363**(4): 926–30.

193. Zhou, H., et al. (2008). Genome-scale RNAi screen for host factors required for HIV replication. *Cell Host Microbe* **4**(5): 495–504.

194. Siolas, D., et al. (2005). Synthetic shRNAs as potent RNAi triggers. *Nat Biotechnol* **23**(2): 227–31.

195. Kim, D. H., et al. (2005). Synthetic dsRNA Dicer substrates enhance RNAi potency and efficacy. *Nat Biotechnol* **23**(2): p. 222–6.

196. Sledz, C. A. and Williams, B. R. (2005). RNA interference in biology and disease [review]. *Blood* **106**(3): 787–94.

197. Sioud, M. and Leirdal, M. (2004). Potential design rules and enzymatic synthesis of siRNAs. *Methods Mol Biol* **252**: 457–69.

198. Reinhart, B. J., et al. (2000). The 21-nucleotide let-7 RNA regulates developmental timing in *Caenorhabditis elegans*. *Nature* **403**(6772): 901–6.

199. Medema, R.H. (2004). Optimizing RNA interference for application in mammalian cells [review]. *Biochem J* **380**(Pt 3): 593–603.

200. Bantounas, I., Phylactou, L. A., and Uney, J. B. (2004). RNA interference and the use of small interfering RNA to study gene function in mammalian systems [review]. *J Mol Endocrinol* **33**(3): 545–57.

201. Walhout, A.J., et al. (2002). Integrating interactome, phenome, and transcriptome mapping data for the *C. elegans* germline. *Curr Biol* **12**(22): 1952–8.

202. Davy, A., et al. (2001). A protein-protein interaction map of the *Caenorhabditis elegans* 26 S proteasome. *EMBO Rep* **2**(9): 821–8.

203. Pothof, J., et al. (2003). Identification of genes that protect the *C. elegans* genome against mutations by genome-wide RNAi. *Genes Dev* **17**(4): 443–8.

204. Kamath, R. S., et al. (2003). Systematic functional analysis of the *Caenorhabditis elegans* genome using RNAi. *Nature* **421**(6920): 231–7.

PART II

DEVELOPMENT OF siRNA FOR THERAPEUTIC APPLICATIONS

CHAPTER 5

DISCOVERY OF NEW siRNA DELIVERY AGENTS

PAUL H. JOHNSON, DIANE FRANK, KUNYUAN CUI, ROGER ADAMI, HARRY WANG, MICHAEL HOUSTON, and STEVEN C. QUAY

5.1 INTRODUCTION

The discovery of RNA interference (RNAi) [1, 2], a fundamental cellular mechanism for silencing gene expression, offers the potential to create a new class of therapeutics with broad applications, high efficacy, low toxicity, and significant potential advantages over other classes of drugs (Table 5.1). Importantly, it also provides a rapid means for target validation and lead identification and optimization, therefore, permitting the development of drugs against targets that have been difficult to exploit by other molecular classes.

There has been a large body of work in applying RNAi technology to the analysis of gene function, investigation of signal transduction pathways, and the identification and validation of new drug targets [3, 4]. Rapid advancements of the technology focused on therapeutic development also have been achieved. Important information is now emerging that indicates there can be significant differences in outcomes obtained with RNAi compared with small molecule drugs against the same target because of their different mechanisms (Table 5.1) [5]. An RNAi therapeutic that significantly reduces the level of a protein in a cell may typically result in disruption of protein complexes. This is a distinctly different mechanism than a small-molecule that competes with an endogenous ligand or substrate for the active site of an enzyme or receptor. When a receptor is removed from the cell by a targeted siRNA, the formerly bound ligands are free to bind other receptors, and some intracellular proteins may be free to become members of other protein complexes. This may

RNA Interference: Application to Drug Discovery and Challenges to Pharmaceutical Development, Edited by Paul H. Johnson

TABLE 5.1 Comparison of Therapeutic Classes

	Small Molecules	Recombinant Proteins, Monoclonal Antibodies	RNAi
Target	Primarily enzymes and cell surface receptors	Extracellular proteins; primarily blood proteins	Broad diversity of intracellular proteins, receptors, including "undrugable" targets
Mechanism	Substrate competition, covalent modification, ligand competition, protein conformational change, allosteric binding	Receptor antagonism, ligand binding	mRNA degradation, inhibition of translation, epigenetic modification
Examples	Lipitor^{TM}, Plavix^{TM}, Vioxx^{TM}	Enbrel^{TM}, Herceptin^{TM}, Rituxan^{TM}	None
Current market	>$175 billion/year with >1000 approved products	>$40 billion/year with >200 approved products	None
Size	Less than 500 Da	50–180 kDa	~13 kDa
Lead identification and optimization	Slow	Slow	Rapid
Manufacturing (cost of goods)	Chemical synthesis; often under $5 per gram	Fermentation; typically $200–650 per gram	Chemical synthesis; unknown but ca $100 per gram is goal
Development challenges	Specificity, potency, target identification, off-target toxicity	Immunogenicity, difficult to purify, unstable, limited delivery options	Primary challenge is delivery; manufacturing costs

have a vastly different effect on a cell than if a small molecule simply inactivates an internal functional domain. This points to the importance of using phenotype-driven cell- and tissue-based screens for lead identification and drug characterization, as these systems utilize endpoints that are related more directly to disease physiology. In some cases, exquisitely high single target specificity may not be as important as having a broader spectrum of effects that take into account redundancy in biological pathway components, which are sometimes mediated by homologous proteins. siRNAs that specifically knock down one protein family member may be less effective in achieving the desired phenotypic outcome than a less specific small molecule that inhibits all the family members, or an siRNA that is targeted to a conserved region of the mRNA (gene) and affects multiple family members simultaneously. Future work must clarify those types of pharmacological targets against which RNAi therapeutics are particularly effective compared with other classes of drugs, as well as the relationship between target(s) specificity and corresponding *in vivo* efficacy and toxicity.

5.1.1 Issues and Challenges

The key challenge and current limitation for successful development of siRNA therapeutics is delivering such drugs efficiently into the cytoplasm of cells *in vivo* [6–8] with a minimum of toxic or immunological side effects [9]. Different delivery formulations will likely be needed for individual therapeutic applications that affect distinct tissue types and that require penetration of various tissue barriers. The barrier that comprises mucosal tissues of the respiratory, gastrointestinal, and urogenital tracts involves transport through tight junctions (TJs), gate-like structures between cells that regulate paracellular passage of various molecules including some types of drugs [10]. Interestingly, biochemical pathways that regulate TJ opening also appear to be important for cellular uptake of siRNA via unique endocytic pathways (P. H. Johnson, 2005, unpublished observations). Penetration of the blood brain barrier also involves traversing a similar endothelial TJ barrier. Treatment of respiratory viral infections will usually involve local delivery to the affected tissue (upper and/or lower respiratory tract), while cancer and inflammation (e.g., arthritis) treatments will generally require systemic administration. A variety of delivery formulation approaches are being pursued, including lipid/liposomal–siRNA complexes, peptide–siRNA complexes and conjugates, and the use of other cationic polymers such as cyclodextrins, chitosans, polyethylenimine (PEI) derivatives, novel lipid/peptide combinations, and new classes of "smart" multifunctional polymers (Table 5.2). Cell type-specific delivery agents using cell surface targeting ligands may enable

TABLE 5.2   Delivery Methods for siRNA Therapeutics

Method	Advantages	Disadvantages	Refs
Cholesterol conjugate	Systemic, stable	Not selective, low efficacy	11,12
SNALP	Systemic, stable	Not selective, toxicity, RES removal	13,14
LipoPlex	Systemic, endothelial cell selective, stable	Toxicity	15–17
Antibody	Systemic, receptor specific	Molecular weight, COGS, immunogenic	18–20
Aptamer	Receptor specific, low immunogenicity	Stability, COGS	21,22
Peptides	Target selective, efficient uptake, biodegradable	Immunogenic, efficacy,	23,24
Cyclodextran, chitosan	Systemic, self-assembling, low toxicity	Complex formulation, not selective	25–28
PEI	Systemic, COGS	Not selective, heterogeneous, toxicity	29,30
"SMART" polymers	Systemic, selective, pH dependant, endosomalytic	New polymers with limited *in vivo* testing	31–34
Hydrodynamic injection	No delivery agent needed, liver specific	Limited applicability, tissue damage	35

lower dosage requirements and fewer toxic side effects than would otherwise result from inhibition of gene expression in nontargeted cells.

Currently, the mechanism(s) of siRNA cellular uptake is poorly understood. There are several possible endocytic pathways that may be involved, each with different efficiencies and compartmentalization often leading to late endosomal processing and degradation. Alternatively, or in addition, membrane fusion of lipid or hydrophobic peptides may be involved. Identifying the most efficient pathway for siRNA uptake and functionality and the ability to optimize siRNA targeting to this route of delivery will be key to successful clinical development of RNAi-based therapeutics.

5.2   CELLULAR UPTAKE MECHANISMS AND TJ DYNAMICS

Organisms including *Caenorhabditis elegans* [1] are able to take up exogenous double-stranded RNA (dsRNA) and mediate its spread to other cells in the body. In general, mammalian cells do not take up dsRNA without a delivery enhancer. However, delivery of siRNA on its own or with a transfection lipid has been shown to result in a clinically relevant knockdown of gene expression when administered directly to mucosal epithelium such as the lung and vagina [36–38]. In addition, there may be specific receptors for dsRNA that could be exploited to improve delivery of siRNA. Interestingly, observations of successful *in vivo* delivery of naked siRNA to cells following intravenous injection [39] may be explained by translocation of siRNA into the cell by a mammalian homologue [40] of the dsRNA-receptor, SID-1. This receptor was first described in *C. elegans*, where it is responsible for the systemic spread of silencing effects [41, 42]. Over expression of the mammalian homologue increases the intracellular uptake of siRNA. In general, however, the lack of activity of "naked" siRNA *in vivo* suggests that not all cell types express the SID-1 homologue at levels that are sufficient to facilitate effective siRNA uptake and gene silencing.

5.2.1 Endocytic Pathways

Most delivery systems for siRNA have cationic residues that enable the formation of a complex with the siRNA and interaction with the cell surface/plasma membrane, which has a negative charge at neutral pH. While it has been thought that delivery of siRNA, antisense oligonucleotides and DNA vectors could be mediated by fusion with the plasma membrane, several recent publications suggest that siRNA uptake may be mediated by one of the endocytotic pathways [43], depending on the type of delivery agent. Four major routes that mediate uptake have been identified: clathrin-mediated, caveolin-mediated, macropinocytosis, and an endocytic route that is clathrin- and caveolae-independent but depends on lipid rafts. The specifics of these pathways have been discussed at length in other reviews [44–46], including the important role that the actin cytoskeleton and associated signaling pathways play in the regulation of endocytosis [47]. Here, we highlight the relevant features and challenges of these pathways with regard to siRNA delivery.

Visualization of siRNA uptake in live cells indicates that the majority is entrapped in punctate perinuclear endosomes and lysosomes [48–50]. While RNAi efficiency has been shown to correlate with perinuclear localization, it is not clear whether this reflects the active population of siRNA. It is possible that the minimal number of siRNA molecules needed to mediate half-maximal RNAi inhibition could be very low and is not detected in fluorescently labeled siRNA microscopy studies. Effective siRNA silencing activity requires siRNA release into the cytoplasm, where it can be loaded into the RNA-induced silencing complex (RISC). Delivery to cells in a manner that supports effective release from the endosome remains one of the major challenges in siRNA delivery.

The clathrin pathway mediates endocytosis of the majority of receptor–ligand complexes and is the endocytic pathway that has been studied most extensively (reviewed in References 51,52). This form of endocytosis occurs in all mammalian cells and ensures the continuous uptake of nutrients including cholesterol-laden low-density lipoprotein and iron-laden transferrin. The clathrin protein is the major constituent of the "coat" of the clathrin-coated pits formed during endocytosis of materials at the cell surface. The formation of vesicles is supported by adaptor proteins that exert their function at different subcellular sites. The coated pits then invaginate, pinch off, and form endocytic vesicles. It is thought that this vesicle cargo is destined for either recycling back to the plasma membrane or for degradation in the lysosome. If targeted to the lysosome, the early endosome becomes acidified and matures to the late endosome. Therefore, successful siRNA delivery into the cytoplasm via this pathway must have a mechanism for endosomal escape.

The caveolae pathway [45] has been shown to internalize pathogen toxins, bacteria, and viruses, presumably as a way to evade trafficking to the lysosome. Therefore, targeting caveolae may provide an efficient means to bypass acidic endosomes and enhance delivery of siRNA to the cytoplasm. It has been shown that particles 200 nm and smaller enter by a clathrin-dependent route, while particles of 500 nm enter by caveolae [44,53]. Larger particles enter by macropinocytosis. Thus, the size of the particle could determine the route of uptake. Macropinocytosis is mediated by actin-driven ruffling and pinching off of irregular sized vesicles. Macropinosomes can undergo acidification but are thought not to traffic to lysosomes. Release of macropinosome contents may be receptor mediated. Therefore, macropinocytosis represents a possible route for increasing siRNA uptake and efficacy of the RNAi effect.

Recent studies on the internalization of receptor tyrosine kinases (RTKs) have described a pathway that is mediated by the actin cytoskeleton and its associated proteins dynamin and cortactin, but is independent of the typical coat proteins (caveolae and clathrin). These endocytic structures are termed dorsal ruffles and form at the dorsal membrane of growth factor-stimulated epithelial cells [51,54,55]. Endocytosis by dorsal ruffles can clear the dorsal membrane of RTKs within minutes, representing a rapid way to downregulate signaling by en masse endocytosis.

5.2.2 TJ Modulation

Epithelial tissue of the respiratory, reproductive, gastrointestinal, renal, and epidermis functions as a selective barrier between the outside environment and the underlying tissue. Epithelial cells are polarized both functionally

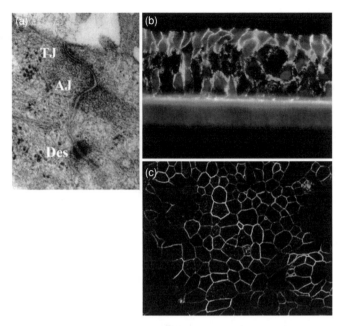

FIGURE 5.1   Epithelial Tight Junctions. A. Transmission electron micrograph of the apical junctional complex in normal human bronchial epithelial cells. Tight junction (TJ), the adherens junction (AJ) and the desmosome (Des). B. Cross-section of immunofluorescent staining of differentiated normal human bronchial epithelial cells for the junctional markers JAM-A (red) and E-Cadherin (green) and DAPI (blue) which marks the nuclei of each cell. C. Confocal image of differentiated normal human bronchial epithelial cells, immunofluorescently labeled for ZO1 (red) and occludin (green). This image is looking down on the apical surface of the cell layer and shows the outlines of the tight junctions which boarder all sides of the apical cells.

and in composition of the lipids and proteins in their apical and basal lateral membranes. This polarity is established in part by the formation of specialized cell–cell junctions referred to as the Apical Junction Complex (AJC) [56]. The AJC is positioned at the apical side of the plasma membrane and is composed of two distinct junctional complexes—the adherens junction (AJ) and the TJ. These junctions are distinct as shown in the electron micrograph in Figure 5.1a, where the TJ is the most apical junction followed by the AJ. Desmosomes provide structural integrity and are dispersed along the basal–lateral junction. The AJ and the TJ are composed of transmembrane proteins that interact directly with the neighboring cells, forming a selective barrier that regulates passage of molecules (reviewed in [57]). The TJ includes occludin, members of the claudin family, and junctional adhesion molecule (JAM-A). The AJ contains E-cadherin and members of the nectin family. Figure 5.1b shows a cross section of immunofluorescent staining of differentiated normal human bronchial epithelial cells for the junctional markers. TJs form a continuous belt of adhesions restricted to the apical membrane, as shown in Figure 5.1c, while E-cadherin is present along the entire basal-lateral membrane but does not provide barrier function. TJs also form between adjacent endothelial cells in the vasculature. The "tightness" of endothelial junctions varies, being very low in the spleen and endocrine glands and very high in the brain and cornea. Therefore, systemic delivery of siRNA and subsequent tissue penetration may vary depending on the target organ.

The AJ and TJ are dynamic structures, undergoing constitutive turnover and recycling. The cytosolic face of the AJC is composed of a large array of distinct proteins that direct the assembly of the AJC [58]. The assembly and disassembly of the AJC is thought to regulate epithelial morphogensis and remodeling processes. Cellular stress such as pathogens, oxidative stress, and cytokines can signal an increase in the endocytosis of the AJC. Studies have shown that endocytosis of the AJ and TJ proteins can occur by clathrin or caveolae endocytic pathways or macropinocytosis (reviewed in Reference 59). Extracellular calcium is required for the formation of the AJC. Modulation of epithelial cell polarity using the calcium chelator ethylene glycol tetraacetic acid (EGTA) has been shown to increase retroviral and adenoviral-mediated gene transfer in rabbit tracheal epithelium [60]. Chelators such as EGTA are capable of disrupting intracellular junctions, decreasing transepithelial resistance and increasing permeability. Evidence from studies in an intestinal epithelial cell line suggests that calcium depletion stimulates endocytosis of the AJC via a clathrin dependent pathway [61]. As mentioned previously, clathrin mediated endocytosis can result in trafficking to an acidic endosome and eventually to the lysosome for degradation. Thus, targeting endocytosis of the AJC via a caveolae or macropinocytic pathway as a means of escaping the degradation route may be an effective way to exploit the ability of TJ modulation to increase siRNA uptake. For example, it has recently been shown that coxsackie virus enters the cell by trafficking to the TJ, where it couples to occludin and induces endocytosis by a macropinocytic and/or caveolar process [62]. A better understanding of the signaling pathways that regulate TJ dynamics and recycling may reveal new approaches to increase RNAi activity through more effective delivery of siRNA to the cytoplasm of epithelial and endothelial cells.

5.3 PEPTIDE-BASED DELIVERY

5.3.1 Cell Penetrating Peptides/Protein Transduction Domains

Cell penetrating peptides (CPPs) are a class of peptides that are of interest due to their ability to be internalized efficiently by cells and to mediate cell uptake of macromolecular cargos including siRNAs, antisense oligonucleotides, gene therapy vectors, and pharmacologically active proteins and peptides. Generally, CPPs are small polybasic and/or amphiphilic molecules up to 40 amino acids in length. CPPs were first discovered in natural proteins containing specific domains called protein transduction domains (PTDs), small cationic peptide regions that can facilitate the uptake of large, biologically active molecules (proteins and polynucleotides) into mammalian cells [24]. Since their discovery more than a decade ago [63, 64], there has been uncertainty about the mechanism(s) by which CPPs/PTDs are internalized into cells.

Most CPPs are derived from sequences of membrane-interacting proteins, such as fusion proteins, signal peptides, transmembrane domains, and antimicrobial peptides. In addition, polycationic peptides such as polylysines, polyarginines, and polyhistidines also have cellular transport properties [65]. Penetratin is a CPP derived from the third helix of the homeodomain of *antennapedia* [66, 67]. Most applications of penetratin are related to protein transfer, such as those involved in the cell cycle progression and induction of apoptosis. This CPP also has been used for transfection of nucleic acids.

The Tat peptide is derived from the transcription-transactivating (Tat) protein of HIV-1 [68]. It is a protein with 101 residues and consists of three functional domains: an acidic N-terminal region required for transactivation activity, a cysteine-rich DNA binding domain, and a basic domain similar to a nuclear localization sequence (NLS). Tat peptide has an ability to cross the plasma membrane and has been used for intracellular transfer of a variety of macromolecules, including fusion proteins and nucleic acids.

Transportan is a CPP designed from the N-terminal fragment of the neuropeptide galanin linked through a lysine residue to mastoparan [69]. This carrier peptide has been used for the cellular transfer of proteins *in vitro*, and peptide nucleic acids (PNAs) both *in vitro* and *in vivo*.

VP22-derived peptide is generated by herpes simplex virus-type 1 [70]. This CPP is expressed in infected cells and then penetrates into neighboring cells and enters their nuclei. Due to its ability to translocate membranes while fused to other peptides or proteins, VP22 peptide has been used for the transfer of functional proteins *in vitro* and *in vivo*.

Calcitonin-derived peptides, especially the 9–32 fragment of human calcitonin (hCT [9–32]), have been used for transfer of green fluorescent protein (GFP) through cellular membranes via covalent carrier-cargo linkage [71]. A hCT derivative with an NLS branched on Lys side chain has been developed to transfer a plasmid through formation of a complex [72].

Many CPPs appear to be amphipathic peptides composed of a polar hydrophilic domain and a nonpolar hydrophobic domain. In general the hydrophobic domain is required for membrane anchoring and the hydrophilic domain is required for solubility and for complex formation with hydrophilic molecules.

5.4 STRUCTURAL FEATURES REQUIRED FOR ACTIVITY

Following internalization of HIV-derived Tat, the protein is subsequently localized to the nucleus where it binds the transactivation response region (TAR) within the long-terminal repeat (LTR) promoter, thereby enhancing transcriptional elongation of HIV [64]. Further studies identified a positively charged sequence between amino acids 48 and 60 that was sufficient for this membrane translocation. The CPPs are generally divided into three different groups depending on the origin of the peptide. The first group is protein-derived peptides, such as Tat and penetratin, which originate from naturally occurring proteins. Another group is the chimeric peptides, in which two or more peptide sequences originating from different proteins are fused together. Examples from this group include TP [69] and MPG [73]. The third group comprises synthetic peptides, of which the polyarginine family [74] and modeled amphipathic peptide (MAP) [75] are the best-studied members. As indicated previously, the polycationic properties of the peptides are important for initiating cellular uptake by binding the cell surface. For delivery of oligonucleotide compounds, such as antisense and siRNA, cationic residues also play an important role in stabilizing complex formation with polyanionic cargos for intracellular delivery. Figure 5.2 shows representative structures of Tat, Penetratin, and Transportin. [76] did a comparative study of several

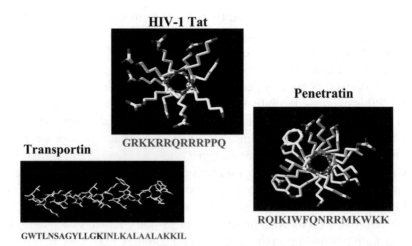

FIGURE 5.2 Cell Penetrating Peptide Structures. Representative amphipathic α-helical structures for Tat, penetratin, and transportin.

cationic polypeptides showing higher cell uptake efficiency for poly-arginines compared with poly-histidines or poly-lysines. Arg7 and Arg9 are the peptides that have been the most widely used for both *in vitro* transfer of peptides and *in vivo* transfer of proteins.

Structurally, amphipathic peptides can be divided into two groups, the so-called primary and secondary amphipathic CPPs. Examples of primary amphipathic peptides include those derived from signal peptides, fusion peptides found in the MPG family and Trp-rich sequences of the Pep family, which consist of amphipathic peptides [65]. Secondary amphipathic peptides are generated by the conformational state in which the hydrophobic and hydrophilic residues are on opposite sides of the molecule and the peptide usually adopts an α-helical structure. Examples include MAP, GALA, JTS-1, and KALA(GALA analog with some A→K mutations) peptides [65, 77]. These peptides adopt an α-helical structure under the acidic conditions of the endosome exposing hydrophobic and hydrophilic faces that can interact with the endosomal membrane to cause pore formation and disruption [65, 77]. The 30 amino acid peptide GALA is an amphipathic peptide that transitions from random coil to α-helical structure as the pH is lowered from 7.6 to 5.0 [78]. It has repeating units of glutamic acid-alanine-leucine-alanine (GALA) that give it its amphipathic character. At physiological pH, the glutamic acid residues exhibit charge repulsion, which is neutralized as the pH is lowered allowing it to adopt the α-helix structure [78–80].

A novel amphipathic peptide, JTS-1, developed by Gottschalk and coworkers, forms an α–helix dominated by strong nonpolar amino acids on the hydrophobic face and glutamic acid residues on the opposite hydrophilic face. It lysed both phosphatidylcholine liposomes and erythrocytes at pH 5, and showed an 8-fold higher hemolysis activity than INF-7 [81]. As with GALA, JTS-1 is negatively charged at neutral pH and is unable to bind the phosphate backbone of DNA. To overcome this problem, all glutamic acid residues of JTS-1 were substituted with either lysine or arginine resulting in the 2 peptides ppTG1 and ppTG20, respectively. Both peptides retained an α-helical conformation along with membrane lytic activity and also were able to compact DNA [82]. It was suggested that cationic fusogenic peptides are optimal for *in vitro* experiments as they are able to condense DNA for transfection. However, anionic fusogenic peptides are preferred *in vivo* because of their greater activity at lower pH than their cationic counterparts, which is necessary in the endosomal environment for more efficient gene delivery [83].

5.4.1 Plasma Membrane Translocation

One of the major obstacles to drug delivery is the difficulty with which active hydrophilic compounds pass through the lipid membrane of cells.

For example, although the cellular uptake of oligonucleotides is very low, it is significantly increased by coupling the antisense oligonucleotide or siRNA to a CPP. Witkowska et al. [84] have characterized several groups of cell-penetrating peptides from published and designed sequences representing a variety of chemical properties for siRNA delivery *in vitro* as well as *in vivo*. Results indicate that CPPs show promise as siRNA delivery agents and, importantly, appear to have low toxicity, particularly compared with cationic lipid based formulations. The 9 L/LacZ cell line and primary cell lines were used to evaluate cellular uptake of the CPPs as determined by fluorescence microscopy, while siRNA knockdown activity was determined by β-galactosidase activity assays as well as endogeneous gene knockdown. eGFP and human TNF-α (hTNF-α) transgenic mouse models were used to evaluate tissue distribution as well as knockdown activities resulting from CPP-mediated delivery of siRNA *in vivo*. They also discovered a peptide, designated PN73, which can deliver siRNA into a variety of cells with almost 100% uptake efficiency. These studies identified the optimal sequences for efficiently delivering siRNA into cells.

Morris et al. [73] described an oligonucleotide delivery system based on the use of a short peptide called MPG. MPG peptide contains a hydrophobic domain, which is derived from HIV gp41 and has a membrane fusion property, as well as a cationic NLS of SV40 T antigen, which appears to mediate nucleic acid interaction. The peptide forms stable "nanoparticles" with siRNA through non-covalent interactions and protects siRNA from degradation. MPG has been reported to deliver siRNA efficiently into a wide variety of mammalian cell lines through a process independent of an endosomal pathway, which enables rapid release of the siRNA into the cytoplasm and promotes robust down regulation of target mRNA. However, this finding appears to be contradicted by later work (described below). MPG has been used for the delivery of siRNA targeting Cyclin B1 into cancer cell lines and a tumor mouse model [85].

Most studies suggest that the positively charged amino acids within the peptide sequence play an important functional role in the activity of cell-penetrating properties [68, 86, 87]. Other studies have further highlighted the importance of arginines over lysines in delivery of peptides and oligonucleotides (M. Houston and P. H. Johnson, 2005, unpublished results) [87]. In particular, the guanidinium group of arginine is pivotal for efficient uptake [76]. A key issue for further study is the extent to which the peptide's membrane translocation activity is compromised when the required cationic residues bind the cargo and are less available for specific cell surface/membrane head group interactions that are necessary for membrane/endocytic transport.

Using Tat as a model CPP, it was shown that initial cell surface binding is to heparin sulfate (HS) proteoglycans; increasing heparin concentration competitively inhibits Tat internalization by binding to the positively charged Tat [88–91]. Consistent with these observations, Tyagi et al. [92] showed that glycosaminoglycan lyases that selectively degrade HS proteoglycans on the cell surface inhibit CPP uptake. They also found that cells genetically impaired in the biosynthesis of fully sulfated proteoglycans were selectively impaired for transduction by a Tat fusion protein (Tat- GFP), suggesting that the interaction of cationic CPPs with cell surface proteoglycans is likely to be the first step mediating cell uptake.

Small molecule hydrophobic drugs can enter cells through a variety of mechanisms, generally characterized as passive diffusion and energy independent. However, most evidence indicates that macromolecules are transported into the cell by endocytosis, a temperature- and energy-dependent process. The mechanism by which CPPs specifically enter cells is not well understood, and the process may differ among peptides. In general, cells rapidly internalize most CPPs in an energy-dependent manner by an endocytic process, but their uptake is unaffected by most inhibitors of classical endocytic pathways (e.g., clathrin and caveloae dependent) (D. Frank and P. H. Johnson 2007, unpublished observations). It appears that the process is not generally mediated by receptors because internalization is also observed by their D-isomers [66, 87, 93, 94]. These data suggest that many CPPs enter cells through a nonclassical endocytic pathway(s). Recently published data suggest that some CPPs enter cells by fluid macropinocytosis, a specialized form of endocytosis that is independent of caveolin, clathrin, and dynamin [95, 96]. Consequently, it appears that some peptides may use a distinct mechanism of translocation or that they have the ability to enter the cells through alternative pathways [97]. Such a pathway has been suggested for penetratin, which is proposed to enter by translocation across the lipid bilayer [96]. Not only does the ability of CPPs to interact with membrane lipids affect the uptake pathway, the endocytosis pathway can also be changed when CPPs are carrying a cargo [95, 97–100]. In another report, it was suggested that MPG and MPG/cargo complexes interact with negatively charged glycosaminoglycans and trigger specific activation of Rac1 GTPase, which is associated with the remodeling of the actin network. This constitutes the "onset" of cellular uptake, wherein increased membrane fluidity promotes entry of MPG or MPG/DNA complexes into the cell. It was also suggested that binding glycosaminoglycans might be a common step for all CPPs, although cell entry of CPPs can follow different pathways [101].

5.4.2 Mechanisms

Early studies appeared to indicate that the internalization of CPPs was not significantly inhibited by incubation at 4°C, depletion of intracellular ATP, or several different inhibitors of endocytosis. Also, cell internalization did not depend on a specific primary sequence, implying that receptor recognition was not involved [66, 68, 94]. Therefore, it was commonly accepted that CPP internalization was neither by endocytosis nor receptor-mediated nor due to a specific transporter. However, subsequent mechanistic studies have shown that both the internalization and nuclear translocation of cell penetratin-containing proteins occurred as an artifact of fixation and should have been evaluated in living cells. The methanol fixation process utilized in these studies induced an artificial influx of both VP22 protein from the herpes Simplex virus and positively charged histone H1 [102, 103]. Several possible mechanisms have been proposed for membrane translocation and the internalization of CPPs. It is likely that the mechanism of entry may be affected by the presence and type of cargo as well as the mode of association, that is, conjugation or complex formation.

In the Carpet Model [104], an example of direct penetration, the positively charged domains of the peptide interact with the negatively charged cell surface, resulting in the disruption of the cell membrane and allowing peptide internalization. The Pore Formation Model [105] also involves direct penetration, but is based on interactions between amphipathic, α-helical peptides and the membrane. The helical peptides lay parallel to the cell membrane and induce a local thinning, resulting in formation of a cylindrical pore structure surrounded by proteins in the lipid bilayer. This is the proposed mechanism of uptake of the antimicrobial peptide melittin. The Inverted Micelle Model [66] was suggested for the cell uptake of penetratin. In this model, penetratin dimer interacts with the negatively charged phospholipids in the plasma membrane. The subsequent interaction of tryptophans in the peptide with the hydrophobic membrane induces invagination in the plasma membrane. The reorganization of the neighboring lipids results in formation of an inverted micelle, and the peptide and cargo are released upon micelle disruption. Thoren et al. [106] have shown that arginine mutation or substitution completely blocks translocation of penetratin. This mechanism may explain the translocation of some amphipathic peptides, while peptides with no hydrophobic amino acids might be taken up through other mechanisms. Recent work, however, has cast doubt on these models as the singular explanation for transmembrane transport of CPPs and their cargos.

Nakase et al. [98] have carried out further investigation of the mechanism of cellular uptake of arginine-rich CPPs and have demonstrated that membrane-associated proteoglycans are indispensable for the induction of the actin organization and macropinocytic uptake. For example, cellular uptake of the Tat peptide is highly dependent on heparan sulfate proteoglycan (HSPG), whereas uptake of the R8 peptide (octaarginine) is less dependent on HSPG. Their studies suggest that the structure of the peptides may determine the specificity for HSPG, and that HSPG is not the sole receptor for macropinocytosis. Comparison of the HSPG specificity of the branched-chain arginine-rich peptides in cellular uptake has suggested that the charge density of the peptides may determine their specificity. The activation of the Rac protein and organization of the actin cytoskeleton were observed within a few minutes after the peptide treatment. These data strongly suggest the possibility that the interaction of the arginine-rich peptides with the membrane-associated proteoglycans quickly activates intracellular signaling and induces actin organization and macropinocytosis.

Structurally, the interaction between a CPP and its nucleic acid cargo takes place primarily between the negatively charged phosphate groups and the positively charged amino acid residues [73]. Such a mechanism, involving electrostatic interactions has been previously suggested for poly-L-lysine- or lysine-rich peptide-mediated oligonucleotide transfection techniques [107, 108]. The importance of polycationic properties in CPPs as they relate to cargo delivery has been highlighted in many studies. The importance of arginine over lysine is suggested from the studies of Wender et al. [87]. In particular, the guanidinium group of arginine seems pivotal for efficient uptake [76]. However, this does not explain the effective uptake demonstrated for KALA and other CPPs lacking arginines in their sequences. Interestingly, changing naturally occurring L-amino acids to D-amino acids in various peptide sequences does not alter the uptake efficiency [66, 87, 93, 94]. But in the case of polyarginines, it increases internalization [76, 87]. No unambiguous definition of CPPs has been proposed, but experiments using D-amino acids indicate that CPPs are not dependent on a chiral receptor for internalization in contrast to ordinary peptide ligands. It suggests that particular residues in a specific CPP sequence may also play an important role in determining the efficacy of CPP as a delivery vector.

5.4.3 CPPs as Delivery Vehicles

Although Tat peptide has shown good cellular uptake, recent results indicate that adding a signal sequence or hydrophobic peptide sequence with membrane crossing activity increases cellular uptake and also enhances endosome release activity (M. Houston and P. H. Johnson, 2006, unpublished results). The same principle may also apply to both penetratin and transportan, for which addition of a hydrophobic region may enhance membrane-penetrating activity. In summary, the ratio of cationic and hydrophobic sequences significantly affects cellular uptake, and in some cases, the strong hydrophobicity in a CPP sequence may decrease the membrane crossing activity because of the affinity of the CPP for the membrane.

CPPs have been utilized for effective delivery of a variety of macromolecules including antisense [73], siRNA [109–113], and proteins [114] by either forming a complex or by covalent conjugation.

Cationic PTDs were shown to enter cells by macropinocytosis [95, 96,98]. Magzoub et al. [115] have studied the mechanism(s) by which CPPs are able to escape from endosomes and macropinosomes and enter the cytosol. Large unilamellar phospholipid vesicles encapsulating different CPPs and an ionophore were produced to create a transmembrane pH gradient (with an acidic interior) similar to the one arising in endosomes *in vivo*. The results indicate different escape mechanisms for different CPPs, which are dependent on acidification of the vesicle interior but do not require lysis of the vesicles. Either heparin sulfate binding or coupling to a cargo inhibited escape.

Most evidence indicates that CPPs enter cells through an endocytic mechanism, perhaps most effectively by macropinocytosis. When the CPP is attached to a cargo, internalization can be affected, particularly, if CPP residues are involved in binding cargo and not free to interact with the cell surface/membrane polar head groups (M. Houston and P. H. Johnson, 2005, unpublished observations). Both macropinosomes and other endosomal structures become acidified through an ATP-dependent proton pump, and the ability of the delivery complex to buffer this pH change may be critical for cargo (e.g., siRNA) release. In an effort to mimic the proton sponge activity similar to PEI [116], histidine has been added to peptide sequences to facilitate release. The imidazole group of histidine has a pK_a of ~6.0, therefore, allowing it to become protonated in acidic environments. At physiological pH, the histidines will remain neutrally charged, thereby imparting selective membrane disruption in the acidic endosome [117–120]. Histidine residues have been incorporated into polylysine and shorter oligolysine peptides or other CPPs to modify their endosome release activities.

Conjugations between CPPs and the delivery cargo have been utilized to increase their cellular uptake. Unlike oligonucleotide complexes with cationic lipids or polymers, peptide–oligonucleotide conjugates are of relatively modest molecular size. Therefore, they are more likely to evade uptake by phagocytosis from the reticuloendothelial system (RES). Successful delivery of antisense-oligonucleotides *in vivo* using CPPs was first shown using a PNA complementary to human galanin receptor 1 (GalR1) mRNA coupled to transportan and penetratin, which resulted in downregulation of these receptors in rat brains [69]. Kilk et al. [121] found new PNA sequences that, when coupled to transportan, resulted in 20-fold higher antisense effects on GalR1 mRNA *in vitro*.

Several commonly used CPPs have demonstrated some cellular toxicity. Neurotoxic effects of Tat peptide were described by Nath et al. [122].

The length of Tat-derived peptides appeared to be important in mediating neurotoxicity, as Tat(31–61) produced significantly higher levels of toxicity than full-length Tat protein. Elongating Tat(31–61) by 10 amino acids to Tat(31–71) decreased the degree of neurotoxicity. Another CPP, penetratin, caused neurotoxic cell death upon 10-μg intrastriatal injection [123]. Drin et al. [87] reported that penetratin starts to induce cell lysis at a concentration of 40 μM. The polycationic CPP, poly-Arginine, induces cell membrane damage resulting in increased permeability and loss of cell–cell contacts in epithelial cells *in vitro* [124].

While studies of CPPs generally indicate cell uptake mechanisms involving endocytic pathways, the mechanism(s) of lipid based drug delivery systems may be different. In studies of standard cationic lipid transfection agents such as lipofectamine, the major route of functional siRNA delivery appears to be by simple fusion, independent of clathrin, caveolin, ATP, and macropinocytosis, but dependent on cholesterol and temperature (J. Lu and J. Chen, 2007, personal communication). The inherent membrane disrupting properties of some types of lipids may account for the higher level of toxicity of liposomal formulations compared with some peptide-based delivery systems.

5.5   TARGETING SPECIFIC CELL TYPES

Successful targeted delivery of siRNA *in vivo* must effectively address three general barriers: junctional barriers of the target tissue, the lipid bilayer membrane of the targeted cell, and the intracellular barriers that separate subcellular compartments and may prevent access to the RNAi machinery (e.g., endosomal trapping). Additional obstacles include competitive binding to circulating macromolecules and nontarget cells, uptake by phagocytic cells, rapid clearance from the circulation by renal excretion, and degradation by nucleases. *In vitro* targeting studies do not represent a realistic evaluation of all the barriers that exist *in vivo* affecting site-specific delivery, although cultured primary cells may be very similar to the corresponding cell type found *in vivo*. Thus, while *in vitro* uptake and knockdown studies are important (particularly using primary cultured cells where possible), screening and optimization of potential delivery agents and formulations must emphasize *in vivo* systems.

5.5.1   Targeting Mechanisms

A variety of ligand-modified complexes have been used to target nucleic acids to cells successfully [125]. For example, mannose receptors on macrophages can be targeted by mannose as a ligand [126], asialoglycoproteins on hepatocytes are targeted by galactoses [127–129], and transferrin receptors and folate receptors on cancer cells are targeted by transferrin and folate, respectively [130, 48].

It is possible that effective cell-specific delivery strategies may involve targeting receptors. A systemic method to deliver siRNAs to specific cells via cell-surface receptors would, in principle, provide a means to introduce siRNAs into desired cell types, decrease the amount of drug required, and avoid nonspecific silencing and toxicity in nontargeted cells, thus achieving maximal therapeutic benefit. There is precedent for this approach, as exemplified by the use of immunoliposomes with an antibody as a targeting ligand-carrying drug within a lipid vesicle [131].

However, the types of receptor(s) desirable for targeting and their specificity for the target cell/tissue type of interest remain key issues in using receptors to target specific cell types. Many types of ligand–receptor complexes cluster in cell-surface clathrin-coated pits, which are internalized to become clathrin-coated endosomes with two possible fates. The receptor may undergo recycling to the plasma membrane or progress to late stage endosomes and finally to primary lysosomes where the receptor and ligand are degraded. Under most circumstances, the degradation route is kinetically favored. For example, the ErbB-1 receptor is rapidly internalized following ligand binding [132, 133], a process requiring receptor tyrosine kinase activity and ubiquitination [26], while other ErbB receptors are endocytosis impaired or exhibit only a very slow endocytic internalization rate. The cytoplasmic domain of the receptor determines whether or not a given ErbB receptor will be rapidly internalized by clathrin-coated pits. Endocytosis may serve a desensitization function by removing the receptor from the plasma membrane leading to degradation and/or facilitate positive signaling during endocytosis, whereby some intracellular signaling pathway(s) is activated. While the clathrin endocytic pathway has been best characterized for its involvement in receptor internalization, it is clear that other pathways such as the caveolar pathway may also be involved for some receptors. In addition, although they have not yet been identified, endocytic pathways have been inferred from internalization processes that are energy and temperature dependent, but are not affected by inhibitors of known pathways [86].

Although CPPs (e.g., penetratin and transportin) are not cell-specific targeting agents, they have been coupled to siRNA to facilitate siRNA intracellular uptake. Use of a reducible disulfide linker permits release of the conjugated peptide, liberating the siRNA in the cytoplasm [112]. Given the likelihood that CPPs can be taken up by an endocytic mechanism (e.g., macropinocytosis) that is not cell type-specific, incorporation of targeting peptides or other ligands into a CPP sequence may facilitate site-specific binding and uptake.

Recently, carbon nanotubes have been shown to traverse cellular membranes by endocytosis, leading to internalization of biological molecules, including DNA, siRNA, and proteins, into immortalized cancer cells. Liu et al. [134] have shown that functionalized single-walled nanotubes (SWNT) can be used as molecular transporters to shuttle short interfering RNA (siRNA) into human T cells and primary cells and to silence the expression of HIV-specific cell-surface receptors and coreceptors. This silencing effect, known to block HIV viral entry and reduce infection, is reported to be superior to that observed with conventional liposome-based nonviral delivery agents. Carbon nanotubes in as-made forms are highly hydrophobic. The authors suggest that SWNTs functionalized with PEG2000 retain a degree of hydrophobicity (because of incomplete coverage of PL-PEG on the tubes), which promotes their binding and association with cells through hydrophobic interactions with nonpolar domains on cell membranes. Again, an increase in cell-specific targeting using this delivery approach will necessitate incorporation of a targeting ligand.

A delivery system consisting completely of RNA was proposed by Guo et al. [135, 136] based on the packaging RNA of the DNA-packaging motor of bacteriophage phi29, which can spontaneously form dimers via interlocking right- and left-hand loops. Attachment of the siRNA to one loop and an RNA aptamer to CD4 to the other loop enabled the development of a cancer cell-targeted system that could silence survivin gene expression *in vitro*. Alternatively, the system also could be targeted by folate.

Schifflelers et al. [137, 138] focused on the cationic polymer PEI coupled to polyethyleneglycol (PEG) as a shielding polymer. The cyclic RGD peptide is a high-affinity ligand for alpha v-integrins that are over expressed on angiogenic endothelial surfaces. This peptide was coupled to the distal end of the PEG-chain and the resulting formulation was effective at directing siRNA uptake to tumor neovasculature.

The iron-binding protein transferrin has been used to target colloids composed of siRNA and cyclodextrin-containing polycations to transferrin receptor-expressing tumor cells [139]. A method to specifically deliver anti-ews-fli1 siRNAs to transferrin receptor-expressing tumors in mice using a cyclodextrin-containing polycation that contains transferrin as a targeting ligand resulted in effective knockdown of target mRNA.

Tissue-specific delivery of siRNAs has been achieved using fusions between protamine and antibodies. In this system, siRNAs were bound by the basic protamine and then targeted to tumor cells via antibodies. In one example, fusion of siRNA to an anti-ERbB2-specific single-chain antibody resulted in targeting of tumor cells expressing the epidermal growth factor receptor ERbB2 [20]. Antibodies that bind cell type-specific cell-surface receptors were fused to protamine and used to deliver siRNAs to cells via endocytosis, resulting in knockdown of target mRNA *in vivo* at a dose of 2 mg/kg in mice.

Peer et al. [19] showed that mixing siRNAs with human integrin LFA-1 (lymphocyte function-associated antigen-1) single-chain antibodies fused to a protamine fragment could specifically deliver siRNAs to, and induce silencing in, primary lymphocytes, monocytes, and dendritic cells, which typically are resistant to lipid-based transfection *in vitro* and are difficult to target *in vivo*. In addition, a fusion protein constructed from an antibody that recognizes activation-dependent conformational changes in LFA-1 was shown to target only activated leukocytes and could be used to suppress gene expression and cell proliferation of activated lymphocytes selectively.

Kumar et al. [23] have demonstrated that a short peptide derived from the rabies virus glycoprotein (RVG) can provide a tool for transvascular delivery of siRNA to the central nervous system. They found that a 29-amino acid RVG peptide specifically binds neuronal cells, including primary neuronal cells, via interaction with the acetylcholine receptor. Moreover, a biotinylated RVG peptide could be localized in brain cells after intravenous (*iv*) administration in mice, suggesting that this peptide can cross the blood brain barrier (BBB), likely by receptor-mediated transcytosis. A chimeric RVG peptide was fused to a positively charged nonamer polyarginine peptide (9R) to enable siRNA binding. The RVG-9R peptide was able to bind siRNA by charge interaction and to transport it selectively into neuronal cells *in vitro* resulting in efficient silencing of a reporter gene.

5.5.2 High-Throughput Screening Systems

While targeting specific receptors may be an effective approach for delivering therapeutic siRNAs, identifying the best receptors for a given application may be laborious and problematical due to the potential for inappropriate receptor activation and undesirable signal transduction. Molecular libraries offer an important approach for identifying delivery agents capable of cell type-specific targeting of siRNAs that may avoid these problems. These libraries can be used to screen specific cells or tissues (either *in vitro* and/or *in vivo*) for selective binding, internalization, and transport of siRNA molecules into the cell so as to permit potent knockdown activity. Recent studies have used two types of high-complexity molecular libraries to select and identify potential siRNA targeting ligands for delivery. The first involves the use of RNA aptamers composed of 25–60 base oligonucleotide libraries. A number of functional RNA aptamers have been selected against a wide range of targets, both protein and nonprotein, through SELEX (systematic evolution of ligands by exponential enrichment) [140, 141]. A second approach for discovering cell-specific drug targeting agents is the use of combinatorial peptide libraries. Phage display technology has been widely used for the screening of such libraries for various drug discovery initiatives [142]. Structurally constrained small proteins or peptide structural motifs can be selected with specific binding/internalization properties suitable for drug delivery.

Both approaches share a common strategy for selecting target-specific ligands that does not require knowledge of specific receptor biology. Cells/tissue of interest are incubated with the molecular library under conditions of defined stringency (to minimize nonspecific binding). After washing at a defined stringency, the binding fraction is recovered, or to select for an internalized molecule, the cells are lysed and the cytoplasmic fraction is recovered. Following amplification of the selected fraction, the process is repeated 3–5 times. The final selected and amplified fraction is typically cloned and subjected to sequencing in order to identify the structure of the oligonucleotide or protein delivery candidate. The potential delivery molecule can be fluorescently labeled and used in cell assays to evaluate uptake properties and intracellular localization, and/or conjugated to an siRNA and evaluated for cell uptake and knockdown activity. Candidates with good knockdown activities can be structurally optimized further to maximize kinetics, stability, and activity properties. The key advantage of both approaches over targeting selected receptors is that the two most important properties of the delivery agent—efficient internalization and mRNA knockdown—are selected for directly.

Aptamers   Aptamers are oligonucleotides that are selected to bind specific targets with high affinity and specificity. They are developed using SELEX to recognize specifically and tightly bind their cognate targets by means of well-defined complementary three-dimensional structures. SELEX is an iterative *in vitro* selection process that starts with a combinatorial library of sequences and consists of two sequential steps (selection and amplification) that can efficiently reduce a complex library of nucleic acids with randomized sequences (complexity 10^{10-14}) to a minimized subset of one or more sequences that bind tightly to the target of choice. Typically, dissociation constants (K_d) for these aptamer–target complexes are in the high picomolar to low nanomolar range. Aptamer libraries can be synthesized chemically, and thus, are attractive reagents for use in therapeutic and delivery applications [143, 144]. Owing to their stability and low toxicity, aptamers targeting surface antigens as well as whole cells have previously been identified as attractive alternatives to antibody and lipid-based delivery formulations.

Aptamer-siRNA chimeras present several advantages for *in vivo* applications. Aptamers and siRNAs have low immunogenicity, can be synthesized in large quantities, and are amenable to a variety of chemical modifications that confer both resistance to degradation and improved pharmacokinetics *in vivo*. Chemically synthesized RNA is amenable to various modifications, such as PEGylation, that can be used to modify its *in vivo* half-life and bioavailability; however, such modifications need to be tested to determine whether they interfere with mechanisms such as uptake and processing by Dicer (described in Section 5.5.3). The smaller size of aptamers compared with that of antibodies (15 vs. 150 kDa) facilitates their *in vivo* delivery by promoting better tissue penetration. In contrast, antibody reagent production in cell culture is considerably more complex and difficult to control. An additional, notable advantage of the chimera over alternative approaches is its simplicity. Like siRNAs, the chimera consists only of RNA, and any nonspecific side effects may, therefore, be limited to those already produced by the siRNAs themselves. As RNA is believed to be less immunogenic than protein, the chimeric RNAs would also be expected to produce less nonspecific activation of the immune system than protein-mediated delivery approaches. However, it remains to be determined whether these chimeric RNAs have an increased potential for inducing an interferon (IFN) response [145]. Two examples of successful use of this approach to deliver siRNA have been reported recently.

McNamara et al. [22] developed aptamer-siRNA chimeras capable of cell type-specific binding and delivery of functional siRNAs into cells. The aptamer portion of the chimeras mediated binding to prostate-specific membrane antigen (PSMA), a cell-surface receptor that is overexpressed in prostate cancer cells and tumor vascular endothelium, whereas the siRNA portion targeted the expression of survival genes. When applied to cells expressing PSMA, these RNAs were internalized and processed by Dicer, resulting in depletion of the siRNA target proteins and cell death. In contrast, the chimeras did not bind to or function in cells that did not express PSMA. These constructs also specifically inhibited tumor growth and mediated tumor regression in a xenograft model of prostate cancer. In a similar study, Chu et al. [21] also developed an aptamer targeting the PMSA antigen, which was coupled to siRNAs via a modular streptavidin bridge. The resulting conjugates could be simply added onto cells without any further preparation, and were taken up within 30 min. In this study, the siRNA-mediated inhibition of gene expression was as efficient as that observed with conventional lipid-based reagents, and was dependent upon conjugation to the aptamer.

Phage Display   Since its development [146], phage display technology has been widely used for the screening of random combinatorial peptide libraries for drug discovery [142]. Peptides displayed as unconstrained linear molecules can adopt numerous conformations; very few of which may represent stable structures. Panning with these unconstrained peptides against targets of interest usually leads to the isolation of peptides with low binding

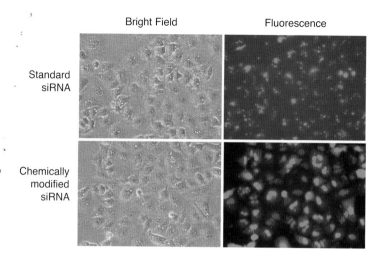

Bright Field   Fluorescence

Standard
siRNA

Chemically
modified
siRNA

Plate 1

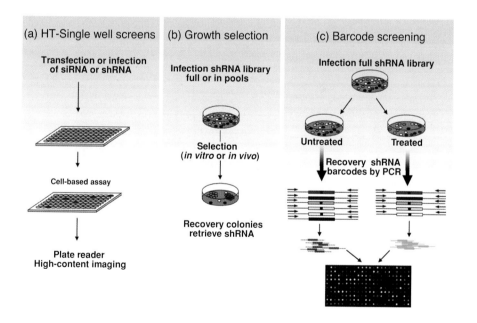

(a) HT-Single well screens

**Transfection or infection
of siRNA or shRNA**

↓

Cell-based assay

↓

**Plate reader
High-content imaging**

(b) Growth selection

**Infection shRNA library
full or in pools**

↓

Selection
(*in vitro* or *in vivo*)

↓

**Recovery colonies
retrieve shRNA**

(c) Barcode screening

Infection full shRNA library

Untreated   Treated

**Recovery shRNA
barcodes by PCR**

Plate 2

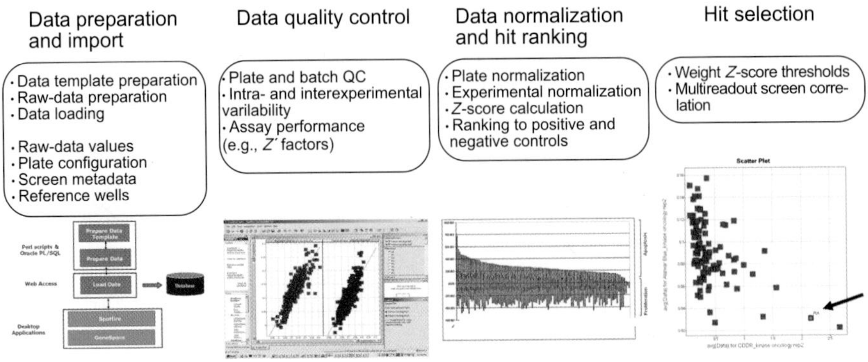

Data preparation and import
· Data template preparation
· Raw-data preparation
· Data loading
· Raw-data values
· Plate configuration
· Screen metadata
· Reference wells
Data quality control
· Plate and batch QC
· Intra- and interexperimental varilability
· Assay performance (e.g., Z′ factors)
Data normalization and hit ranking
· Plate normalization
· Experimental normalization
· Z-score calculation
· Ranking to positive and negative controls
Hit selection
· Weight Z-score thresholds
· Multireadout screen correlation
Scatter Plot

Plate 3

(a)
TJ
AJ
Des
(b)
(c)

Plate 4

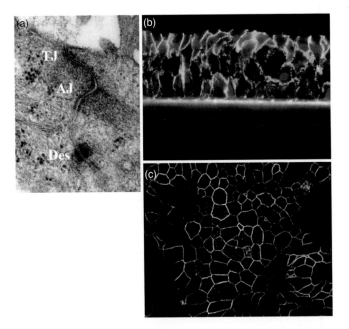

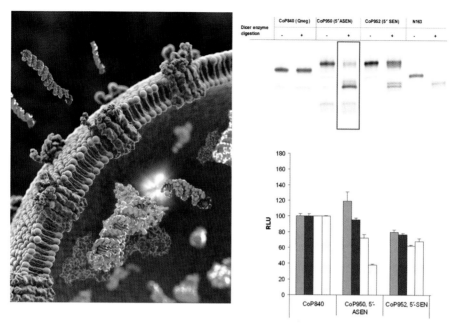

Plate 5

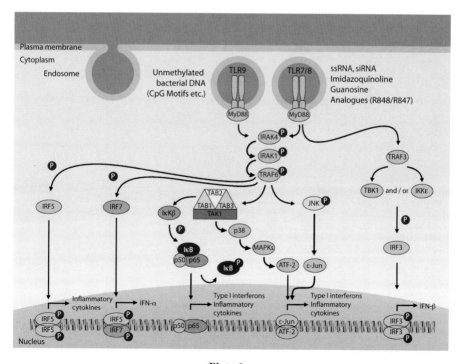

Plate 6

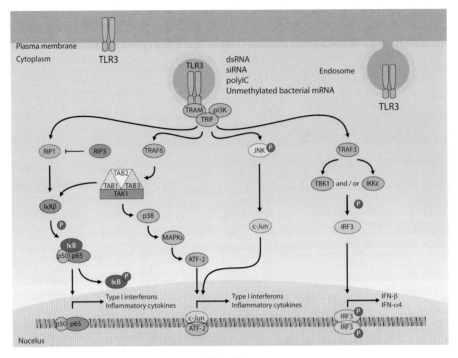

Plate 7

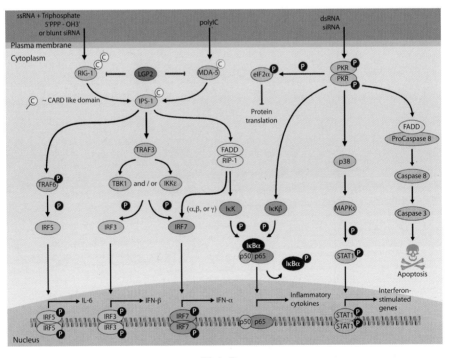

Plate 8

affinity. Reducing the conformational freedom of the displayed peptides is necessary to decrease entropy and increase the binding affinity [147, 148]. Constrained libraries have often achieved a reduction in conformational freedom by incorporating a pair of cysteine residues at both ends of linear peptides. This results in disulfide bridges that form peptide loops, yielding cyclic peptide libraries that have been reported to increase binding affinity [149] and stability in biological fluids [150]. The use of defined protein scaffolds for the generation of random libraries has the potential to increase binding affinity further by providing a more rigid conformation [151]. Examples of folded protein scaffolds that have been used for peptide display include the zinc finger motif, which has been used to construct a degenerate library for the isolation of peptides that bind to DNA and RNA [152, 153], and Kunitz domains, which have been used as a scaffold for libraries designed for the discovery of improved serine protease inhibitors [154].

Herman et al. [155] developed a new peptide library technology based on a 20 amino acid Trp cage miniprotein, with multiple variable positions, displayed on bacteriophage T7. They demonstrated that the library could be used to identify peptides that bind to specific cell types and that may be suitable for the delivery of therapeutic siRNAs. The Trp cage is a hydrophobic cluster with Trp-25 buried in a central location where it is shielded from solvent exposure. The residues that form the cage around Trp-25 include multiple proline residues (Pro-31, 36–38) that are oriented so that the proline rings are located on both faces of the indole ring of Trp 25, as well as a Phe side chain that completes the hydrophobic cluster [156, 157]. The optimized Trp cage miniprotein TC5b (NLYIQWLKDGGPSSGRPPPS) has been extensively studied because it is an ultra fast, cooperatively folding system [158]. Within the optimized Trp cage sequence, there are several positions where the substitution of amino acids does not compromise folding of the miniprotein. Some of those positions are solvent exposed, making them ideal for the display of random amino acids in a highly diverse library. Utility of the library was demonstrated by identification of specific binding ligands including AAADPYAQWLQSMGPHSGRPPPR, which bound to human bronchial epithelial cells. A high complexity library based on the Trp cage miniprotein has demonstrated potential for identifying novel cell- and protein-binding peptides that could be used for the delivery of therapeutic molecules or as target-specific therapeutic agents.

5.5.3 Dicer Substrate Conjugates

The affinity of delivery agents that bind siRNAs noncovalently must not be so strong that they inhibit RNAi activity. Conjugation of macromolecular targeting agents to siRNAs can result in inhibition due to effects on RISC.

One solution to this problem is to conjugate the delivery moiety to an extended form of the siRNA that can be processed intracellularly by the enzyme Dicer and effectively loaded into the RISC.

Witkowska et al. [84] have described methods for synthesis and conjugation of peptides to siRNA. Peptides can be efficiently synthesized by

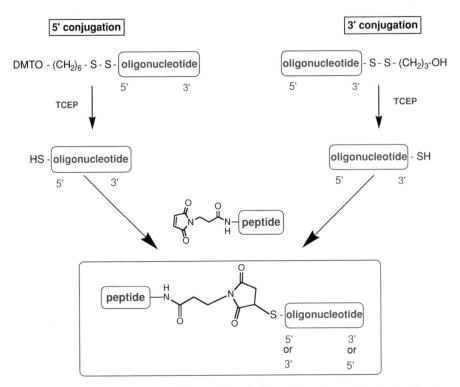

FIGURE 5.3 Methods for Synthesis of 5′ and 3′ siRNA-Peptide Conjugates. For conjugation, the N-termini of the peptides are functionalized with 3-maleimidopropionic acid while the 5′ siRNA sense or antisense strands are modified with a 1-O-dimethoxytrityl-hexyl-disulfide linker. Peptides are then conjugated to the 5′ end of the siRNA sense or antisense strands via a thioether bond. The thiol is liberated by reduction of the disulfide bond of the 5′-linker of the oligonucleotide using aqueous TCEP hydrochloride [tri(2-carboxyethyl)phosphine hydrochloride] and reacted with the maleimide groups attached to the N-termini of the peptides. Conjugates are synthesized under high denaturing conditions (50% formamide) to prevent aggregation and precipitation and then purified by ion exchange chromatography (IEX). Products are analyzed by liquid chromatography coupled with electrospray ionization mass spectrometry (LC-MS) using hexafluoroisopropanol/triethylamine as ion pairing agents and methanol as the organic modifier at 65°C. Single stranded conjugates are annealed to the antisense strands by heating to 90°C for 3 minutes followed by gradual cooling to ambient temperature over 1 hour.

the solid phase methods using standard Fmoc chemistry and conjugated to duplex RNA as described in Figure 5.3.

The enzyme Dicer, involved in the natural processing of long duplex RNA molecules to siRNAs, helps to load siRNAs into RISC. Synthetic Dicer substrates, at a size of 25–30 nucleotide pairs, can be significantly more effective at silencing genes at lower dose compared with many first generation siRNAs [159, 160]. A major potential therapeutic advantage in using Dicer substrates for delivery is that targeting and uptake functions can be covalently attached to the RNA; Dicer processing inside the cell removes potential inhibitory effects of the delivery agent on RISC. Figure 5.4 shows that conjugation of a 30-residue peptide to the 5'-end of the sense strand of an siRNA leads to inefficient Dicer-mediated cleavage of a 27-mer extended siRNA compared with a nonconjugated control, and the siRNA is not active. However, a peptide conjugate formed at the 5'-end of the antisense strand is efficiently cleaved by Dicer to produce an active siRNA.

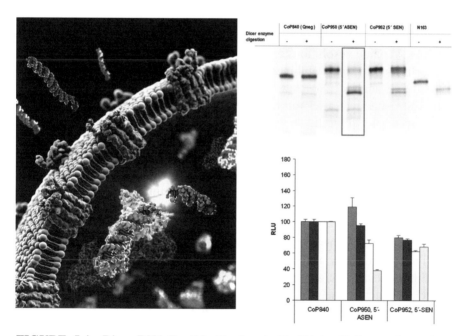

FIGURE 5.4   Dicer RNA-Peptide Conjugate Facilitates Delivery. A covalent conjugate consisting of a peptide (purple) and a 27 base pair duplex RNA (green) that targets a specific cell-surface receptor (purple), is transported into the cell and binds to the Dicer enzyme (orange), which cleaves the RNA to the correct size (~21 base pairs) for RNA interference. Drawn to molecular scale based on the crystal structure of Dicer [187] and the NMR structure of the Trp-Cage miniprotein [156,157].

5.6   FORMULATION DISCOVERY AND DEVELOPMENT

5.6.1   General Screening Strategies and Analysis Methods

The challenge with any formulation screening effort is understanding the *in vitro/in vivo* correlations for the models used. It is important to recognize that a testing paradigm that screens for activity of a formulation relative to the performance of a transfection reagent may not always provide a relevant benchmark for comparison. This is especially true when evaluating different classes of reagents for activity, such as peptides or polymers compared with lipids. Screening models usually involve *in vitro* cell-based assays. While the ability to screen for properties indicative of cellular internalization is important, such screening may not lead to a definitive answer regarding actually efficacy. The ultimate measure is gene expression (protein) knockdown, but this is also subject to the caveats stated previously regarding correlation of *in vitro* and *in vivo* systems [161].

Screening for siRNA delivery agents is similar to small molecule discovery. It involves a combination of *in vitro* and *in vivo* testing strategies, with an iterative feedback loop for selection and optimization (Figure 5.5). The screening process begins with stocks of candidate delivery agents and siRNAs prepared in solutions or simple formulations of excipients and buffer. The solutions are then combined to achieve an appropriate N/P ratio (cationic nitrogen to anionic phosphate) or a range of N/P ratios for testing. The initial measurement after mixing is an evaluation of solubility and particle size. Generally, solubility may be determined by visual means with careful observation of particulates in the solution. Once the prototype screening formulations pass any solubility and particle size requirements, they are dosed onto cell-line models for determination of biological activity. The initial *in vitro* cell-line screens provide a preliminary estimate of activity and toxicity. Lead compounds identified by these analyses are then advanced to primary cell screens. These may be one or more cell types that are relevant to the intended *in vivo* therapeutic application. It is important to begin evaluating specific requirements, such as biological stability, as the progression of a lead candidate occurs. *In vivo* screening of primary cells provides a more effective model in which to identify and evaluate toxicities that are relevant to a particular cell type compared with immortalized cell lines. Taken together, the data from knockdown, toxicity, and stability studies can provide a roadmap for successful development. Incorporating the findings of these studies into subsequent iterations of the process should support continued progress toward a therapeutically viable formulation. The cycle can then be repeated to optimize further the selection and initial formulation screening of promising delivery candidates.

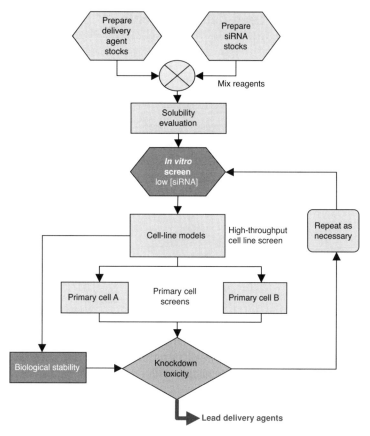

FIGURE 5.5 *In vitro* **Delivery Agent Screening**. An *in vitro* screening strategy consists of preparing formulations of the delivery agents with low concentrations (10 to 100 nM) of siRNA. The formulations are evaluated for solubility on the basis of particle size, which is kept below 200 nm. The knockdown activity and toxicity of formulations are initially tested in cell lines. In parallel, the biological stability in serum-based media is evaluated to determine the stability of the siRNA in the formulation. Formulations showing activity and low toxicity in the cell lines are then tested in primary cell lines relevant to the therapeutic application. The results define the activity of the delivery system, the cellular uptake properties of the formulation, and toxicity. Success criteria for these assays will depend on the cell and target gene and the screening agent being tested. Lead formulations meeting the activity criteria may be recycled through the screen, reformulated, and further optimized. Specific mechanistic questions and hypotheses may be postulated and tested. Candidate formulations meeting all assigned criteria will advance to *in vivo* testing.

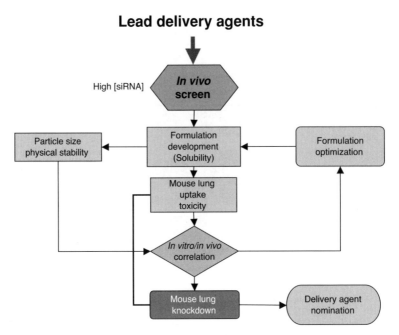

FIGURE 5.6 *In vivo* **Delivery Agent Screening**. Lead formulations identified in the *in vitro* screening operation are initially reformulated to meet the requirements of *in vivo* testing. A major factor that changes with this transition is the concentration required in *in vivo* studies. This is usually in the mg/kg dose level, which translates to several hundred ugs to mgs per mL concentrations. The initial formulation is then evaluated for its particle size and short-term physical stability. Dosing studies commence in parallel in a mouse model evaluating the uptake and toxicity in a localized tissue model, which in this example is lung. In parallel, the knockdown of a target gene is evaluated in the model. Both the uptake and knockdown data are used to derive potential correlations with the data obtained in the previously described *in vitro* screen. The formulation is optimized as necessary to provide the highest level of knockdown with the lowest toxicity.

The use of high-throughput *in vitro* testing schema can rapidly generate data needed to understand critical issues relevant to specific delivery agents, including, efficacy, toxicity, cost-of-goods (COGS), and intellectual property (IP). Subsequently, low-throughput *in vivo* delivery screening (Figure 5.6) is performed to evaluate a formulation's ability to knockdown the target mRNA in an animal model effectively, the toxicity of the delivery vehicle, tissue distribution, and pharmacokinetic properties. The *in vivo* screening paradigm begins with the candidates and formulations that result from the *in vitro* screens. The lead delivery agents need to be formulated for attributes different from those required for *in vitro* testing. This usually consists of higher concentrations of siRNA and better protection of the siRNA from nuclease degradation, as well as optimization of the delivery system to avoid complement activation and opsonization. Such alterations may include chemical modifications to the siRNA and the use of PEG to reduce immunogenicity and improve pharmacokinetic properties of the siRNA-delivery complex. Once an initial *in vivo* formulation is developed, it is important to determine its longer-term physical and chemical stability and its stability in biological fluids, so as to ensure that it has the basic properties necessary for clinical and commercial development. Initially, the formulation can be screened *via* multiple routes. Pulmonary delivery to airway epithelial cells is one route that offers an opportunity for direct delivery of siRNA formulations and also enables comparisons with naked siRNA. This system enables direct administration of siRNA to a tissue that already has been validated as a target for drug delivery. Moreover, direct administration to airway epithelia may avoid toxicity and instability that are likely to result from systemic administration. Comparing data from the initial *in vivo* screen with the *in vitro* data may identify correlations between the two methodologies that improve the understanding of specific formulation and screening issues. Several cycles of testing and reformulation should yield a formulation candidate suitable for further preclinical development. Further optimization of such candidates should in turn support the initiation of clinical testing with a formulation that has the greatest likelihood to demonstrate acceptable safety, tolerability, and efficacy profiles.

The extent to which the structure of the siRNA (including chemical modifications) affects its delivery properties using a given formulation is not well understood. Strategies for selection of an siRNA molecule usually begin with a bioinformatics-based selection of sequences using homology and thermodynamic criteria [162] including the 3'- and 5'-UTR (untranslated regions) [163] and results in selecting various 21-mer duplex RNAs against the target gene of interest. Other possible siRNA structures are blunt ended 19-mers, which have been shown to be efficacious despite some earlier concerns regarding IFN response [164]. In addition, it has been hypothesized that 25/27-mer Dicer substrates may be a more effective form of siRNA because they are believed to increase the efficiency of RISC incorporation [160]. Short hairpin siRNA structures can also be effective knockdown agents [165, 166].

Usually, cell lines are the first screening line, as they represent the most inexpensive and rapid means to grow cells quickly and screen activity rapidly. Delivery studies can be performed using commercial transfection reagents that are simple to use, can be formulated by mixing the siRNA at low concentration and are added directly to cells. An IC_{50} curve across several orders of magnitude, typically from 0.01 to 100 nM, is sufficient to accurately rank order the knockdown capability of the different candidate siRNAs [167]. The top three to five lead sequences identified on the basis of lowest IC_{50} can then be evaluated for uptake and knockdown in a primary cell culture model. Once candidate sequences have been tested using a reference cell line and transfection agent under single concentration conditions and lead compounds have been identified and optimized for stability by chemical modification, the preliminary *in vitro* evaluation of dose-dependent knockdown efficacy of the different sequences in various cell types is typically completed.

Transitioning to *in vivo* studies is challenging, and there is not always a direct correlation between the formulations that are successful *in vitro* and those that show promise *in vivo*. This is due to differences in the formulations used in each system. *In vitro* models are appropriate primarily for screening delivery agents in simple surrogate formulations to identify specific candidate excipients and their properties, rather than the entire formulation. One of the most significant challenges initially faced in moving to *in vivo* screening involves the dose levels required, which translates directly to the siRNA concentration required. High concentrations of siRNA impact the formulation in several ways, most significantly on the colloidal stabilization of a dosable particle. This property also directly impacts the preparation and assembly of the particle due to the challenge in creating colloidal or nanosuspensions that have solids content appropriate for dosing. In order to provide colloidal stability to siRNA-containing particles, a steric stabilizer such as PEG may be added to the formulation. The use of PEG for *in vitro* studies may actually hinder cell uptake and result in loss of knockdown activity (R. Costantino and P. H. Johnson, 2006, unpublished observations), whereas the same formulation may work well *in vivo*. This is a challenge for *in vivo* screening and there currently are no published *in vivo* delivery agents that effectively deliver siRNA to tissues of interest across a broad spectrum of primary cell types [168], although this is likely to be an achievable goal.

An example of a commercially developed *in vivo* siRNA formulation is based on SNALP (stabilized nucleic acid lipid particles) technology, developed by Tekmira Pharmaceutical Corporation, Vancouver, BC, for *in vivo* delivery to liver. It is a PEGylated cationic lipid particle that has been shown to be effective for hepatitis C knockdown in monkeys and against ApoB [13,14]. The formulation appears to be primarily limited to RES clearance by liver and lungs and may require additional modification, including the incorporation of targeting ligands to deliver siRNA efficiently to other cell types. Another effective formulation, which is composed of novel lipids, is Silence Therapeutics' (formerly Atugen AG) AtuPlex. This formulation contains a modified N-palmityl-N-oleyl tail with a β-L-arginyl-2,3-L-diaminopropionic acid tricationic head group, complemented with a phytanoyl helper lipid and a PEGylated DSPE-PEG2000. Upon formulation, the resulting nanoparticle, which can be produced in the 50–200 nm diameter range in an siRNA lipoplex, effectively transfects vascular endothelial cells *in vivo* [16, 17].

The use of high-throughput liquid handling systems is an effective way to screen small molecule, lipid, and peptide libraries for molecules that may constitute a single delivery agent or comprise a formulation. Examples include cationic lipids and peptides that may serve a primary function in cell surface targeting, binding, and surface activation (e.g., actin mobilization) leading to siRNA uptake; fusogenic lipids and peptides that may enhance endosomal escape; PEGylated lipids that may enhance pharmacokinetic particle stability; other excipients that may be required as tonicifiers, solubilizers, and buffer; and agents to stabilize the shelf life of a formulation from physical and chemical degradation processes. Molecules may be screened individually or in combination using specific assays that measure individual steps in the delivery process such as cell binding, surface activation, membrane association, specific endocytic pathway utilization (defined by using pathway-specific drug inhibition), compartmentalization, specific endosomal localization, endosomal escape, and mRNA knockdown. Other important assays relate to toxicity measurements including cell viability, membrane lytic properties (e.g., red blood cell hemolysis), and nontarget related pathway stimulation, including toll-like receptor (TLR) activation and IFN response. While the knockdown efficacy of the siRNA delivery formulation is clearly most important, understanding the ways in which intermediate steps in the delivery process are inefficient or rate limiting helps to identify areas for further optimization. Improving the efficiency of these intermediate steps ultimately improves the ability of the formulation to achieve maximal knockdown of the target.

5.6.2 Delivery Agent Selection Criteria

The selection of a delivery agent from screens will depend on the overall screening strategy being implemented, the ultimate application of the siRNA therapeutic, and its intended route of administration. The most important criteria for both *in vitro* and *in vivo* models will be efficacy (knockdown), toxicity, and the associated therapeutic index (LD_{50}/ED_{50}: the ratio given by the dose required to produce the toxic effect divided by the therapeutic dose), particularly in the animal model of greatest relevance. Rather than relying exclusively on mRNA knockdown data, the primary evaluation should focus on knockdown of the specific target protein. *In vitro/in vivo* correlations are limited for nucleic acid delivery, and in some situations, correlate poorly [111]. Making relevant correlations between these analyses will be critical to the success of rapid screening efforts that have the potential to improve the development of siRNA delivery systems.

Identifying the appropriate intracellular transport route(s) and optimizing the efficiency of internalization of the siRNA are critical factors involved in evaluating the potential effectiveness of a delivery agent. Similarly, the nature and strength of the siRNA-delivery agent(s) complex, which must dissociate once inside the cell, will influence siRNA efficacy. There are several different materials that can be selected to promote effective delivery including cationic lipids and liposomal formulations, cationic polymers such as dendrimers, PEI, chitosan, peptides and peptide-based compounds [169] and acrylic acid-based polymers. There are also combinations that provide unique properties and novel functionalities, such as combining lipids and peptides [170]. Figure 5.7 shows an example of the potential synergy between peptides and lipids. Some cationic peptides are very efficient at internalizing siRNA, but have low knockdown activity. Although neutral lipids alone generally are not active delivery agents, some exhibit good knockdown activity when combined with certain cationic peptides.

There are two broad categories of delivery agent functions: those based on biological effects and those resulting from biophysical properties. Biological properties reflect specific interactions with the cell for initial binding and targeting, subcellular trafficking and compartmentalization, as well as properties affecting dissociation leading to siRNA activity. These can be peptide, protein, carbohydrate, or other biologically derived material that is intended to serve as a biological ligand for a specific intended property [171]. Physicochemical properties provide structure and shape to the delivery system, stability to the particle and the siRNA, colloidal properties such as nanoparticle suspension stability, and physical and chemical stability [172]. The choice of materials will influence nonspecific protein binding, such as opsonization and complement activation, for example, which occur in response to a significant excess of unneutralized positive charge (high zeta potential). Ideally, the delivery system will comprise the simplest combination of materials that provides the intended biological activity, stability and safety profile, and that also is amenable to production and scale-up, and has an acceptable COGS profile.

The selection criteria used for screening can be identified using a combination of tests and assays to determine the ability of the material to meet desired specifications within the two main categories of delivery properties (biological and biophysical). General principles for selecting an agent are based primarily on an evaluation of efficacy and toxicity. Efficacy will be ranked by the level of knockdown of the target gene. Toxicity is determined by viability of the cells and plasma stability *in vitro* [173, 174] and pharmacokinetic properties *in vivo*.

Physical properties can be characterized using particle sizing (e.g., dynamic light scattering), binding assays, (using RNA duplex denaturation temperature, Tm, gel mobility shift, dye exclusion assays, zeta potential

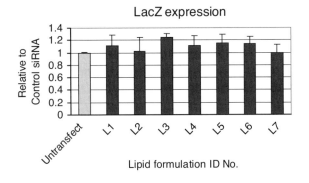

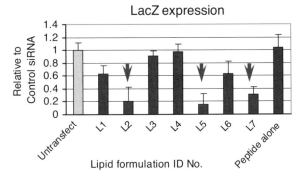

FIGURE 5.7   Lipid-Peptide Synergy. The top panel shows the knockdown activity of seven different lipid formulations. There is no effect of the formulations compared to the untransfected control seen on the left. In the lower panel, the impact of the same lipid formulations combined with a peptide agent shows > 70% knockdown in formulations L2, L5, and L7, while L3, L4, and L6 do not show any significant effect. The peptide alone, seen in the right hand bar, does not result in effective knockdown. This synergy is a key outcome of the combination of different classes of delivery agents.

measurement), differential scanning calorimetry (DSC) and purity criteria (using LC-MS). The size of the particles should be submicron and the goal is to achieve particles that can readily traverse capillary beds. The size most often strived for is a particle less than 100 nm in diameter. The condensation of siRNA is dissimilar to plasmid DNA condensation because the 21–27-mer length scale of most siRNAs is shorter than the 50 base pair persistence length typically required for charge neutralized condensation to occur [175]. Therefore, particle formation is driven by charge properties of the neutralized species and mainly by their hydrophobic effect. Interactions with siRNA can be identified using techniques such as dye exclusion or DSC. These studies can provide information related to the binding of the different materials, and can provide an estimate of the ability of the siRNA to interact, and remain complexed with these materials under different solution conditions [172].

5.6.3 Choosing Appropriate *in vitro* and *in vivo* Screening Systems

In vitro/in vivo correlations are not yet well established for siRNA delivery. There are many differences, as discussed above, most significantly those due to *in vivo* tissue and circulatory barriers that are absent in *in vitro* systems. In principle, however, cellular uptake and intracellular processing pathways may be similar for *in vivo* and at least some *in vitro* systems (e.g., certain primary cells in culture and monolayers of polarized cells).

Bartlett and Davis [176] demonstrated that the kinetics of siRNA knockdown is strongly affected by cell division and its associated dilution, rather than the siRNA half-life. Using an *in vitro* luciferase-based model system, it was shown that rapidly dividing cells recover to their pretreatment levels within about 1 week of knockdown, but nondividing fibroblasts required more than 3 weeks to return to steady state levels. Similar results were also shown *in vivo* with A/J mice resulting in 10 days of sustained knockdown in a subcutaneous tumor model.

An *in vitro* screen using immortalized cell lines (instead of primary cells that are more typical of *in vivo* response) represents a static environment. This alone may result in significant biological differences compared with an *in vivo* system that affects the activity of the delivery system. For therapeutic applications, it is accepted that the appropriate standard for efficacy is demonstrated by *in vivo* activity. This is because the *in vivo* conditions involve a myriad of obstacles that can hinder effective delivery, including circulation half-life, stability, immune response, effective uptake in the target cell or tissue type, and the appropriate intracellular trafficking to ensure optimal activity in the RISC complex [177]. However, whether a given animal model is adequately representative of human biology is always an issue. It is advantageous to pursue *in vivo* screening in animal models whenever possible, but cost, time, and availability generally limit *in vivo* analyses to a relatively small number of lead candidates, rather than as a primary lead identification tool.

An example where screening strategy can make a significant difference is in the use of PEG. Typically, PEGylation is performed to improve colloidal stability of siRNA particles, reduce opsonization and increase persistence of the particles in circulation. Unfortunately, PEG modification for *in vitro* studies may actually result in loss of measurable activity by adversely affecting cellular uptake, whereas the same formulation may work well *in vivo* [15]. This example highlights the need to evaluate candidate formulations early in *in vivo* models, rather than relying solely on *in vitro* testing.

5.6.4 Formulation Optimization

Nanoparticles may be the most effective physical form for siRNA delivery, as each particle typically contains multiple siRNA molecules (as high as several thousands). Each binding event between a nanoparticle and a cell, thus, has the potential to deliver many siRNA simultaneously. Single-molecule complexes may be inherently less efficient. Nanoparticles may involve either noncovalent or covalent interactions in the physical association of the siRNA with the delivery agent(s) [178]. Ultimately, multiple components including the siRNA are combined into a system that self-assembles into a nanoparticle that serves to stabilize the siRNA from enzymatic degradation, shields the siRNA from opsonization and complement activation, interacts with the cell to enable internalization, and finally releases the siRNA inside the cell [179]. In addition to identifying the components used to deliver siRNA, the process used to assemble and optimize the nanoparticle is equally important. Nanoparticle-based delivery systems are usually composed of polyionic materials, with siRNA having a negatively charged phosphate backbone and the delivery agents (e.g., cationic polymers, peptides, and lipids) being cationic in nature. The interactions between these materials is complex and is difficult to stabilize. Because the systems are dependent on their ability to self-assemble [180,181], particle size ranges from approximately 20 to 200 nm and may exhibit considerable heterogeneity. There is often a need to apply an external force to enable assembly into the appropriate size, for example, using pressure, heat, pH, or ionic gradients. Examples are the extrusion of lipids to create liposomal systems and dialysis procedures required to prepare the formulation [182, 183].

Formulation optimization can occur only after all the necessary components of the formulation, including siRNA, delivery agents, and other formulation excipients, have been determined. The optimization of multicomponent formulations can often benefit from the use of a Design of Experiments (DOE) approach [184–186] in which specific experimental designs and statistical methods for data analysis are used to optimize formulation performance. A series of structured tests are designed in which multiple input variables are systematically changed and the effects on output are evaluated. DOE is important as a formal way of maximizing information gained, while minimizing resources required. It is more powerful than "one change at a time" experimental methods, because it enables the evaluation of the impact that single or combinatorial inputs have on output. A matrix representing a full set of possible combinations of factors and levels is used to draw the maximum amount of information from the data available. DOE plans for all possible dependencies in the first place, and then prescribes exactly what data are needed to assess them, that is, whether input variables change the response on their own, when combined, or not at all.

5.7 SUMMARY AND FUTURE DIRECTIONS

RNAi-based therapeutics have the potential to provide a new class of broadly applicable therapies with clinically relevant efficacy and safety. Efficient delivery and cost-effective manufacturing are major challenges that must be met to achieve success. While current manufacturing processes are far from cost-effective, they are likely to show significant improvement over time. No current delivery system appears to have both the desired efficiency and safety profile necessary for an RNAi therapeutic to have a clear clinical advantage over other classes of drugs. However, based on recent results and promising new systems under development, there is reason to believe that this will change in the near future. Specific research areas critical for establishing the most effective methods of siRNA delivery and maximum clinical therapeutic potential include the following: (1) Future work must clarify those types of pharmacological targets against which RNAi therapeutics are particularly effective compared with other classes of drugs and the relationship between target(s) specificity and corresponding *in vivo* efficacy and toxicity. (2) Identifying the most efficient pathway(s) for siRNA uptake and functionality and optimizing siRNA targeting to this route(s) of delivery will be key for clinical success. (3) A better understanding of the signaling pathways that regulate TJ dynamics may reveal new approaches to increase RNAi activity through more effective tissue penetration and enhanced intracellular delivery of siRNA. (4) CPPs/PTDs have potential as effective siRNA delivery agents. Most CPPs appear to enter cells through an endocytotic mechanism, perhaps most effectively by macropinocytosis. The guanidinium group of arginine is important for efficient uptake. A key issue for further study is the extent to which the peptide's membrane translocation activity may be compromised when the required cationic residues bind the siRNA and are less available for specific cell surface/membrane head group interactions that are necessary for membrane/endocytic transport. (5) Several technologies, including aptamer and phage display molecular libraries, may provide effective strategies for identifying new cell targeting RNA or peptide sequences. Cell-type specific delivery agents may enable lower dosage requirements and fewer toxic side effects.

REFERENCES

1. Fire, A., Xu, S., Montgomery, M. K., Kostas, S. A., Driver, S. E., and Mello, C. C. (1998). Potent and specific genetic interference by double-stranded RNA in *Caenorhabditis elegans*. *Nature* **391**: 806–11.

2. Elbashir, S. M., Harborth, J., Lendeckel, W., Yalcin, A., Weber, K., and Tuschl, T. (2001). Duplexes of 21-nucleotide RNAs mediate RNA interference in cultured mammalian cells. *Nature* **411**: 494–8.

3. Dillon, C. P., Sandy, P., Nencioni, A., Kissler, S., Rubinson, D. A., and Van Parijs, L. (2005). RNAi as an experimental and therapeutic tool to study and regulate physiological and disease processes. *Annu Rev Physiol* **67**: 147–73.

4. Kim, D. H. and Rossi, J. J. (2007). Strategies for silencing human disease using RNA interference. *Nat Rev Genet* **8**: 173–84.

5. Fitzgerald, K. (2005). RNAi versus small molecules: different mechanisms and specificities can lead to different outcomes. *Curr Opin Drug Discov Devel* **8**: 557–66.

6. Behlke, M. A. (2006). Progress towards in vivo use of siRNAs. *Mol Ther* **13**: 644–70.

7. Dykxhoorn, D. M. and Lieberman, J. (2006). Running interference: prospects and obstacles to using small interfering RNAs as small molecule drugs. *Annu Rev Biomed Eng* **8**: 377–402.

8. Quay, S. C. and Johnson, P. H. (2007). RNAi therapeutics: the future of medicine. *Pharma* **3**: 18–21.

9. Sledz, C. A. and Williams, B. R. (2005). RNA interference in biology and disease. *Blood* **106**: 787–94.

10. Johnson, P. H. and Quay, S. C. (2005). Advances in nasal drug delivery through tight junction technology. *Expert Opin Drug Deliv* **2**: 281–98.

11. Kim, W. J., Christensen, L. V., Jo, S., Yockman, J. W., Jeong, J. H., Kim, Y. H., and Kim, S. W. (2006). Cholesteryl oligoarginine delivering vascular endothelial growth factor siRNA effectively inhibits tumor growth in colon adenocarcinoma. *Mol Ther* **14**: 343–50.

12. Soutschek, J., Akinc, A., Bramlage, B., Charisse, K., Constien, R., Donoghue, M., Elbashir, S., Geick, A., Hadwiger, P., Harborth, J., John, M., Kesavan, V., Lavine, G., Pandey, R. K., Racie, T., Rajeev, K. G., Rohl, I., Toudjarska, I., Wang, G., Wuschko, S., Bumcrot, D., Koteliansky, V., Limmer, S., Manoharan, M., and Vornlocher, H. P. (2004). Therapeutic silencing of an endogenous gene by systemic administration of modified siRNAs. *Nature* **432**: 173–8.

13. Morrissey, D. V., Lockridge, J. A., Shaw, L., Blanchard, K., Jensen, K., Breen, W., Hartsough, K., Machemer, L., Radka, S., Jadhav, V., Vaish, N., Zinnen, S., Vargeese, C., Bowman, K., Shaffer, C. S., Jeffs, L. B., Judge, A., MacLachlan, I., and Polisky, B. (2005). Potent and persistent in vivo anti-HBV activity of chemically modified siRNAs. *Nat Biotechnol* **23**: 1002–7.

14. Zimmermann, T. S., Lee, A. C., Akinc, A., Bramlage, B., Bumcrot, D., Fedoruk, M. N., Harborth, J., Heyes, J. A., Jeffs, L. B., John, M., Judge, A. D., Lam, K., McClintock, K., Nechev, L. V., Palmer, L. R., Racie, T., Rohl, I., Seiffert, S., Shanmugam, S., Sood, V., Soutschek, J., Toudjarska, I., Wheat, A. J., Yaworski, E., Zedalis, W., Koteliansky, V., Manoharan, M., Vornlocher, H.

P., and MacLachlan, I. (2006). RNAi-mediated gene silencing in non-human primates. *Nature* **441**: 111–4.

15. Li, W. and Szoka, F. C. Jr,. (2007). Lipid-based nanoparticles for nucleic acid delivery. *Pharm Res* **24**: 438–49.

16. Santel, A., Aleku, M., Keil, O., Endruschat, J., Esche, V., Durieux, B., Loffler, K., Fechtner, M., Rohl, T., Fisch, G., Dames, S., Arnold, W., Giese, K., Klippel, A., and Kaufmann, J. (2006a). RNA interference in the mouse vascular endothelium by systemic administration of siRNA- lipoplexes for cancer therapy. *Gene Ther* **13**: 1360–70.

17. Santel, A., Aleku, M., Keil, O., Endruschat, J., Esche, V., Fisch, G., Dames, S., Loffler, K., Fechtner, M., Arnold, W., Giese, K., Klippel, A., and Kaufmann, J. (2006b). A novel siRNA-lipoplex technology for RNA interference in the mouse vascular endothelium. *Gene Ther* **13**: 1222–34.

18. Hogrefe, R. I., Lebedev, A. V., Zon, G., Pirollo, K. F., Rait, A., Zhou, Q., Yu, W., and Chang, E. H. (2006). Chemically modified short interfering hybrids (siHYBRIDS): nanoimmunoliposome delivery in vitro and in vivo for RNAi of HER-2. *Nucleosides Nucleotides Nucleic Acids* **25**: 889–907.

19. Peer, D., Zhu, P., Carman, C. V., Lieberman, J., and Shimaoka, M. (2007). Selective gene silencing in activated leukocytes by targeting siRNAs to the integrin lymphocyte function-associated antigen-1. *Proc Natl Acad Sci U S A* **104**: 4095–100.

20. Song, E., Zhu, P., Lee, S. K., Chowdhury, D., Kussman, S., Dykxhoorn, D. M., Feng, Y., Palliser, D., Weiner, D. B., Shankar, P., Marasco, W. A., and Lieberman, J. (2005). Antibody mediated in vivo delivery of small interfering RNAs via cell-surface receptors. *Nat Biotechnol* **23**: 709–17.

21. Chu, T. C., Twu, K. Y., Ellington, A. D., and Levy, M. (2006). Aptamer mediated siRNA delivery. *Nucleic Acids Res* **34**: e73.

22. McNamara, J. O. 2nd, Andrechek, E. R., Wang, Y., Viles, K. D., Rempel, R. E., Gilboa, E., Sullenger, B. A., and Giangrande, P. H. (2006). Cell type-specific delivery of siRNAs with aptamer-siRNA chimeras. *Nat Biotechnol* **24**: 1005–15.

23. Kumar, P., Wu, H., McBride, J. L., Jung K-E, Hee Kim, M., Davidson, B. L., Kyung Lee, S., Shankar, P., and Manjunath, N. (2007). Transvascular delivery of small interfering RNA to the central nervous system. *Nature* **448**: 39–43.

24. Meade, B. R. and Dowdy, S. F. (2007). Exogenous siRNA delivery using peptide transduction domains/cell penetrating peptides. *Adv Drug Deliv Rev* **59**: 134–40.

25. Heidel, J. D., Yu, Z., Liu, J. Y., Rele, S. M., Liang, Y., Zeidan, R. K., Kornbrust, D. J., and Davis, M. E. (2007). Administration in non-human primates of escalating intravenous doses of targeted nanoparticles containing ribonucleotide reductase subunit M2 siRNA. *Proc Natl Acad Sci U S A* **104**: 5715–21.

26. Dikic, I. (2003). Mechanisms controlling EGF receptor endocytosis and degradation. *Biochem Soc Trans* **31**: 1178–81.

27. Pille, J. Y., Li, H., Blot, E., Bertrand, J. R., Pritchard, L. L., Opolon, P., Maksimenko, A., Lu, H., Vannier, J. P., Soria, J., Malvy, C., and Soria, C. (2006). Intravenous delivery of anti-RhoA small interfering RNA loaded in nanoparticles of chitosan in mice: safety and efficacy in xenografted aggressive breast cancer. *Hum Gene Ther* **17**: 1019–26.

28. Liu, X., Howard, K. A., Dong, M., Andersen, M. O., Rahbek, U. L., Johnsen, M. G., Hansen, O. C., Besenbacher, F., and Kjems, J. (2007). The influence of polymeric properties on chitosan/siRNA nanoparticle formulation and gene silencing. *Biomaterials* **28**: 1280–8.

29. Grzelinski, M., Urban-Klein, B., Martens, T., Lamszus, K., Bakowsky, U., Hobel, S., Czubayko, F., and Aigner, A. (2006). RNA interference-mediated gene silencing of pleiotrophin through polyethylenimine-complexed small interfering RNAs in vivo exerts antitumoral effects in glioblastoma xenografts. *Hum Gene Ther* **17**: 751–66.

30. Thomas, M., Lu, J. J., Ge, Q., Zhang, C., Chen, J., and Klibanov, A. M. (2005). Full deacylation of polyethylenimine dramatically boosts its gene delivery efficiency and specificity to mouse lung. *Proc Natl Acad Sci U S A* **102**: 5679–84.

31. Stayton, P. S. and Hoffman, A. S. (2008). "Smart" pH-responsive carriers for intracellular delivery of biomolecular drugs. In: V. Torchilin (ed.), *Multifunctional Pharmaceutical Nanocarriers*. Springer, New York.

32. El-Sayed, M. E., Hoffman, A. S., Stayton, P. S. (2005). Smart polymeric carriers for enhanced intracellular delivery of therapeutic macromolecules. *Expert Opin Biol Ther* **5**: 23–32.

33. Convertine, A. J., Benoit, D. S., Duvall, C. L., Hoffman, A. S., Stayton, P. S. (2009). Development of a novel endosomolytic diblock copolymer for siRNA delivery. *J Control Release* **133**: 221–9.

34. Benoit, D. S., Henry, S. M., Shubin, A. D., Hoffman, A. S., Stayton, P. S. (2010). pH-responsive polymeric sirna carriers sensitize multidrug resistant ovarian cancer cells to doxorubicin via knockdown of polo-like kinase 1. *Mol Pharm* **7**: 442–55.

35. Lewis, D. L. and Wolff J. A. (2007). Systemic siRNA delivery via hydrodynamic intravascular injection. *Adv Drug Deliv Rev* **59**: 115–23.

36. Zhang, W., Yang, H., Kong, X., Mohapatra, S., San Juan-Vergara, H., Hellermann, G., Behera, S., Singam, R., Lockey, R. F., and Mohapatra, S. S. (2005). Inhibition of respiratory syncytial virus infection with intranasal siRNA nanoparticles targeting the viral NS1 gene. *Nat Med* **11**: 56–62.

37. Zhang, Y., Cristofaro, P., Silbermann, R., Pusch, O., Boden, D., Konkin, T., Hovanesian, V., Monfils, P. R., Resnick, M., Moss, S. F., and Ramratnam, B. (2006). Engineering mucosal RNA interference in vivo. *Mol Ther* **14**: 336–42.

38. Bitko, V., Musiyenko, A., Shulyayeva, O., and Barik, S. (2005). Inhibition of respiratory viruses by nasally administered siRNA. *Nat Med* **11**: 50–5.

39. Duxbury, M. S., Matros, E., Ito, H., Zinner, M. J., Ashley, S. W., and Whang, E. E. (2004). Systemic siRNA- mediated gene silencing: a new approach to targeted therapy of cancer. *Ann Surg* **240**: 667–74.

40. Duxbury, M. S., Ashley, S. W., and Whang, E. E. (2005). RNA interference: a mammalian SID-1 homologue enhances siRNA uptake and gene silencing efficacy in human cells. *Biochem Biophys Res Commun* **331**: 459–63.

41. Feinberg, E. H. and Hunter, C. P. (2003). Transport of dsRNA into cells by the transmembrane protein SID-1. *Science* **301**: 1545–7.

42. van Roessel, P. and Brand, A. H. (2004). Spreading silence with Sid. *Genome Biol* **5**: 208.

43. Saleh, M. C., van Rij, R. P., Hekele, A., Gillis, A., Foley, E., O'Farrell, P. H., and Andino, R. (2006). The endocytic pathway mediates cell entry of dsRNA to induce RNAi silencing. *Nat Cell Biol* **8**: 793–802.

44. Conner, S. D. and Schmid, S. L. (2003). Regulated portals of entry into the cell. *Nature* **422**: 37–44.

45. Cheng, Z. J., Singh, R. D., Marks, D. L., and Pagano, R. E. (2006). Membrane microdomains, caveolae, and caveolar endocytosis of sphingolipids. *Mol Membr Biol* **23**: 101–110.

46. Bathori, G., Cervenak, L., and Karadi, I. (2004). Caveolae–an alternative endocytotic pathway for targeted drug delivery. *Crit Rev Ther Drug Carrier Syst* **21**: 67–95.

47. Smythe, E. and Ayscough, K. R. (2006). Actin regulation in endocytosis. *J Cell Sci* **119**: 4589–98.

48. Chiu, S. J., Marcucci, G., and Lee, R. J. (2006). Efficient delivery of an antisense oligodeoxyribonucleotide formulated in folate receptor-targeted liposomes. *Anticancer Res* **26**: 1049–56.

49. Medina-Kauwe, L. K., Xie, J., and Hamm-Alvarez, S. (2005). Intracellular trafficking of nonviral vectors. *Gene Ther* **12**: 1734–51.

50. Lingor, P., Michel, U., Scholl, U., Bahr, M., and Kugler, S. (2004). Transfection of "naked" siRNA results in endosomal uptake and metabolic impairment in cultured neurons. *Biochem Biophys Res Commun* **315**: 1126–33.

51. McNiven, M. A. (2006). Big gulps: specialized membrane domains for rapid receptor-mediated endocytosis. *Trends Cell Biol* **16**: 487–92.

52. Royle, S. J. (2006). The cellular functions of clathrin. *Cell Mol Life Sci* **63**: 1823–32.

53. Rejman, J., Oberle, V., Zuhorn, I. S., and Hoekstra, D. (2004). Size-dependent internalization of particles via the pathways of clathrin- and caveolae-mediated endocytosis. *Biochem J* **377**: 159–69.

54. Kirkham, M. and Parton, R. G. (2005). Clathrin-independent endocytosis: new insights into caveolae and non-caveolar lipid raft carriers. *Biochim Biophys Acta* **1746**: 349–63.

55. Orth, J. D. and McNiven, M. A. (2006). Get off my back! Rapid receptor internalization through circular dorsal ruffles. *Cancer Res* **66**: 11094–6.

56. Tsukita, S., Furuse, M., and Itoh, M. (2001). Multifunctional strands in tight junctions. *Nat Rev Mol Cell Biol* **2**: 285–93.

57. Blaschuk, O. W. and Rowlands, T. M. (2002). Plasma membrane components of adherens junctions. *Mol Membr Biol* **19**: 75–80.

58. Matter, K. and Balda, M. S. (2003). Signalling to and from tight junctions. *Nat Rev Mol Cell Biol* **4**: 225–36.

59. Ivanov, A. I., Nusrat, A., and Parkos, C. A. (2005). Endocytosis of the apical junctional complex: mechanisms and possible roles in regulation of epithelial barriers. *Bioessays* **27**: 356–65.

60. Wang, G., Zabner, J., Deering, C., Launspach, J., Shao, J., Bodner, M., Jolly, D. J., Davidson, B. L., and McCray, P. B. Jr. (2000). Increasing epithelial junction permeability enhances gene transfer to airway epithelia In vivo. *Am J Respir Cell Mol Biol* **22**: 129–38.

61. Ivanov, A. I., Nusrat, A., and Parkos, C. A. (2004). Endocytosis of epithelial apical junctional proteins by a clathrin-mediated pathway into a unique storage compartment. *Mol Biol Cell* **15**: 176–88.

62. Coyne, C. B. and Bergelson, J. M. (2006). Virus-induced Abl and Fyn kinase signals permit coxsackievirus entry through epithelial tight junctions. *Cell* **24**: 119–31.

63. Frankel, A. D. and Pabo, C. O. (1988). Cellular uptake of the tat protein from human immunodeficiency virus. *Cell* **55**: 1189–93.

64. Green, M. and Loewenstein, P. M. (1988). Autonomous functional domains of chemically synthesized human immunodeficiency virus tat trans-activator protein. *Cell* **55**: 1179–88.

65. Deshayes, S., Morris, M. C., Divita, G., and Heitz, F. (2005). Cell-penetrating peptides: tools for intracellular delivery of therapeutics. *Cell Mol Life Sci* **62**: 1839–49.

66. Derossi, D., Calvet, S., Trembleau, A., Brunissen, A., Chassaing, G., and Prochiantz, A. (1996). Cell internalization of the third helix of the Antennapedia homeodomain is receptor-independent. *J Biol Chem* **271**: 18188–93.

67. Derossi, D., Chassaing, G., and Prochiantz, A. (1998). Trojan peptides: the penetratin system for intracellular delivery. *Trends Cell Biol* **8**: 84–7.

68. Vives, E., Brodin, P., and Lebleu, B. (1997). A truncated HIV-1 Tat protein basic domain rapidly translocates through the plasma membrane and accumulates in the cell nucleus. *J Biol Chem* **272**: 16010–7.

69. Pooga, M., Hallbrink, M., Zorko, M., and Langel, U. (1998). Cell penetration by transportan. *FASEB J* **12**: 67–77.

70. Elliott, G. and O'Hare, P. (1997). Intercellular trafficking and protein delivery by a herpes virus structural protein. *Cell* **88**: 223–33.

71. Machova, Z., Muhle, C., Krauss, U., Trehin, R., Koch, A., and Merkle, H. P. (2002). Cellular internalization of enhanced green fluorescent protein ligated to a human calcitonin-based carrier peptide. *Chembiochem* **3**: 672–7.

72. Krauss, U., Muller, M., Syahl, M., and Beck-Sickinger, A. G. (2004). In vitro gene delivery by a novel human calcitonin (hCT)-derived carrier peptide. *Bioorg Med Chem Lett* **14**: 51–4.

73. Morris, M. C., Vidal, P., Chaloin, L., Heitz, F., and Divita, G. (1997). A new peptide vector for efficient delivery of oligonucleotide into mammalian cells. *Nucleic Acid Res* **25**: 2730–6.

74. Rothbard, J. B., Garlington, S., Lin, Q., Kirschberg, T., Kreider, E., McGrane, P. L., Wender, P. A., and Khavari, P. A. (2000). Conjugation of arginine oligomers to cyclosporin A facilitates topical delivery and inhibition of inflammation. *Nat Med* **6**: 1253–7.

75. Oehlke, J., Scheller, A., Wiesner, B., Krause, E., Beyermann, M., Klauschenz, E., Melzig, M., and Bienert, M. (1998). Cellular uptake of an alpha-helical amphipathic model peptide with the potential to deliver polar compounds into the cell interior non-endocytically. *Biochim Biophys Acta* 1414: 27–39.

76. Mitchell, D. J., Kim, D. T., Steinman, L., Fathman, C. G., and Rothbard, J. B. (2000). Polyarginine enters cells more efficiently than other polycationic homopolymers. *J Pept Res* **56**: 318–25.

77. Mahat, R. I., Monera, O. D., Smith, L. C., and Rolland, A. (1999). Peptide-based gene delivery. *Curr Opin Mol Ther* **1**: 226–43.

78. Subbarao, N. K., Parente, R. A., Szoka, F. C., Jr., Nadasdi, L., and Pongracz, K. (1987). pH-Dependent bilayer destabilization by an amphipathic peptide. *Biochemistry* **26**: 2964–72.

79. Parente, R. A., Nadasdi, L., Subbarao, N. K., and Szoka, F. C. Jr., (1990). Association of a pH-sensitive peptide with membrane vesicles: role of amino acid sequence. *Biochemistry* **29**: 8713–9.

80. Parente, R. A., Nir, S., and Szoka, F. C. Jr,. (1990). Mechanism of leakage of phospholipid vesicle contents induced by the peptide GALA. *Biochemistry* **29**: 8720–8.

81. Gottschalk, S., Sparrow, J. T., Hauer, J., Mims, M. P., Leland, F. E., Woo, S. L., and Smith, L. C. (1996). A novel DNA-peptide complex for efficient gene transfer and expression in mammalian cells. *Gene Ther* **3**: 448–57.

82. Rittner, K., Benavente, A., Bompard-Sorlet, A., Heitz, F., Divita, G., Brasseur, R., and Jacobs, E. (2002). New basic membrane-destabilizing peptides for plasmid-based gene delivery in vitro and in vivo. *Mol Ther* **5**: 104–14.

83. Martin, M. E. and Rice, K. G. (2007). Peptide-guided gene delivery. *AAPS J* **9**: E18–29.

84. Witkowska, R. T., Ahmadian, M., Dattilo, J. W., Purvis, L. J., Mayer, S. J., Chen, L., Chen, Y., Cui, K., Farber, K. W., Roth, S. E., Houston, M. E., Johnson, P. H., and Quay, S. C. (2007). Peptide-mediated delivery of siRNA via noncovalent complexes and covalent conjugates. In: Rolka K., Rekowski P., and Silberring J. (Eds), Peptides, Proc. 29th Eur. Pep. Sym., Gdansk, Poland, p 78.

85. Crombez, L., Charnet, A., Morris, M. C., Aldrian-Herrada, G., Heitz, F., and Divita, G. (2007). A non-covalent peptide-based strategy for siRNA delivery. *Biochem Soc Trans* **35**: 44–6.

86. Drin, G., Cottin, S., Blanc, E., Rees, A. R., and Temsamani, J. (2003). Studies on the internalization mechanism of cationic cell-penetrating peptides. *J Biol Chem* **278**: 31192–201.

87. Wender, P. A., Mitchell, D. J., Pattabiraman, K., Pelkey, E. T., Steinman, L., and Rothbard, J. B. (2000). The design, synthesis, and evaluation of molecules that enable or enhance cellular uptake: peptoid molecular transporters. *Proc Natl Acad Sci U S A* **97**: 13003–8.

88. Mann, D. A. and Frankel, A. D. (1991). Endocytosis and targeting of exogeneous HIV-1 Tat protein. *EMBO J* **10**: 1733–9.

89. Rusnati, M., Coltrini, D., Oreste, P., Zoppetti, G., Albini, A., Noonan, D., d'Adda Di Fagagna, F., Giacca, M., and Presta, M. (1997). Interaction of HIV-1 Tat protein with heparin. Role of backbone structure, sulfation, and size. *J Biol Chem* **272**: 11313–20.

90. Rusnati, M., Tulipano, G., Urbinati, C., Tanghetti, E., Giuliani, R., Giacca, M., Ciomei, M., Corallini, A., and Presta, M. (1998). The basic domain in HIV-1 Tat protein as a target for polysulfonated heparin-mimicking extracellular Tat antagonists. *J Biol Chem* **273**: 16027–37.

91. Hakansson, S., Jacobs, A., and Caffrey, M. (2001). Heparin binding by the HIV-1 tat protein transduction domain. *Protein Sci* **10**: 2138–9.

92. Tyagi, M., Rusnati, M., Presta, M., and Giacca, M. (2001). Internalization of HIV-1 requires cell surface heparan sulfate proteoglycans. *J Biol Chem* **276**: 3254–61.

93. Elmquist, A., Lindgren, M., Bartfai, T., and Langel, U. (2001). VE-cadherin-derived cell-penetrating peptide, pVEC, with carrier functions. *Exp Cell Res* **269**: 237–44.

94. Futaki, S., Suzuki, T., Ohashi, W., Yagami, T., Tanaka, S., Ueda, K., and Sugiura, Y. (2001). Arginine-rich peptides. An abundant source of membrane-permeable peptides having potential as carriers for intracellular protein delivery. *J Biol Chem* **276**: 5836–40.

95. Wadia, J. S., Stan, R. V., and Dowdy, S. F. (2004). Transducible TAT-HA fusogenic peptide enhances escape of TAT-fusion proteins after lipid raft macropinocytosis. *Nat Med* **10**: 310–5.

96. Kaplan, I. M., Wadia, J. S., and Dowdy, S. F. (2005). Cationic TAT peptide transduction domain enters cells by macropinocytosis. *J Control Release* **102**: 247–53.

97. Console, S., Marty, C., Garcia-Echeverria, C., Schwendener, R., and Ballmer-Hofer, K. (2003). Antennapedia and HIV transactivator of transcription (TAT) "protein transduction domains" promote endocytosis of high molecular weight cargo upon binding to cell surface glycosaminoglycans. *J Biol Chem* **278**: 35109–14.

98. Nakase, I., Tadokoro, A., Kawabata, N., Takeuchi, T., Katoh, H., Hiramoto, K., Negishi, M., Nomizu, M., Sugiura, Y., and Futaki, S. (2007). Interaction of arginine-rich peptides with membrane-associated proteoglycans is crucial

for induction of actin organization and macropinocytosis. *Biochemistry* **46**: 492–501.

99. Richard, J. P., Melikov, K., Brooks, H., Prevot, P., Lebleu, B., and Chernomordik, L. V. (2005). Cellular uptake of unconjugated TAT peptide involves clathrin-dependent endocytosis and heparan sulfate receptors. *J Biol Chem* **280**: 15300–6.

100. Suzuki, T., Futaki, S., Niwa, M., Tanaka, S., Ueda, K., and Sugiura, Y. (2002). Possible existence of common internalization mechanisms among arginine-rich peptides. *J Biol Chem* **277**: 2437–43.

101. Gerbal-Chaloin, S., Gondeau, C., Aldrian-Herrada, G., Heitz1, F., Gauthier-Rouvière, C., and Divita, G. (2007). First step of the cell penetrating peptide mechanism involves Rac1 GTPase-dependent actin-network remodelling. *Biol Cell* **99**: 223–38.

102. Lundberg, M. and Johansson, M. (2002). Positively charge DNA binding proteins cause apparent cell membrane translocation. *Biochem Biophys Res Commun* **291**: 367–71.

103. Falnes, P. O., Wesche, J., and Olsnes, S. (2001), Ability of the Tat basic domain and VP22 to mediate cell binding, but not membrane translocation of diphtheria toxin A fragment. *Biochemistry* **40**: 4349–58.

104. Oren, Z. and Shai, Y. (1998). Mode of action of linear amphipathic alpha-helical antimicrobial peptides. *Biopolymers* **47**: 451–63.

105. Matsuzaki, K., Yoneyama, S., and Miyajima, K. (1997). Pore formation and translocation of melittin. *Biophys J* **73**: 831–8.

106. Thoren, P., Persson, D., Esbjorne, E., Gokso, M., Lincoln, P., and Norden, P. (2004). Membrane binding and translocation of cell-penetrating peptides. *Biochemistry* **43**: 3471–89.

107. Michael, S. J. and Curiel, D. T. (1994). Strategies to achieve targeted gene delivery via the receptor-mediated endocytosis pathway. *Gene Ther* **1**: 223–32.

108. Bordier, B., Perala-Heape, M., Degols, G., Lebleu, B., Litvak, S., Sarih-Cottin, L., and Helene, C. (1995). Sequence-specific inhibition of human immunodeficiency virus (HIV) reverse transcription by antisense oligonucleotides: comparative study in cell-free assays and in HIV-infected cells. *Proc Natl Acad Sci U S A* **92**: 9383–7.

109. Utku, Y., Dehan, E., Ouerfelli, O., Piano, F., Zuckermann, R. N., Pagano, M., and Kirshenbaum, K. (2006). A peptidomimetic siRNA transfection reagent for highly effective gene silencing. *Mol Biosyst* **2**: 312–7.

110. Bayer, T. S., Booth, L. N., Knudsen, S. M., and Ellington, A. D. (2005). Arginine-rich motifs present multiple interfaces for specific binding by RNA. *RNA* **11**: 1848–57.

111. Veldhoen, S., Laufer, S. D., Trampe, A., and Restle, T. (2006). Cellular delivery of small interfering RNA by a non-covalently attached cell-penetrating peptide: quantitative analysis of uptake and biological effect. *Nucleic Acids Res* **34**: 6561–73.

112. Muratovska, A. and Eccles, M. R. (2004). Conjugate for efficient delivery of short interfering RNA (siRNA) into mammalian cells. *FEBS Lett* **558**: 63–8.

113. Zatsepin, T. S., Turner, J. J., Oretskaya, T. S., and Gait, M. J. (2005). Conjugates of oligonucleotides and analogues with cell penetrating peptides as gene silencing agents. *Curr Pharm Des* **11**: 3639–54.

114. Tunnemann, G., Martin, R. M., Haupt, S., Patsch, C., Edenhofer, F., and Cardoso, M. C. (2006). Cargo-dependent mode of uptake and bioavailability of TAT-containing proteins and peptides in living cells. *FASEB J* **20**: 1775–84.

115. Magzoub, M., Pramanik, A., and Graslund, A. (2005). Modeling the endosomal escape of cell-penetrating peptides: transmembrane pH gradient driven translocation across phospholipid bilayers. *Biochemistry* **44**: 14890–97.

116. Gebhart, C. L. and Kabanov, A. V. (2001). Evaluation of polyplexes as gene transfer agents. *J Control Release* **73**: 401–16.

117. Kichler, A., Leborgne, C., Marz, J., Danos, O., and Bechinger, B. (2003). Histidine rich amphipathic peptide antibiotics promote efficient delivery of DNA into mammalian cells. *Proc Natl Acad Sci U S A* **100**: 1564–8.

118. Pichon, C., Goncalves, C., and Midoux, P. (2001). Histidine-rich peptides and polymers for nucleic acids delivery. *Adv Drug Deliv Rev* **53**: 75–94.

119. Midoux, P., Kichler, A., Boutin, V., Maurizot, J. C., and Monsigny, M. (1998). Membrane permeabilization and efficient gene transfer by a peptide containing several histidines. *Bioconjug Chem* **9**: 260–67.

120. Midoux, P., LeCam, E., Coulaud, D., Delain, E., and Pichon, C. (2002). Histidine containing peptides and polypeptides as nucleic acid vectors. *Somat Cell Mol Genet* **27**: 27–47.

121. Kilk, K., Elmquist, A., Saar, K., Pooga, M., Land, T., Bartfai, T., Soomets, U., and Langel, U. (2004). Targeting of antisense PNA oligomers to human galanin receptor type 1 mRNA. *Neuropeptides* **38**: 316–24.

122. Nath, A., Psooy, K., Martin, C., Knudsen, B., Magnuson, D. S., Haughey, N., and Geiger, J. D. (1996). Identification of a human immunodeficiency virus type 1 Tat epitope that is neuroexcitatory and neurotoxic. *J Virol* **70**: 1475–80.

123. Bolton, S. J., Jones, D. N., Darker, J. G., Eggleston, D. S., Hunter, A. J., and Walsh, F. S. (2000). Cellular uptake and spread of the cell-permeable peptide penetratin in adult rat brain. *Eur J Neurosci* **12**: 2847–55.

124. Shahana, S., Kampf, C., and Roomans, G. M. (2002). Effects of the cationic protein poly-L-arginine on airway epithelial cells *in vitro*. *Mediators Inflamm* **11**: 141–8.

125. Davis, B. G. and Robinson, M. A. (2002). Drug delivery systems based on sugar-macromolecule conjugates. *Curr Opin Drug Discov Dev* **5**: 279–88.

126. Hattori, Y., Kawakami, S., Suzuki, S., Yamashita, F., and Hashida, M. (2004). Enhancement of immune responses by DNA vaccination through targeted gene delivery using mannosylated cationic liposome formulations following intravenous administration in mice. *Biochem Biophys Res Commun* **317**: 992–9.

127. Hattori, Y., Kawakami, S., Yamashita, F., and Hashida, M. (2000). Controlled biodistribution of galactosylated liposomes and incorporated probucol in hepatocyte-selective drug targeting. *J Control Release* **69**: 369–77.

128. Managit, C., Kawakami, S., Nishikawa, M., Yamashita, F., and Hashida, M. (2003). Targeted and sustained drug delivery using PEGylated galactosylated liposomes. *Int J Pharm* **266**: 77–84.

129. Sato, A., Takagi, M., Shimamoto, A., Kawakami, S., and Hashida, M. (2007). Small interfering RNA delivery to the liver by intravenous administration of galactosylated cationic liposomes in mice. *Biomaterials*. **28**: 1434–42.

130. Cardoso, A. L., Simoes, S., de Almeida, L. P., Pelisek, J., Culmsee, C., Wagner, E., and Pedroso de Lima, M. C. (2007). siRNA delivery by a transferrin-associated lipid-based vector: a non-viral strategy to mediate gene silencing. *J Gene Med* **9**: 170–83.

131. Kontermann, R. E. (2006). Immunoliposomes for cancer therapy. *Curr Opin Mol Ther* **8**: 39–45.

132. Carpenter, G. (2000). The EGF receptor: a nexus for trafficking and signaling. *Bioessays* **22**: 697–707.

133. Linggi, B. and Carpenter, G. (2006). ErbB receptors: new insights on mechanisms and biology. *Trends Cell Biol* **16**: 649–56.

134. Liu, Z., Winters, M., Holodniy, M., and Dai, H. (2007b). siRNA delivery into human T cells and primary cells with carbon-nanotube transporters. *Angew Chem Int Ed Engl* **46**: 2023–7.

135. Guo, S., Tschammer, N., Mohammed, S., and Guo, P. (2005). Specific delivery of therapeutic RNAs to cancer cells via the dimerization mechanism of phi29 motor pRNA. *Hum Gene Ther* **16**: 1097–109.

136. Guo, S., Huang, F., and Guo, P. (2006). Construction of folate-conjugated pRNA of bacteriophage phi29 DNA packaging motor for delivery of chimeric siRNA to nasopharyngeal carcinoma cells. *Gene Ther* **13**: 814–20.

137. Schiffelers, R. M., Ansari, A., Xu, J., Zhou, Q., Tang, Q., Storm, G., Molema, G., Lu, P. Y., Scaria, P. V., and Woodle, M. C. (2004). Cancer siRNA therapy by tumor selective delivery with ligand-targeted sterically stabilized nanoparticle. *Nucleic Acids Res* **32**: e149.

138. Schiffelers, R. M. and Storm, G. (2006). ICS-283: a system for targeted intravenous delivery of siRNA. *Expert Opin Drug Deliv* **3**: 445–54.

139. Hu-Lieskovan, S., Heidel, J. D., Bartlett, D. W., Davis, M. E., and Triche, T. J. (2005). Sequence-specific knockdown of EWS-FLI1 by targeted, nonviral delivery of small interfering RNA inhibits tumor growth in a murine model of metastatic Ewing's sarcoma. *Cancer Res* **65**: 8984–92.

140. Nimjee, S. M., Rusconi, C. P., and Sullenger, B. A. (2005). Aptamers: an emerging class of therapeutics. *Annu Rev Med* **56**: 555–83.

141. Pestourie, C., Tavitian, B., and Duconge, F. (2005). Aptamers against extracellular targets for in vivo applications. *Biochimie* **87**: 921–30.

142. Lowman, H. B. (1997). Bacteriophage display and discovery of peptide leads for drug development. *Annu Rev Biophys Biomol Struct* **26**: 401–24.

143. Farokhzad, O. C., Cheng, J., Teply, B. A., Sherifi, I., Jon, S., Kantoff, P. W., Richie, J. P., and Langer, R. (2006a). Targeted nanoparticle-aptamer bioconjugates for cancer chemotherapy in vivo. *Proc Natl Acad Sci U S A* **103**: 6315–20.

144. Farokhzad, O. C., Karp, J. M., and Langer, R. (2006b). Nanoparticle-aptamer bioconjugates for cancer targeting. *Expert Opin Drug Deliv* **3**: 311–24.

145. Reynolds, A., Anderson, E. M., Vermeulen, A., Fedorov, Y., Robinson, K., Leake, D., Karpilow, J., Marshall, W. S., and Khvorova, A. (2006). Induction of the interferon response by siRNA is cell type- and duplex length-dependent. *RNA* **12**: 988–93.

146. Smith, G. P. (1985). Filamentous fusion phage: novel expression vectors that display cloned antigens on the virion surface. *Science* **228**: 1315–7.

147. Ladner, R. C. (1995). Constrained peptides as binding entities. *Trends Biotechnol* **13**: 426–30.

148. Uchiyama, F., Tanaka, Y., Minari, Y., and Tokui, N. (2005). Designing scaffolds of peptides for phage display libraries. *J Biosci Bioeng* **99**: 448–56.

149. Giebel, L. B., Cass, R. T., Milligan, D. L., Young, D. C., Arze, R., and Johnson, C. R. (1995). Screening of cyclic peptide phage libraries identifies ligands that bind streptavidin with high affinities. *Biochemistry* **34**: 15430–5.

150. Nakamura, G. R., Starovasnik, M. A., Reynolds, M. E., and Lowman, H. B. (2001). A novel family of hairpin peptides that inhibit IgE activity by binding to the high-affinity IgE receptor. *Biochemistry* **40**: 9828–35.

151. Ladner, R. C. and Ley, A. C. (2001). Novel frameworks as a source of high-affinity ligands. *Curr Opin Biotechnol* **12**: 406–10.

152. Rebar, E. J. and Pabo, C. O. (1994). Zinc finger phage: affinity selection of fingers with new DNA-binding specificities. *Science* **263**: 671–3.

153. Friesen, W. J., and Darby, M. K. (1998). Specific RNA binding proteins constructed from zinc fingers. *Nat Struct Biol* **5**: 543–6.

154. Dennis, M. S., Herzka, A., and Lazarus, R. A. (1995). Potent and selective Kunitz domain inhibitors of plasma kallikrein designed by phage display. *J Biol Chem* **270**: 25411–7.

155. Herman, R. E., Badders, D., Fuller, M., Makienko, E. G., Houston, M. E., Quay, S. C., and Johnson, P. H. (2007). The TRP cage motif as a scaffold for the display of a randomized peptide library on bacteriophage T7. *J Biol Chem* **282**: 9812–24.

156. Neidigh, J. W., Fesinmeyer, R. M., Prickett, K. S., and Andersen, N. H. (2001). Exendin-4 and glucagon-like-peptide-1: NMR structural comparisons in the solution and micelle-associated states. *Biochemistry* **40**: 13188–200.

157. Neidigh, J. W., Fesinmeyer, R. M., and Andersen, N. H. (2002). Designing a 20-residue protein. *Nat Struct Biol* **9**: 425–30.

158. Qiu, L., Pabit, S. A., Roitberg, A. E., and Hagen, S. J. (2002). Smaller and faster: the 20-residue Trp-cage protein folds in 4 micros. *J Am Chem Soc* **124**: 12952–3.

159. Kim, D. H., Behlke, M. A., Rose, S. D., Chang, M. S., Choi, S., and Rossi, J. J. (2005). Synthetic dsRNA Dicer substrates enhance RNAi potency and efficacy. *Nat Biotechnol* **23**: 222–6.

160. Amarzguioui, M., Lundberg, P., Cantin, E., Hagstrom, J., Behlke, M. A., and Rossi, J. J. (2006). Rational design and in vitro and in vivo delivery of Dicer substrate siRNA. *Nat Protoc* **1**: 508–17.

161. Perrimon, N. and Mathey-Prevot, B. (2007). Applications of high-throughput RNA interference screens to problems in cell and developmental biology. *Genetics* **175**: 7–16.

162. Reynolds, A., Leake, D., Boese, Q., Scaringe, S., Marshall, W. S., and Khvorova, A. (2004). Rational siRNA design for RNA interference. *Nat Biotechnol* **22**: 326–30.

163. Rossi, J. J. (2005). RNAi and the P-body connection. *Nat Cell Biol* **7**: 643–4.

164. Czauderna, F., Fechtner, M., Dames, S., Aygun, H., Klippel, A., Pronk, G. J., Giese, K., and Kaufmann, J. (2003). Structural variations and stabilising modifications of synthetic siRNAs in mammalian cells. *Nucleic Acids Res* **31**: 2705–16.

165. Harborth, J., Elbashir, S. M., Vandenburgh, K., Manninga, H., Scaringe, S. A., Weber, K., and Tuschl, T. (2003). Sequence, chemical, and structural variation of small interfering RNAs and short hairpin RNAs and the effect on mammalian gene silencing. *Antisense Nucleic Acid Drug Dev* **13**: 83–105.

166. Wang, Q., Contag, C. H., Ilves, H., Johnston, B. H., and Kaspar, R. L. (2005). Small hairpin RNAs efficiently inhibit hepatitis C IRES-mediated gene expression in human tissue culture cells and a mouse model. *Mol Ther* **12**: 562–8.

167. Judge, A. D., Bola, G., Lee, A. C., and MacLachlan, I. (2006). Design of noninflammatory synthetic siRNA mediating potent gene silencing in vivo. *Mol Ther* **13**: 494–505.

168. Barton, G. M. and Medzhitov, R. (2002). Retroviral delivery of small interfering RNA into primary cells. *Proc Natl Acad Sci U S A* **99**: 14943–5.

169. Pack, D. W., Hoffman, A. S., Pun, S., and Stayton, P. S. (2005). Design and development of polymers for gene delivery. *Nat Rev Drug Discov* **4**: 581–93.

170. Duzgunes, N., De Ilarduya, C. T., Simoes, S., Zhdanov, R. I., Konopka, K., and Pedroso de Lima, M. C. (2003). Cationic liposomes for gene delivery: novel cationic lipids and enhancement by proteins and peptides. *Curr Med Chem* **10**: 1213–20.

171. Yang, J., Chen, H., Vlahov, I. R., Cheng, J. X., and Low, P. S. (2006). Evaluation of disulfide reduction during receptor-mediated endocytosis by using FRET imaging. *Proc Natl Acad Sci U S A* **103**: 13872–77.

172. Adami, R. C., Collard, W. T., Gupta, S. A., Kwok, K. Y., Bonadio, J., and Rice, K. G. (1998). Stability of peptide-condensed plasmid DNA formulations. *J Pharm Sci* **87**: 678–83.

173. Matsui, K., Horiuchi, S., Sando, S., Sera, T., and Aoyama, Y. (2006). RNAi silencing of exogenous and endogenous reporter genes using a macrocyclic

octaamine as a "compact" siRNA carrier. Studies on the nonsilenced residual activity. *Bioconjug Chem* **17**: 132–8.

174. Almofti, M. R., Harashima, H., Shinohara, Y., Almofti, A., Li, W., and Kiwada, H. (2003). Lipoplex size determines lipofection efficiency with or without serum. *Mol Membr Biol* **20**: 35–43.

175. Bloomfield, V. A., Crothers, D. M., and Tinoco, I. (2000). Nucleic acids structures, properties, and functions. *University Science Books*. Sausalito, CA.

176. Bartlett, D. W. and Davis, M. E. (2006). Insights into the kinetics of siRNA-mediated gene silencing from live-cell and live-animal bioluminescent imaging. *Nucleic Acids Res* **34**: 322–33.

177. Shankar, P., Manjunath, N., and Lieberman, J. (2005). The prospect of silencing disease using RNA interference. *JAMA* **293**: 1367–73.

178. Toub, N., Malvy, C., Fattal, E., and Couvreur, P. (2006). Innovative nanotechnologies for the delivery of oligonucleotides and siRNA. *Biomed Pharmacother* **60**: 607–20.

179. Sinha, R., Kim, G. J., Nie, S., and Shin, D. M. (2006). Nanotechnology in cancer therapeutics: bioconjugated nanoparticles for drug delivery. *Mol Cancer Ther* **5**: 1909–17.

180. Jonkheijm, P., Van Der Schoot, P., Schenning, A. P., and Meijer, E. W. (2006). Probing the solvent-assisted nucleation pathway in chemical self-assembly. *Science* **313**: 80–3.

181. Khaled, A., Guo, S., Li, F., and Guo, P. (2005). Controllable self-assembly of nanoparticles for specific delivery of multiple therapeutic molecules to cancer cells using RNA nanotechnology. *Nano Lett* **5**: 1797–808.

182. Niculescu-Duvaz, D., Heyes, J., and Springer, C. J. (2003). Structure-activity relationship in cationic lipid mediated gene transfection. *Curr Med Chem* **10**: 1233–61.

183. Harvie, P., Wong, F. M., and Bally, M. B. (1998). Characterization of lipid DNA interactions. I. Destabilization of bound lipids and DNA dissociation. *Biophys J* **75**: 1040–51.

184. Tye, H. (2004). Application of statistical "design of experiments" methods in drug discovery. *Drug Discov Today* **9**: 485–91.

185. Singh, B., Kumar, R., and Ahuja, N. (2005). Optimizing drug delivery systems using systematic "design of experiments." Part I: fundamental aspects. *Crit Rev Ther Drug Carrier Syst* **22**: 27–105.

186. Singh, B., Dahiya, M., Saharan, V., and Ahuja, N. (2005). Optimizing drug delivery systems using systematic "design of experiments." Part II: retrospect and prospects. *Crit Rev Ther Drug Carrier Syst* **22**: 215–94.

187. Macrae, I. J., Zhou, K., Li, F., Repic, A., Brooks, A. N., Cande, W. Z., Adams, P. D., and Doudna, J. A. (2006). Structural basis for double-stranded RNA processing by Dicer. *Science* **311**: 195–8.

CHAPTER 6

siRNA DELIVERY VEHICLES

ALIASGER K. SALEM and MARK A. BEHLKE

6.1 INTRODUCTION

RNA interference (RNAi) has become the method of choice to suppress gene expression *in vitro*. It is also emerging as a powerful tool for *in vivo* research. In this chapter, we discuss the potential for use of delivery systems for synthetic small interfering RNAs (siRNAs) to overcome the limitations of siRNAs and enhance therapeutic efficacy.

Altering the expression levels of genes using specialized molecules is an approach that has received increasing interest within the scientific and clinical community. A significant milestone in this technology was reported by Fire and Mello in 1998, where double-stranded RNAs (dsRNAs) that were several hundred bases long initiated suppression of complementary genes in the nematode *Caenorhabditis elegans*. The process was coined RNAi [1]. Antiviral defense mechanisms in higher organisms are complex and similar long dsRNAs stimulate interferon (IFN) release, triggering a cascade of interferon-stimulated genes in addition to RNAi. As a result, long dsRNAs are not suitable for use as triggers of RNAi in mammalian cells. It was later determined that long dsRNAs did not directly cause gene suppression; rather, the long dsRNAs were processed by an endoribonuclease called Dicer into smaller 21–23 base pair (bp) duplexes with 2-base 3′-overhangs. These species were called siRNAs and are the actual molecules responsible for suppression [2–4]. SiRNAs prepared synthetically can be transfected into cells and provide specific suppression of complementary genes. They do not usually trigger the IFN responses associated with long dsRNAs [5]. SiRNAs enter a multimember protein complex called the RNA-induced silencing complex (RISC). One strand of the duplex (the passenger strand) is cleaved and

RNA Interference: Application to Drug Discovery and Challenges to Pharmaceutical Development, Edited by Paul H. Johnson
Copyright © 2011 John Wiley & Sons, Inc.

discarded. The other strand (the guide strand) is retained and directs the sequence specificity of RISC and thus the specificity of the RNAi silencing [6,7].

SiRNAs can be very potent. Transfections at subnanomolar concentrations are able to achieve greater than 90% reduction in mRNA levels. [8]. The use of siRNAs has virtually superseded antisense oligonucleotides as the most prominent gene knockdown tool used *in vitro* and is showing increasing promise for *in vivo* applications. This chapter focuses on the formulation and delivery of siRNA duplexes *in vivo*. Other chapters and recent reviews consider *in vivo* use of siRNA from different perspectives including chemical modification [9–20].

6.1.1   Current Limitations to Delivery of siRNAs *in Vivo*

Delivery of siRNAs is a critical issue for ensuring efficacy *in vivo*. Viral vectors are very efficient for delivery of siRNAs. However, viral vectors also have several concerns associated with immunogenicity. Viral vectors have been associated with instigating leukemia and anaphylaxis. In addition, production of viral vectors can be time-consuming and costly due to increased safety requirements. Although duplex RNA is more resistant to nuclease attack than single-stranded DNA, unmodified siRNAs are nevertheless rapidly degraded when administered intravenously (IV) in mammals. SiRNAs can also stimulate undesirable immune responses as detailed below. Degradation of siRNA and stimulation of an immune response can be delayed or avoided by chemical modification of the oligonucleotides and/or by complexation with a carrier/delivery particle [21].

6.1.2   IFN Induction and the Innate Immune System

One significant barrier in the use of antisense DNA oligonucleotides was a sequence-specific induction of the innate immune system. This effect resulted from interaction of DNAs bearing unmethylated CpG motifs with Toll-like receptor 9 (TLR9). As discussed above, it was well known that long dsRNA results in strong type-1 IFN responses *in vivo*, but it was originally anticipated that the shorter siRNAs would be safe to use. Unfortunately, short siRNAs can also induce IFN responses. IFN responses are not always generated following siRNA administration since stimulation is both sequence and cell type specific. TLR3, 7, and 8 specifically recognize RNAs. TLR3, 7, and 8 are found in intracellular locations such as endosomes or lysosomes. Other members of the TLR family are found on the cell surface [22–24]. IFN responses can also be triggered by the dsRNA-dependent protein kinase (PKR), $2',5'$-oligoadenylate synthetase (OAS), and retinoic acid inducible gene I (RIG-I) pathways [25, 26]. Because TLR3, 7, and 8 are all found in intracellular compartments such as endosomes, ligands for these TLRs must reach these locations for activation to take place. Thus, use of cationic lipid type delivery tools, which provide access to these compartments, maximizes the risk of triggering IFN responses. More information about siRNA activation of innate immunity via TLR signaling can be found in a review by Marques and Williams [27]. From a delivery perspective, it has been shown that extensive 2'-modification of a sequence that is otherwise strongly immunostimulatory as unmodified RNA can prevent an immune response when that same sequence is administered IV in mice using a lipid-based particle delivery system [21]. In addition, formulation strategies allow for the co-encapsulation of endosomal inhibitors such as chloroquine that might blunt innate immune responses to siRNAs.

6.1.3 siRNA Administration Without Delivery Assistance

In spite of the relative susceptibility of unmodified siRNA duplexes to degradation in serum, several groups have reported positive results using unmodified siRNAs administered by low volume IV injection in mice without the use of any facilitated delivery system [28–32]. Before discussing delivery strategies to enhance siRNA delivery efficacy, we should make note of these results. For example, unmodified siRNAs that target vascular endothelial growth factor (*VEGF*) were delivered to nude mice bearing subcutaneous (SC) implants of rat fibrosarcoma cJ4 cells that express luciferase [29]. SiRNAs (125 μg/kg/day) in Phosphate Buffered Saline (PBS) were injected IV, IP, or SC at a dose of 3 μg per injection. Regardless of the route of administration, a single anti-*VEGF* siRNA dose given to the mice showed 40–50% suppression of luciferase activity in the tumor implants by day 3 postinjection in comparison with controls. Those mice that were given intraperitoneal (IP) injections of siRNAs in PBS every day showed a 66% reduction in tumor volume and a 70% reduction in tumor-associated VEGF levels compared with controls after day 16. The effects that changes in levels of ribonucleotide reductase (RR) have on the efficacy of gemcitabine treatment of pancreatic tumor cells implants in nude mice have also been studied [30]. Higher levels of RR have been linked as a cause of resistance to gemcitabine chemotherapy. SiRNAs targeting the M2 subunit of RR (*RRM2*) can reduce the RR levels, which, therefore, increases tumor cell susceptibility to gemcitabine *in vitro*. For example, MIAPaCa2 pancreatic tumor cells were implanted in nude mice and were given control treatments, an anti-*RRM2* siRNA (150 μg/kg IV), and/or gemcitabine (150 mg IP) twice weekly for 6 weeks. The anti-*RRM2* siRNA-treated mice showed reduced RRM2 levels in tumor extracts compared with control siRNA-treated mice. Treatment with gemcitabine or the anti-*RRM2* siRNA alone resulted in a modest reduction in tumor volume while treatment with the combination of gemcitabine with anti-*RRM2* siRNA showed a synergistic effect with 87% reduction in tumor size. Mice receiving combination treatment had no detectable liver metastasis whereas 80% of the control and 40% of gemcitabine or siRNA monotherapy animals had significant tumor burden in their livers. Similarly, CEACAM6 is a cell surface adhesion molecule linked with pancreatic adenocarcinoma tumor progression and metastasis. Anti-*CEACAM6* siRNAs, therefore, have potential as a therapy for reducing tumor growth. As with the anti-*RRM2* siRNA study, unmodified siRNAs were dosed at 150 µg/kg in PBS IV twice weekly. BxPC3 cells were implanted in the pancreas of nude mice and animals were given either PBS alone, a control siRNA, or an anti-*CEACAM6* siRNA for 6 weeks. Mice treated with target-specific siRNAs had smaller tumors, 46% lower CEACAM6 levels, reduced evidence for angiogenesis, and reduced hepatic metastasis than control mice. Survival after 6 weeks of treatment was 0/10 for PBS-treated mice, 0/10 for control siRNA-treated mice, and 9/10 for anti-*CEACAM6*-treated mice [31].

Although some researchers have reported success in use of unmodified siRNAs without delivery vehicles, due to the current limitations of siRNA delivery described in Section 6.1.1, the majority of studies have reported that improved uptake and efficacy can be seen when siRNAs are administered as a complex with some kind of polymer that facilitates delivery and/or tissue targeting.

6.2 NONVIRAL siRNA DELIVERY VEHICLES

Chemical modifications, can be used to provide stabilization to duplexes and protect against degradation. However, plasma clearance can still happen quickly. Using a delivery vehicle can help to protect against degradation and improve the pharmacokinetics. For example, in one study the plasma half-life of an unmodified siRNA duplex in mice was 0.03 h and the half-life of a modified duplex was 0.8 h, which was improved to 6.5 h by delivering the modified duplex in a stabilized nucleic acid lipid particle (SNALP) [21]. In a similar study, unconjugated duplexes injected in rats had an elimination half-life of 0.1 h but conjugating cholesterol to the duplex increased the half-life to 1.5 h. As discussed above, unmodified duplexes have shown some potential for *in vivo* applications but these studies suggest that increased therapeutic benefit will be achieved by utilizing a delivery system. Optimally, the system would combine use of chemically modified duplexes with the delivery strategies described in this chapter or peptide delivery tools.

In the following sections, we describe some of the nonviral drug delivery vehicles that have shown the most promise for delivery of siRNA. Nonviral delivery is favorable for siRNA delivery because of ease of use, potential for large-scale production, and reduced specific immune responses. Nonviral siRNA delivery broadly falls into two categories: physical methods and synthetic methods.

6.2.1 Physical Methods

Direct injection is a facile and safe method to deliver unmodified duplexes to the target location. However, siRNA delivered by this technique remains susceptible to degradation by nucleases. As a result, direct injection is most effective when combined with physical methods that improve the efficiency of delivery and thus duplex activity.

Electroporation   Electroporation permeabilizes the membranes of cells when an electrical current is applied. The siRNA is usually delivered in high ionic strength mediums. Skin and muscle are the most common targets for electroporation. Optimization of electroporation includes factors such as siRNA dose, electrode shape and number, and electrical field strength and duration [33]. Electroporation is a useful method for delivering siRNAs *in vitro* to cell lines that are resistant to alternative methods of delivery such as cationic lipid mediated transfection. It is a technique that is also being investigated for siRNA delivery *in vivo*. For example, electroporation has been used to deliver unmodified anti-*EGFP* siRNA into mouse muscles in conjunction with EGFP expression plasmids [34]. Significant inhibition of EGFP fluorescence was observed for the anti-*EGFP* but not for the control siRNA. Electroporation has also been used to deliver unmodified siRNAs targeting TNF-α in mice with collagen-induced arthritis (CIA) [35]. Local expression of EGFP in knee joints of mice was only observed if electroporation was employed to deliver EGFP expression plasmids. In addition, luciferase expression plasmids were delivered with siRNAs that suppressed luciferase or siRNAs that suppress EGFP. Only the combination with the siRNA that suppresses luciferase showed 90% suppression of luciferase activity. To induce arthritism, mice were injected with 2 doses of type-II collagen. Inflammation was initiated by IP injection of LPS 3 days after the second dose. Three days after the LPS injection, mice were given 3 weekly 10 μg doses of anti-*TNF*-α siRNA into the knee joint using direct injection with electroporation. Anti-*TNF*-α siRNA treatment significant reduced inflammation and arthritis scores in comparison with controls. Similar observations were seen when electroporation was used to deliver unmodified siRNA targeting TNF-α complexed with cationic lipid (siPORT Amine) in rats with collagen-induced arthritis [36].

Significant reduction of TNF-α mRNA levels in synovial tissue and inflammation was observed using paw swelling and histological examination relative to controls.

Gene Gun Delivery of siRNAs   Gene guns can be used for the direct delivery of siRNAs into cells. Commercially supplied gold particles with spermidine on the surface are coated with siRNA and then fired at cells, resulting in direct penetration through the cell membrane and delivery of the nucleic acid cargo. Typical pressures for delivery of the gold particles are in the region of 400 psi allowing for shallow subdermal penetration [37, 38]. The gene gun can be used to improve immune responses in mice treated with DNA vaccines [39]. Human papillomavirus type 16 (HPV-16) virus infection is associated with development of cervical cancer. In one study, mice were immunized against HPV-16 using a plasmid expressing the *E7* gene of HPV-16; however, a robust immune response was not generated in part as a result of the transient nature of gene expression when delivered by the gene gun. Delivering the HPV-16 E7 plasmid with siRNAs targeting the proapoptotic genes *BAX* and *BAK* increased the number of antigen-specific IFN-γ^+ CD8$^+$ T-cell precursors. The combined vaccine significantly reduced TC-1 tumor load in comparison with vaccines delivered with a control siRNA.

Sonoporation Delivery of siRNAs   Cell membrane permeability to siRNAs can also be increased using ultrasound. Ultrasound contrast agents such as microbubbles help to reduce the energy threshold for cavitation. For example, microbubbles from focused ultrasound (aka sonoporation) have been used to deliver siRNAs to cells *in vitro* [40]. Sonoporation was used to deliver an EGFP expression plasmid with or without an unmodified anti-*EGFP* siRNA to cardiac tissue in mice [41]. Injection of the EGFP-expression plasmid was targeted to the left ventricle of anesthetized mice and transthoracic ultrasound stimulation was applied. Only the injection with the anti-*EGFP* siRNA inhibited EGFP fluorescence in the cardiac ventricular wall and in the coronary arteries.

Administration Using Hydrodynamic Delivery   High-pressure hydrodynamic intravascular injection involves quick delivery of relatively big volumes to enhance delivery of siRNAs. Parameters that can be optimized in this method are the injection rate and volume. Volumes range in values equivalent to 1/10th of an animal's body weight. The injection rates for 0.1 mL/g are typically in the range of 0.3–0.4 mL/s [33]. Volumes or rates below these critical values tend to result in significant decreases in delivery efficiency. Using the hydrodynamic (HD) method, siRNAs predominantly accumulate in the liver and lesser proportions are also found distributed in the kidney, spleen, lung, and heart. The mechanism of cellular uptake is purported to be due to membrane disruption. An alternative hypothesis states that the HD method results in extravasation in hepatocytes combined with receptor mediated endocytosis. For example, luciferase expression plasmids with unmodified controls were delivered to mice using the HD delivery method and assessed using *in vivo* bioluminescence imaging 3 days after injection [42]. Luciferase activity in the liver was only significantly reduced (by 81%) when the plasmids were codelivered with the anti*luciferase* siRNAs. Although IFN levels (or other cytokines) were not measured, the hAAT marker was utilized as a control for nonspecific effects. RNAi activity was detected in several tissues, including liver, kidney, spleen, lung, and pancreas [43]. Duration of silencing determined using expression plasmids encoding secreted human placental alkaline phosphatase (SEAP) and an anti-*SEAP* siRNA delivered by HD injection showed 83% suppression on day 1 postinjection, 32% on day 4, and were at control levels by day 14.

The HD method has been used to deliver siRNAs that protect mice from liver damage triggered by Fas-mediated apoptosis [44]. Three doses of 50 µg Anti-*Fas* siRNAs or control anti-*EGFP* siRNAs were delivered. A 10-fold reduction in *Fas* mRNA and Fas protein levels was observed in the mouse hepatocytes in comparison with controls with suppression lasting approximately 10 days. The anti-*Fas* siRNA did not stimulate fulminant hepatitis or hepatic fibrosis in mice after treatment with Concanavalin A, which is a known inducer of hepatitis. Delivery of the anti-*Fas* siRNA also protected mice from a dose of anti-Fas antibody (Jo2), which normally kills in a few days and can protect mice from renal ischemia-reperfusion injury [45]. In these studies, renal ischemia was triggered by clamping one renal pedicle for 35 min and the other kidney was removed. For mice treated with the anti-*Fas* siRNA, 8/10 survived in comparison with 2/10 for those receiving a control siRNA or saline.

Caspase 8 is an essential enzyme in the Fas-apoptosis pathway. The HD method has been used to deliver siRNAs that target *caspase 8* to block hepatic necrosis following challenge with the agonist anti-Fas antibody (Jo2) or recombinant adenoviruses encoding Fas ligand [46]. SiRNAs were administered using HD tail vein or portal vein injections. A fourfold reduction in *Caspase 8* mRNA levels was observed following siRNA delivery to mouse hepatocytes, with 5/11 mice surviving in comparison with the 0/17 mice treated with controls. Anti-*caspase 8* and anti-*caspase 3* siRNAs have shown protection for mice from hepatic ischemia-reperfusion injury [47]. Hydrodynamic delivery has also been used to demonstrate the antiviral potential of siRNAs *in vivo*.

For example, a plasmid encoding the Hepatitis B virus (HBV) genome that was codelivered with anti-HBV siRNAs to the livers of mice using the HD method was able to reduce HBV titers generated in transfected livers by 10^5 on day 2 and 10^2 on day 3 at the dose studied [48]. A similar HBV plasmid model system was employed in another report, which similarly studied use of anti-HBV siRNAs in mice using HD delivery [49]. When modified RNAs were compared with unmodified RNAs, the modified duplexes displayed a 1.5 log greater reduction in HBV DNA and surface antigen levels 72 h after injection than unmodified siRNAs. Only the modified duplexes (albeit at a higher dose) were able to inhibit HBV when injected 3 days after initiation of infection by HBV plasmid injection.

HD delivery does have some potential adverse consequences, which must be considered. The HD delivery method results in a rise in serum alanine aminotransferase that is linked to low degrees of hepatocytes necrosis. Liver toxicity may be a potential limitation for human use [33]. As a result, HD has largely been viewed as a research tool. However, some success for HD delivery of siRNAs and other nucleic acids to skeletal muscle in rats, dogs, and Rhesus macaques have been reported [50]. In a modification of the original HD delivery methods, a limb is isolated by application of a blood pressure cuff or tourniquet and a large volume of the siRNA solution is administered IV. Therapeutic delivery of plasmids or siRNAs in humans using this approach may be possible with only moderate reversible tissue damage if care is taken in application of the technique [51].

6.2.2 Synthetic siRNA Delivery Systems

As mentioned earlier, unmodified siRNAs are rapidly degraded when administered IV in mammals. Many of the delivery tools developed for plasmid DNA can be adapted to siRNA. It should be noted that cationic polymers can bind to phosphate backbones of siRNA but cannot condense them to the same extent as plasmid DNA. As a result, any formulation developed for siRNA delivery cannot simply be extrapolated from plasmid DNA studies but must undergo separate optimization experiments [52]. The following sections describe some of the most promising formulations and delivery approaches for siRNA.

Liposomes The vast majority of delivery systems developed for siRNAs have focused on liposomes, lipids, and variations thereof. Liposomes are spherical vesicles composed of a membrane that is formed from cholesterol and phospholipid bilayers. Liposomes can be formed from mixed lipid chains such as phosphatidylethanolamine or from pure lipids such as dioleolylphosphatidyl ethanolamine (DOPE). Liposomes have a central aqueous core that is suitable for transporting a nucleic acid cargo. In addition to the hydrophilic core, liposomes form a hydrophobic membrane shell. Because hydrophilic solutes cannot pass through lipids very easily, entrapping them in these cores masks their hydrophilicity, allowing them to pass through hydrophobic environments (like membranes) more readily. The versatility of liposomes means that in converse, hydrophobic compounds can be entrapped in the membrane allowing for delivery of both hydrophobic and hydrophilic compounds. To deliver the siRNA to an intracellular location, the liposomal lipid bilayer can fuse with other lipid bilayers, such as cell membranes, thus delivering the liposome contents. Cationic liposomes are composed of positively charged lipid bilayers and can be complexed with negatively charged siRNA duplexes. Studies on cationic liposome-DNA complexes have shown that a two-dimensional columnar phase exists in the lipid composition regime that is substantially more effective at delivering nucleic acids when compared with the lamellar structured cationic liposome–DNA complexes. Optical microscopy studies showed that the lamellar structured complexes could bind stably to model anionic cellular membranes, while the hexagonal lattice complexes were less stable and rapidly fused and released the DNA once they had bound to the model anionic cellular membrane [53].

Although cationic lipids are routinely used as transfection reagents *in vitro*, their use *in vivo* is limited by toxicity. This toxicity is highest with IV administration; successful *in vivo* use of cationic lipids to deliver siRNAs has been reported using IP administration, intrathecal, or direct CNS injection, and topical applications [54–60]. Toxicity can be reduced by careful control over the dose, chemical composition and other parameters. For example, liposomes have been specifically formulated to have decreased toxicity when delivered IV. However, care must be taken when changing the chemical composition because it can also change the properties and efficacy of the delivery system [61]. Liposomes are attractive as drug delivery vehicles because they already have FDA approval for use [62]. Attaching ligands such as folate can enhance their targeting efficiency and provide more desirable and/or specific biodistribution [63, 64]. The use of targeting ligands will be discussed in greater detail in Section 6.4. Conjugation of hydrophilic polyethylene glycol (PEG) onto the surface of liposomes can provide greater steric stabilization in an aqueous environment and imbue "stealth" like properties to the particles. PEG can reduce the relative "stickiness" of liposomes to serum proteins, which are detected by reticuloendothelial cells and macrophages and can trigger opsonization and clearance of liposome/protein aggregates. A PEG coating can therefore reduce/delay clearance and enhance the pharmokinetic profiles [65, 66]. The use of PEG modifications will be discussed in greater detail in Section 6.3. Liposomes have been successfully utilized for delivery of antisense oligonucleotides and siRNAs *in vivo* [21, 67–69].

While a significant number of reports have shown successful *in vivo* delivery of siRNAs using liposome or polyplex reagents, toxicity remains a concern that must be addressed. For example, a direct comparison of the relative toxicity in mice of siRNAs delivered in cationic 1,2-dioleoyl-3-trimethylammonium-propane (DOTAP) liposomes versus the cardiolipin analogue CCLA:DOPE liposomes was performed using IV injection. The CCLA liposomes were found to be significantly less toxic [69]. A single dose of 100 mg/kg of DOTAP liposomes killed 2/3 mice in comparison with 0/3 mice treated with the CCLA liposomes. However, multiple doses of the CCLA liposomes at the same concentration still resulted in a 1/3 mortality rate. This suggests that some toxicity and morbidity may still be occurring even though the mice survive treatment. Toxicity of cationic lipids is associated with electrostatic effects and as a result the ratio of the lipid to siRNA can have a significant impact on adverse effects. Serum can lead to aggregation and inactivation of lipid delivery complexes, which is an issue that has plagued gene delivery for many years. Particle aggregation can result in clumping in capillary beds, another potential barrier to use. Cationic particles can interact with serum proteins that can trigger an inflammatory cascade, including a Type-1 IFN response. Higher doses of liposomes can incur hepatic necrosis, thrombocytopenia, and lymphopenia [70]. Liposomal systems that present a neutral stabilized surface have lower toxicity, increase circulation times and enhance stability [71]. Reviews by Dass [72], Audouy [73], and Simberg [74] discuss in greater detail cationic liposome delivery methods and *in vivo* toxicity issues.

As discussed earlier, the synthetic cardiolipin analogue (CCLA) is a cationic liposome that displays sevenfold higher efficiency and lower toxicity than DOTAP liposomes in IV administration of siRNAs [69]. The Ras/Raf/MAPK signaling pathway is involved in approximately 1/3 of human cancers. An unmodified siRNA specific for *c-raf* was injected IV to Severe Combine Immune Deficiency (SCID) mice that had a SC breast cancer tumor MDA-MB-231. By day 8, liposomal formulations of the siRNA resulted in tumors that were 73% smaller than mice treated with the siRNA alone. These results emphasize the importance of a delivery vehicle for anti-*c-Raf* siRNA treatment. In a related study, the anti-*Raf-1* siRNA was delivered with or without the chemotherapy agent Taxotere to inhibit growth of SC implants of the prostate cancer cell line PC-3 in SCID mice [68]. The siRNA was also delivered with or without liposomal formulation. Delivery of the siRNA alone reduced Raf-1 protein levels by 37% and had no effect on tumor growth. Delivery of the liposomal formulation of siRNA reduced Raf-1 levels by 89% and suppressed tumor growth by 49%. Delivery of the liposomal formulation of siRNA in combination with Taxotere reduced Raf-1 levels by 98% and inhibited tumor growth by 89%.

As discussed earlier, neutral liposomes are attractive for IV delivery of siRNAs. For example, neutral liposomes composed of 1,2-dioleoyl-*sn*-glycero-3-phosphatidylcholine (DOPC) resulted in an approximately 10-fold increase in delivery efficiency when compared with DOTAP liposomes and a 30-fold improvement in efficacy in comparison with nucleic acids with no delivery vehicle. The highest uptake of siRNA was observed in liver, kidney, and lungs [75]. Some human cancers overexpress the tyrosine kinase receptor EphA2. This overexpression is correlated with poor prognosis in ovarian cancer. An anti-*EphA2* siRNA with or without liposomal formulation was administered to nude mice with IP implants of the ovarian cancer cell line HeyA8 or SKOV3ip1, with or without the chemotherapeutic agent paclitaxel. The average tumor size was reduced by 35–50% using the anti-*EphA2* siRNA, by 45–68% using paclitaxel, and by 86–91% with combination therapy. As discussed with the anti-*c-Raf* siRNA studies, several reports have shown that the combination of siRNA with a cytotoxic chemotherapeutic agent works synergistically in reducing tumor size.

A promising lipid particle for siRNA delivery is the SNALP that is composed of cationic, neutral, and fusogenic lipids, which fully encapsulate the nucleic acid cargo [21]. Liposomes that encapsulate siRNA are typically prepared by mixing lipids (DSPC:Chol:PEG-C-DMA: DLinDMA = 20:48:2:30 molar ratio) in ethanol with an aqueous solution of siRNA in a controlled, stepwise manner. SNALPs were formed after an instantaneous dilution of ethanol and a second stepwise dilution. SNALPs have previously been reported to improve delivery of antisense oligonucleotides in mice [76]. Tekmira Pharmaceuticals, British Columbia, Canada (previously Protiva Biotherapeutics) has utilized SNALP technology to introduce RNAi-based therapeutics for liver-related diseases, such as hepatitis B and hypercholesterolemia [77–79]. Unmodified siRNAs administered using this delivery method strongly stimulated innate immune responses, while the highly modified duplexes (including $2'$-O-methyl, $2'$-F, DNA, and PS bonds) did not. When siRNAs were delivered using SNALPs, the highest levels of RNAs were found in the liver and spleen but displayed limited accumulation in the lung. Modified siRNAs delivered in SNALPs had a plasma half-life 6.5 h compared with 2 min for unmodified naked siRNAs.

Delivering siRNAs with cationic lipids is also advantageous because it can lower the dose needed for efficacy. For example, an unmodified control siRNA or a siRNA specific for the delta opioid receptor (DOR) was delivered as an implanted intrathecal catheter in the lumbar spine of rats [58]. Low doses of siRNA (2.5–20 µg/kg) were delivered using the cationic lipid i-Fect™. Fluorescence signals could be seen from the dye-labeled siRNA in the spinal cord and dorsal root ganglia only when delivered with the lipid. An anti-*DOR* siRNA generated significant reductions in DOR protein levels but not in the control-treated animals. Confirmation of specificity was supported by the absence of any detectable change in levels of the related mu opioid receptor. Although the use of siRNAs in CNS studies has been shown to be efficacious, a few groups have encountered limited benefits *in vivo* even when the same siRNAs were effective *in vitro* [80, 81].

We have discussed IP and IV routes of administration. Cationic lipids can also be employed to facilitate delivery through epithelial or mucosal surfaces. For example, unmodified siRNAs have been delivered topically in a murine deafness model system [59]. The *GJB2* gene (gap junction protein, beta-2) encodes a transmembrane protein that is involved in potassium recycling during auditory signaling. Some severe forms of hereditary deafness are caused by allelic variants of this gene. DOTAP/cholesterol liposomes (GeneSHUT-TLE^{TM}) were used to deliver anti-*GJB2$_{R75W}$* siRNAs to the cochleae of mice in a mixture using 0.5 μg siRNA in 2 μL soaked in a piece of gel foam which was surgically placed against the round window membrane. SiRNA delivered in this fashion reversed the auditory impairment caused by expression of the mutant human gene in mouse cochleae with an associated reduction in expression of *GJB2$_{R75W}$* mRNA by 70%. Cationic lipid carriers have also been used as a topical paste intravaginally to block herpes simplex virus-2 (HSV2) infection in mice [60]. Mice that were vaginally infected with HSV2 and treated with the optimal anti-HSV2 siRNAs using lipid delivery had ~80% survival at day 15. In contrast, those mice that received the control or no siRNA had 20–25% survival. In these studies, no activation of the immune response was observed. Therefore delivery of siRNAs in liposomal or cationic lipid pastes or paints should have potential for other epithelial surfaces, such as oral or rectal mucosa.

Naked siRNAs or siRNAs complexed with cationic lipids have been used to treat respiratory viruses. Direct delivery can be achieved by intranasal or intratracheal administration; alternatively, siRNAs can be given IV. For example, unmodified siRNAs specific to viral NP and PA proteins have been shown to protect mice from lethal infection with influenza virus injected IV using the HD delivery method [82]. Viral titers in lung tissue were 63-fold lower when antiinfluenza siRNAs were administered in comparison with control siRNAs. Using intranasal administration, the use of cationic lipids may improve results. For example, unmodified siRNAs with or without complexation with the cationic lipid TransIT-TKO^{TM} were used to treat pulmonary infection with respiratory syncytial virus (RSV) and parainfluenza virus (PIV) in mice by targeting the viral "*P*" gene for both viruses [83]. Delivery of siRNAs without the cationic lipid had 70% of the efficacy in comparison with delivery with the cationic lipid.

There are some drawbacks to the use of cationic lipids as delivery vehicles for siRNAs. Cationic lipid transfection agents deliver nucleic acids to endosomal compartments in cells *in vitro* whereas electroporation or other physical delivery approaches do not, and siRNA delivery done using electroporation is less likely to stimulate IFN secretion [84]. These observations appear to translate *in vivo*. Unmodified siRNAs complexed with lipids/liposomes delivered IV are more likely to cause IFN pathway activation [21] when compared with unmodified "naked" siRNAs using the HD delivery method [85–87]. A note of caution has also been advised when using liposomal mediated delivery of siRNAs because of reports that the stability of reporter mRNAs is independent of multiple modifications including the AUUUA instability element, poly(A) tails and 5′ methylated caps when delivered in a liposomal formulation. Even typically hyper-unstable nonadenylated mRNAs remain stable when delivered in liposomes with limited degradation over a 4-h period. One explanation for this was that the transfected RNAs remained confined in a cellular compartment that removed the mRNAs from mechanisms responsible for degradation. Under these circumstances, a significant proportion of the delivered RNA molecules would not be used and would have the potential to induce toxicity [88].

In work originating from Alnylam Pharmaceuticals and Protiva Biotherapeutics (now Tekmira Pharmaceuticals), Zimmerman and colleagues demonstrated that siRNAs delivered systemically in a liposomal formulation can silence the target apolipoprotein B (ApoB) in nonhuman primates. ApoB-specific siRNAs were encapsulated in SNALPs and dosed to cynomolgus monkeys by IV injection at 1 or 2.5 mg/kg. A single siRNA injection resulted in dose-dependent silencing of APOB messenger RNA expression in the liver 48 h after administration, with maximal silencing of >90%. Significant reductions in ApoB protein, serum cholesterol and low-density lipoprotein (LDL) levels were observed as early as 24 h after treatment and lasted for at least 11 days at the highest siRNA dose [79].

More recently, teams from Massachusetts Institute of Technology (MIT) including Anderson, Langer, and colleagues (working together with Alnylam Pharmaceuticals) have been aggressively pursuing new derivatives of liposome-based technologies for siRNA delivery using a novel combinatorial lipid library approach. Akinc and colleagues described a new class of liposome RNAi delivery systems called "lipidoids." The authors created a collection of more than 1200 structurally different lipidoids. They then identified compounds that could induce significant silencing when prepared with either siRNA or single-stranded antisense 2′-O-methyl (2′-OMe) oligoribonucleotides targeting microRNA (miRNA) [89]. They showed that linking to bile acids or long-chain fatty acids and cholesterol resulted in siRNA uptake into cells and efficient *in vivo* silencing. Tissue distribution for siRNAs uptake was influenced by whether high- or low-density lipoprotein was used. High-density lipoprotein (HDL) resulted in siRNA accumulation in the liver, gut, kidney, and steroidogenic organs. In contrast, use of LDL led to accumulation mainly in the liver. The organ-specificity was due to varying expression of LDL-receptor and SR-B1 receptor (for HDL) [90]. Improvements in lipid content and formulation ratios have led to newer generation of lipid nanoparticles that can achieve significant liver gene silencing in mice even after a

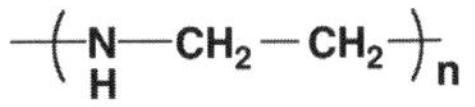

$$-\left(\begin{array}{c}N\\H\end{array}-CH_2-CH_2\right)_n$$

FIGURE 6.1   Base chemical structure of PEI.

single injection at doses below 0.01 mg/kg. In nonhuman primates, doses as low as 0.03 mg/kg effectively silenced the *transthyretin* gene [91]. In other recent studies, researchers from Alnylam Pharmaceuticals, Tekmira Pharmaceuticals, and the University of British Columbia developed novel lipid agents (different from the lipidoids) that showed excellent potential for use in delivery of siRNA. In these studies, potent *in vivo* activity was achieved using siRNA doses as low as 0.01 mg/kg in rodents and 0.1 mg/kg in nonhuman primates [92]. Lipid-based technologies have advanced far beyond the older, highly toxic reagents that are well known and commonly used in research labs; these new generation compounds have tremendous potential for therapeutic use.

Polyethyleneimine   A wide variety of methods have been used to facilitate delivery of nucleic acids which do not employ cationic lipids. Nucleic acids have a high negative charge density and some kind of cationic polymer is usually employed to bind the nucleic acid, neutralize charge, and assist with transport across the cell membrane. Polyethyleneimine (PEI) (Figure 6.1) has been used for many years to facilitate nucleic acid delivery [93]; however, due to toxicity and variable performance it has not found widespread acceptance as a delivery tool for either antisense oligonucleotides or siRNAs.

The cationic polymer PEI comes in two forms: linear and branched. The repeat unit of the polymer is two carbon atoms followed by a nitrogen atom. In the branched form, PEI has 1°, 2°, and 3° amines that can be protonated, allowing PEI to serve as a buffer through a wide pH range. The positive charge of the PEI gives effective binding to the negatively charged nucleic acids, and complexation/condensation protects the nucleic acids from digestion in serum and as the complex enters cells. Once in the endosomal compartment, PEI might act as a buffer to induce osmotic swelling and cause release from the endosome, which is necessary to avoid degradation of the nucleic acids when the endosome fuses with the lysosome. Previous studies have found that PEI/DNA complexes with higher buffering capacities give better transfection efficiencies [94].

PEI has drawn interest for nucleic acid delivery applications because of its endosomolytic activity and strong nucleic acid compaction ability. However, cell viability has been shown to be adversely affected by exposure to PEI, possibly because of membrane permeabilization by PEI. We have previously observed in cell culture that PEI has an LD50 value (value at which 50% of the cells die) of around 25 μg/m. The LD_{50} of linear PEI is around 4 mg/kg in mice [95], significantly limiting *in vivo* utility. When bound to a ligand, the cytotoxic effects of PEI appear to be lessened. Lower molecular weight PEI has lower toxicity than higher molecular weight PEI, most likely because of aggregation of the larger molecules on the outer cell membrane.

Several studies have suggested that the branched form of the molecule gives greater success in delivery of nucleic acids [96, 97]. However, some reports suggest that PEI22, a linear version of the molecule, had greater delivery efficiencies than the branched molecules PEI25 or PEI800 when applied to neuroblastoma and colon carcinoma cell lines *in vitro* [98]. It has been reported that the molecular weight of the PEI affects transfection efficiencies, with lower molecular weight PEI (25 kDa) giving better uptake than higher molecular weight PEI (800 kDa), possibly because of aggregation of higher molecular weight particles [96, 97]. The ratio of the nitrogen atoms in PEI to the phosphate atoms in the siRNA is called the N:P ratio. Complexes with a higher charge ratio give better siRNA activity efficiency, but also show higher toxicity effects.

The nitrogen atoms in the polymer have the ability to accept hydrogen atoms, allowing PEI to potentially serve as a buffer through a wide range of pH values. As previously mentioned, this buffering capacity of the PEI conjugate enhances transfection efficiency and makes PEI a good potential candidate for siRNA delivery vehicles. When PEI accepts protons in the endosomal compartment, osmotic swelling occurs which may cause the endosome to burst, releasing the PEI and its cargo before reaching the degradative compartment of the lysosome. This mechanism is often referred to as "the proton sponge effect," although it has been disputed by a number of investigators whether PEI is responsible for this endosomolytic activity. PEI can be used as a "base" for formulation of more complex particles with improved properties. For example, a pegylated PEI particle with a vasculature-targeting "RDG" peptide has been shown to successfully delivery siRNAs in a mouse xenograft tumor model as will be discussed in Section 6.4.2 [99]. Deacylation of PEI lowers toxicity and improves pulmonary delivery of siRNAs in mice [100], and folate-modified pegylated PEI is being tested for siRNA delivery in tumor cells [101].

PEI has been used to deliver siRNAs targeting influenza virus via retroorbital IV injection in mice [102]. Unmodified siRNAs specific for genes encoding nucleocapsid protein (*NP*) or viral transcriptase (*PA* and *PB1*) complexed to PEI were delivered IV (using an N:P ratio of 5). No apparent innate immune response (IFN-α) was detected in the lungs of mice using either influenza-specific or control siRNAs with PEI. Administration of the influenza-specific siRNAs reduced viral titers in infected mouse lungs. Reductions of viral titers ranged from 1 to 3 $\log_{10}$ even when administered 5–24 h after infection.

Deacylated PEI (PEI187) improved delivery of nucleic acid in mice by IV administration 10^4-fold and dramatically improved pulmonary targeting [100]. For example, deacylated PEI187 was used to deliver anti-*NA* siR-NAs in mice by retroorbital IV injection in an *in vivo* influenza model. Viral titers were reduced by 94% using a single dose of siRNA. However, it should be noted that the differences between these results and those obtained with the unmodified PEI were not large. Care must be taken when interpreting results in systems studying viral infections as the immunostimulatory potential of the siRNA delivered can contribute to changes in viral titer as much as RISC-mediated gene silencing [103].

Linear low-molecular weight PEI has been used as a carrier to deliver unmodified siRNAs by IP administration in nude mice with SC implants of SKOV-3 tumors [104]. PEI was able to protect unmodified siRNAs from degradation in serum in comparison with siRNAs that were not complexed with PEI. The naked siRNAs degraded within 15 min of exposure to serum. In contrast, approximately 2/3 of the siRNAs complexed with PEI were intact after 6 h incubation. Delivering the siRNA–PEI complexes IP led to the highest accumulation in muscle and tumor and to a lesser extent in liver. SKOV-3 tumors were implanted into the flanks of nude mice and a siRNA specific for the *HER-2* oncogene was administered three times a week until tumors reached a size of 10 mm^2. The anti-*HER-2* siRNA administered with PEI resulted in a significant reduction in tumor size as well as an average of 50% reduction in *HER-2* mRNA in excised tumors while control or naked siRNAs did not influence tumor growth.

Cyclodextrin-PEI Conjugates   Cyclodextrin-modified PEI is significantly less toxic than unmodified PEI and can be used as a nucleic acid delivery tool. Addition of an adamantine-PEG additionally stabilizes the complex under physiological conditions and improves its performance *in vivo* [105]. Cyclodextrin copolymers are much less toxic (LD$_{50}$ of ∼200 mg/kg in mice) than PEI (LD$_{50}$ of 4 mg/kg in mice); grafting β-cyclodextrin onto PEI reduces toxicity [106]. However, there is a tradeoff between reducing toxicity and decreasing efficacy of delivery, so empiric testing must be done to optimize relative ratios of each group [105]. For an overview of issues involved with the design of polyplex delivery agents, see reviews by Davis and colleagues and Putnam and colleagues [33, 107, 108].

Dendrimers   PAMAM dendrimers (Figure 6.2) are an exciting new class of macromolecular architecture called starburst polymers. Unlike classical polymers, dendrimers display a significant level of molecular uniformity, narrow molecular weight distribution, specific size and shape characteristics, and a highly functionalized terminal surface. PAMAM dendrimers have primary

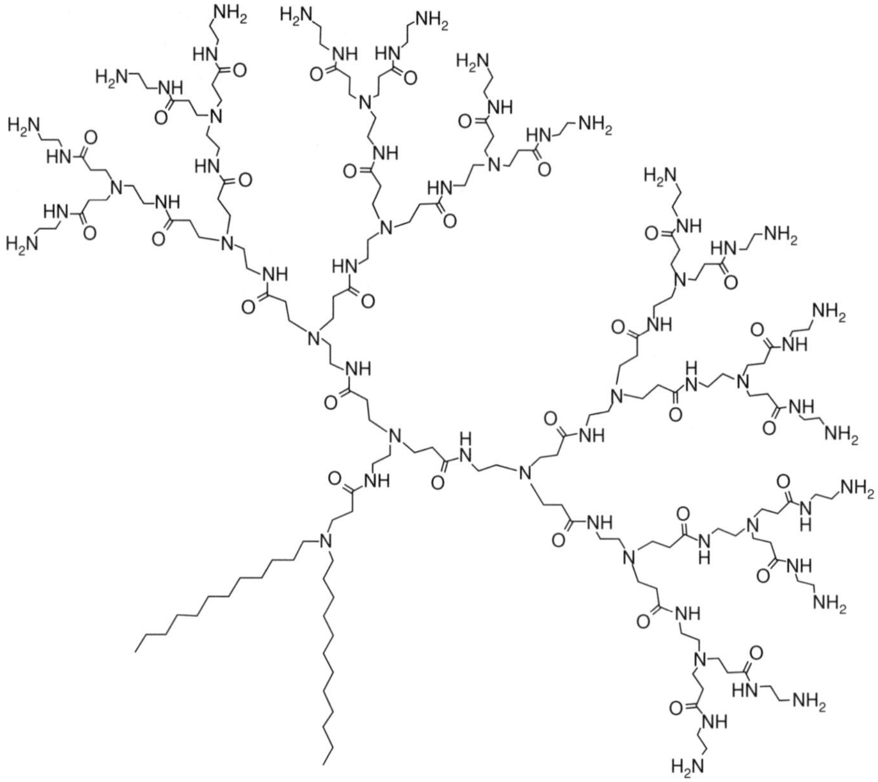

FIGURE 6.2   Chemical structure of polyamidoamine (PAMAM) dendrimer.

amine groups on their surface and tertiary amine groups present on the inside. The primary amine groups facilitate siRNA binding and promote cellular uptake of siRNAs, while the internal tertiary amino groups act as a proton sponge in endosomes as discussed for PEI in Section Polyethyleneimine thus enhancing the release of siRNA into the cytoplasm.

Polypropylenimine (PPI) dendrimers appear to be attractive nonviral vectors for the delivery of siRNAs. However, just like other delivery tools, dendrimers have their own toxicity profile. The toxicity of generation 2 and generation 3 PPI dendrimers was examined in two human cell lines. Using concentrations and protocols typical for siRNA delivery, PPI dendrimers induced significant changes in gene expression in A431 epithelial cells. The number of genes affected was greater with G3 PPI compared with G2 PPI dendrimers in A431 cells. Gene expression changes varied with cell type. Further, a dendrimer–DNA complex resulted in gene expression signatures that were different from the polymer alone. Alterations in expression of a variety of pathways were examined using microarray methods and included changes in defense responses, cell proliferation and apoptosis [109].

A G3 polyamidoamine (PAMAM) dendrimer was complexed with alpha-cyclodextrin (alpha-CyD) (alpha-CDE conjugate) and tested as a siRNA carrier [110]. Cotransfection of a luciferase reporter plasmid with or without an anti-Luc siRNA was compared using the alpha-CDE-dendrimer and three commercial cationic lipids. Superior delivery with lower toxicity was observed for the dendrimer complexes than the cationic lipids. However, it is important to note that this assay required cotransfection of both plasmid DNA + siRNA. Reagents can be excellent delivery vehicles for siRNAs yet perform relatively poorly when delivering large plasmid DNAs. Therefore, this assay would be insensitive to differences in reagent performance that related to siRNA alone.

Dimethylaminoethyl Methacrylate-Propylacrylic Acid   Stayton and colleagues have reported on the development of a diblock copolymer that can promote intracellular release of siRNA. The diblock copolymers are synthesized by reversible addition fragmentation chain transfer polymerization and have a positively charged block of dimethylaminoethyl methacrylate (DMAEMA) to condense siRNA, and a second component made of DMAEMA, propylacrylic acid (PAA), and butyl methacrylate (BMA) that can promote intracellular release of the siRNA. The diblock copolymers have strong hemolytic properties at endosomal pH. The copolymers condensed siRNA into particles below 250 nm with slightly positive zeta potentials and generated reasonable knockdown of GAPDH in HeLa cells [111]. While these diblock copolymers have significant potential for siRNA delivery, additional *in vivo* studies are necessary to determine how useful this chemistry will prove to be.

Chitosan   Chitosan (Figure 6.3) is a biodegradable polysaccharide extracted from crustacean shells. It has been shown to be nontoxic in animals and humans. In addition to numerous biomedical applications such as wound

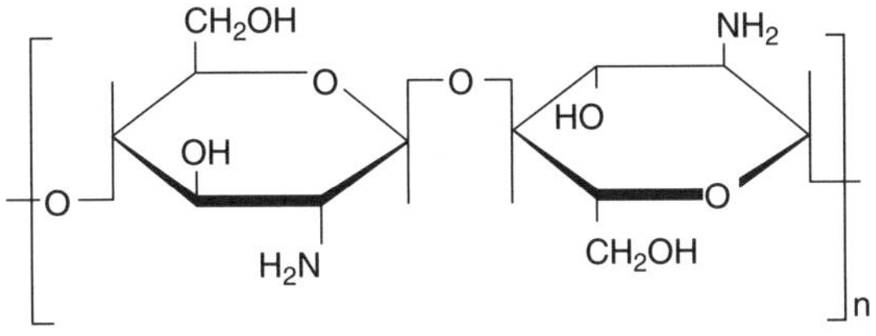

FIGURE 6.3   Chemical structure of chitosan.

healing, chitosan has shown potential for delivery of DNA and nucleic acids because of its ability to electrostatically bind to the nucleic acids and partially protect the nucleic acids from nuclease degradation [112–116].

Chitosan–siRNA delivery systems have been used to treat RSV [117]. To prepare the nanoparticles, siRNA was added to filtered chitosan while stirring and left for 1 h. The nanoparticles formed between siRNA duplexes and chitosan polymer and ranged in size from 40 to 600 nm. As discussed with PEI, the size of nanoparticle formation is dependent on the N:P ratio, with an increase in size seen at lower N:P ratios. At low chitosan concentrations, smaller nanoparticles form at higher N:P ratios and larger nanoparticles form at lower N:P ratios. Similarly, at high chitosan concentrations, the nanoparticle hydrodynamic radius increases with decreasing N:P ratio. Nanoparticle-induced suppression of EGFP was seen in H1299 human lung carcinoma cells (77.9%) and murine peritoneal macrophages (89.3%). Efficient *in vivo* RNAi of up to 43% reduction was achieved in bronchiole epithelial cells of transgenic EGFP mice after nasal administration of chitosan/siRNA formulations in comparison with controls [118]. The importance of siRNA formulation conditions with chitosan was further highlighted in a study that showed that high Molecular Weight (MW) and degrees of deacetylation are necessary to form stable nanoparticles in the 200 nm size range. Chitosan/siRNA formulations that were prepared with low MW chitosan below 10 kDa or with N:P ratios less than 50 resulted in negligible knockdown of GFP in H1299 human lung carcinoma cells. These results are in stark contrast to the reports of plasmid DNA and chitosan formulations in which low MW chitosan (4.7 kDa) could produce stable nanoparticles effective at transfection, further highlighting the need for formulations optimized for siRNA instead of simply translating systems that work for plasmid DNA [113]. Chitosan/siRNA nanoparticles prepared from high MW chitosans ranging from 65 to 170 kDa, and higher than 80% degrees of deacetylation showed gene silencing between 45% and 65%. The highest GFP suppression of 80% was achieved using chitosan/siRNA formulations at an N:P ratio of 150, high MW between 114 and 170 kDa, and an 84% degree of deacetylation [119]. It has been suggested that the excess of chitosan loosely associated with the nanoparticles at higher N:P ratios contributes to increased stability and gene silencing. It should be noted that while stable chitosan–DNA complexes are beneficial for protecting DNA, it can also limit release of DNA to the nucleus [120, 121].

Overexpression of RhoA in cancer is associated with increased tumor cell proliferation and tumor angiogenesis. When an anti-*RhoA* siRNA is complexed with chitosan, it inhibits xenografted aggressive breast cancer more efficiently than conventional blockers of Rho-mediated signaling pathways. An anti-*RhoA* siRNA was encapsulated in chitosan-coated polyisohexylcyanoacrylate (PIHCA) nanoparticles and administered every

3 days at a dose of 150 or 1500 µg/kg body weight in nude mice. This formulation inhibited the growth of tumors by a minimum of 90%. After 30 days, the higher doses resulted in necrosis associated with angiogenesis inhibition but was without other toxic effects as determined by body weight gain; biochemical markers of hepatic, renal, and pancreatic function; and macroscopic appearance of organs [122].

In another study, anti-*TNF*α siRNA were complexed in chitosan nanoparticles and administered via IP injection to treat CIA in mice. While knockdown of *TNF*α using unmodified siRNA with this delivery system improved arthritis scores, 2′OMe-modified duplexes performed far better, presumably due to decreased immune recognition and improved stability [123]. Thus chemical modification of the siRNA cargo is important in other carrier systems such as chitosan and not just when using lipid-based delivery tools.

Protamine   Protamines are small, arginine-rich, nuclear proteins that replace histones late in the haploid phase of spermatogenesis and are believed essential for sperm head condensation and DNA stabilization and represents another class of polycation that can be complexed with siRNAs to facilitate delivery. Protamine has been employed as a carrier for nucleic acids and can be conjugated to a variety of molecules that improve its performance, including lipids [124]. Protamine can be conjugated to antibody Fab fragments to selectively target delivery to specific cell types and this approach has been successfully used to deliver siRNAs in mice as discussed in Section 6.4.5 [125].

Atelocollagen   Atelocollagen is a purified type I collagen of calf dermis with pepsin treatment. A collagen molecule has an amino acid sequence called a telopeptide at both N and C termini, which confers most of the collagen's antigenicity. Atelocollagen obtained by pepsin treatment is low in immunogenicity because it is free from telopeptides. Atelocollagen has found wide utility in clinical applications including wound healing and vessel prosthesis and as a bone cartilage substitute and haemostatic agent. siRNA binds to atelocollagen directly to form siRNA–atelocollagen fiber complexes [126]. Atelocollagen complexed with siRNA is reported to be resistant to nucleases and is efficiently transduced into cells, thereby allowing long-term gene silencing. For example, atelocollagen has been used to assist in IV delivery of siRNAs in a bone tumor-metastasis model system in mice [127]. Luciferase-expressing PC-3M-luc-C6 cells were injected into nude mice. After 4 weeks, unmodified siRNAs were administered by IV injection either with or without 0.05% atelocollagen. Luciferase expression was measured by *in vivo* bioluminescence 24 h later. The control siRNA or the siRNA without atelocollagen had no effect. The anti-*Luc* siRNA administered with atelocollagen showed a 90% reduction in luciferase activity. In contrast, the control siRNA or anti-*Luc* siRNA without atelocollagen showed no reduction in luciferase activity. Atelocollagen distributed siRNA into the liver, lung, spleen, and kidney. SiRNAs delivered by this approach did not result in a detectable increase in IL-12 or α-IFN levels, although measurements beyond the 2 h postinjection studied here would be necessary to provide definitive confirmation of this. The zeste homolog 2 (*EZH2*) and 3′-hydroxykinase p110-α-subunit (*p110-α*) are two genes reported to be involved in metastasis. Anti-*EZH2* or anti-*p110*-α siRNAs were injected IV after injection of tumor cells, and animals were imaged for the presence of bone implants. Anti-*EZH2* and anti-*p110*-α siRNAs resulted in significant inhibition in the number of bone lesions when administered with atelocollagen, while a control siRNA or siRNAs delivered without atelocollagen did not affect tumor development.

Atelocollagen has also been injected directly into tumors. For example, an unmodified anti-*VEGF* siRNA in a solution of atelocollagen in PBS was injected into established human prostate cancer PC-3 cell implants in nude mice [128]. The anti-*VEGF* siRNA delivered with atelocollagen reduced tumor volume in a dose-dependent fashion with the highest dose-treated mice having tumors that were ~80% smaller than controls. A proportional 80% reduction in VEGF protein was also observed by day 17. Tumors injected with ^{32}P-labeled siRNA and atelocollagen were detectable by day 7, while the siRNA delivered without atelocollagen was undetectable after only one day.

Midkine (MK) is a heparin-binding growth factor that is a product of the retinoic acid-responsive gene. MK-deficient mice exhibit a striking reduction of neointima formation in a restenosis model, which is reversed on systemic MK administration. It has been observed that the intima–media ratio and the intima thickness at 28 days after grafting were both reduced over 90% when compared with controls following perivascular application of MK siRNA using atelocollagen. This strategy has potential as a treatment against human vein graft failure [129].

Single-Walled Carbon Nanotubes Carbon nanotubes (CNT) have shown potential utility in a variety of biological applications including use as DNA and protein biosensors, ion channel blockers, bioseparators, and biocatalysts [130]. This potential stems from their specific surface or adaptable size-dependent properties in combination with their anisotropic character. Their anisotropy is of consequence since it influences their electronic, photonic, mechanical, and chemical properties [131]. The chemical modification and solubilization of carbon nanotubes is essential to their successful application in drug delivery. Atomically ordered, carbon nanotubes demonstrate low chemical reactivity. However, many researchers have reported successful

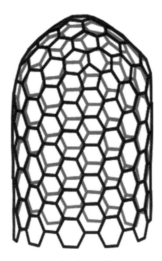

FIGURE 6.4   Schematic of single-walled carbon nanotube structure.

functionalization of both the ends and sidewalls of single-walled carbon nanotubes (SWCNTs) (Figure 6.4) and multi-walled carbon nanotubes (MWCNTs). In addition, nanotubes have the advantage of facile DNA, peptide, or other molecular incorporation into their hollow space [130, 132].

Ideal SWCNTs contain two separate regions, each with a unique reactivity toward covalent chemical modification. The intermittent five-membered rings on the caps increase reactivity at these points to levels similar to fullerenes [133]. The functionalization of carbon nanotubes can broadly be divided into two categories: (a) direct attachment of functional groups to the graphitic surface and (b) the use of the nanotube-bound carboxylic acids [130]. For example, functionalization of CNTs using polyethylene-oxide chains has been achieved by using carboxylic acid end groups [134]. This imparts the nanotubes with enhanced water solubility and nonspecific protein-resistant properties. Surface functionalization in this manner enables adsorption or attachment of various molecules or antigens. This provides a mechanism for specific recognition and cell targeting [131].

In the only study to date to have used carbon nanotubes for siRNA delivery, the SWNTs were shown to be a promising approach for DC-based immunotherapy. The SWNTs were modified using 1,6-diaminohexane to prepare positively charged SWNTs (SWNTs+) which could electrostatically bind to siRNAs to form complexes of siRNA with SWNTs. These complexes were found to be internalized by antigen presenting cells including splenic CD11 c+ DCs and CD11b+ cells for silencing of the target cytokine signaling 1 (SOCS1) gene. *SOCS1* restricts the ability of DCs to break self-tolerance and induce antitumor immunity. It should be noted that neither the T nor the

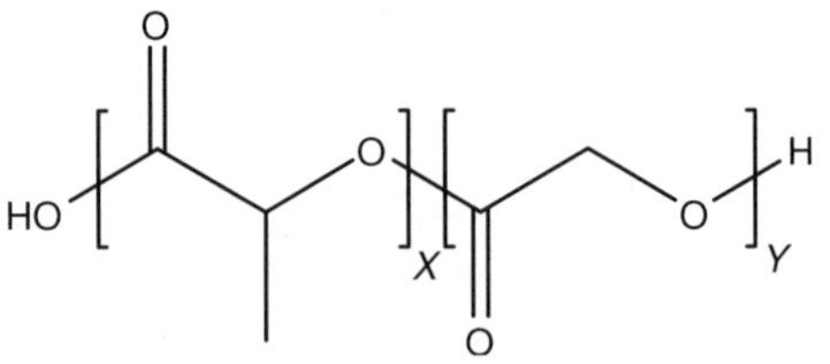

FIGURE 6.5   Structure of polylactic-co-glycolic acid (PLGA). X is the number of units of lactic acid, and Y is the number of units of glycolic acid.

B cells showed significant uptake of SWNTs. IV injection of SWNTs complexed with the *SOCS1*siRNA reduced *SOCS1* expression and significantly retarded the growth of established B16 tumors in mice after 15 days [135].

Polylactic-co-Glycolic Acid   Sustained-release delivery of siRNA may be achieved using poly (lactic-co-glycolic acid) (PLGA; Figure 6.5), which already has a demonstrated track record as a vehicle for small molecule drug and protein delivery [136, 137]. Therapeutic agents, either entrapped, adsorbed, or chemically coupled onto a PLGA matrix, show rapid endolysosomal escape and sustained intracytoplasmic delivery [136]. Biodegradable PLGA microparticles loaded with bioactive agents are biocompatible [138], although some reports have shown that hemolysis of red blood cells can occur [139]. PLGA microparticles have the capacity to protect siRNAs from nuclease degradation and increase RNA stability [140, 141]. The lack of toxicity of PLGA microparticles and the burst release associated with early availability of nucleic acids followed by more sustained release represent important factors in prolonging the time span of siRNA activity [142]. One study reported that PLGA nanoparticles loaded with siRNAs inhibit GFP expression. Delivery of siRNA into 293 T cells resulted in visual reduction of GFP expression [143]; however; there was no attempt to quantify or perform statistical analysis of the biological activity of the nanoparticles.

A significant hurdle in the development of these PLGA delivery systems has been the difficulty of entrapping hydrophilic nucleic acids within the hydrophobic PLGA [144, 145]. Methods used to entrap DNA into PLGA particles include spray-drying and oil-in-water solvent evaporation methods [140, 146, 147]. However, the nucleic acid can be damaged during these encapsulation procedures. The encapsulated DNA is exposed to an acidic environment within the particles, which can lead to depurination and strand scission. These limitations require addition of cationic excipients and modification of the formulation methodology to overcome these issues [140, 146]. A recent study by Saltzman and colleagues has made stronger progress in the utility of PLGA nanoparticles in siRNA delivery. A single dose of siRNA-loaded PLGA nanoparticles to the mouse female reproductive tract generated strong longer term silencing. Silencing was located in the vaginal lumen and the uterine horns, and the PLGA nanoparticles were able to enter the epithelial tissue [148].

6.3 PEGYLATION OF DELIVERY VECTOR

When siRNA is delivered by polymers such as protamine and PEI, the net positive charge of the nucleic acid/polymer polyplex can result in aggregation and can interact with negatively charged serum proteins. Addition of PEG(pegylation) to a siRNA-cationic polymer polyplex can shield the positive charge, reducing aggregation, increasing circulation time, and reducing toxicity. In addition, pegylated polyplexes appear to accumulate to a greater extent in tumor tissue. Tumors often contain a complex vascular network in order to feed their rapid growth. Coupled with inadequate lymphatic drainage, this allows an enhanced permeation and retention effect (EPR effect). This EPR effect is thought to be the mechanism by which polyplexes accumulate in the tumor even in the absence of any specific targeting ligand [149]. In one study, PEG was attached to a polycation using low pH cleavable pyridylhydrazines. Such systems allow for intracellular endosomal targeted cleavage [150]. It took only 10 min for the polymer to become 90% hydrolyzed and completely deshielded at pH 5. In contrast, at pH 7.4 the half-life was $1\frac{1}{2}$ h and the shield was intact. These pH sensitive delivery systems generated high transfection efficiencies when injected IV into tumor bearing mice. A limitation to this system, however, was that significant nonspecific gene expression changes were detected in liver and lung. In a recent study by Dassie and colleagues, pegylation of aptamer-siRNA chimeras significantly increased the half-life of the chimeras and as a result improved their antitumor activity [151].

6.4 CELL TARGETING LIGAND CONJUGATION TO siRNA DELIVERY VEHICLES

Cell targeting ligands directly linked to siRNAs can significantly improve their efficacy. Targeting ligands can also be added to the siRNA delivery vehicle to reduce nonspecific uptake while promoting tissue specific targeting and uptake. A variety of different conjugates that facilitate delivery of nucleic acids have been characterized [152], and novel small molecule libraries are under development that assist targeting of a wide range of different and specific cell types [153]. Here, we discuss some of the cell targeting ligands that are increasingly being explored for conjugation to siRNA delivery vehicles, including transferrin, folate, RGD, and TAT.

6.4.1 Transferrin

Transferrin was one of the first proteins exploited for receptor-mediated nucleic acid delivery, as all metabolic cells take in iron through receptor-mediated endocytosis of the transferrin–iron complex. Transferrin receptors are also present in higher concentrations on many tumor cells [37]. For example, it has been shown that transferrin-PEI conjugates provided transfection to several lines of tumor cells, in several cases resulting in a 30- to 1000-fold enhanced transfection [154]. Additionally, transfection efficiency was improved at lower N:P ratios that are more suitable for *in vivo* applications (lower toxicity). After several different cell lines were examined, a trend was observed in which improved delivery was achieved in cells with elevated levels of transferrin receptors. One complication is that transferrin receptors are also present on many other cell types; this study did not evaluate uptake in nontumor cells. Consistent with a receptor mediated process, B16 melanoma cells, which have low expression of the transferrin receptor, did not show an increase in transfection efficiency for the transferrin–PEI complex [154]. To demonstrate that uptake was specific, blocking experiments were done with free transferrin as competitor. The transfection efficiency of the polyplexes was inhibited by the presence of free transferrin, while a PEI complex used as control showed no inhibition.

In another example, conjugation of transferrin to a cyclodextrin/adamantine/PEG-cationic polyplex improved tumor targeting and was successfully employed to deliver siRNAs *in vivo* in mice [155]. Transferrin was chemically linked to the cyclodextrin-polyplex to enhance siRNA uptake into tumor cells in a mouse model of Ewing's sarcoma. Ewing's sarcoma tumors produce an aberrant transcript *EWS-FL11*, which has been linked to oncogenesis. An anti-*EWS-F11* siRNA complexed with the transferrin delivery complex was injected into SCID mice with tumors formed from TC71 cells. This treatment resulted in a 60% decrease in *EWS-F11* mRNA levels. The siRNA was coinjected with the TC71-Luc tumor cells followed by twice weekly dosing for 8 weeks and tumor growth was assessed. SiRNA delivered with transferrin-polyplexes had minimal tumor formation. SiRNA delivered with polyplexes without the transferrin targeting moiety had delayed onset of tumor formation, while mice treated with control siRNA or siRNA without any delivery vehicle showed the most rapid tumor development. Alternative strategies include the potential use of transferrin and epidermal growth factor (EGF) as ligands, which have been shown to improve targeting of DNA-polyplexes

(PEGylated-PEI) to tumor cells in mice [156]. When possible, employing some kind of specific cell surface marker or receptor targeting technique generally improves *in vivo* delivery of nucleic acid polyplexes and concomitantly improves specificity.

6.4.2 RGD

Adenoviruses have five RGD motifs (amino acid triplet) in their viral penton base that they use to bind to $\alpha_v \beta_3$ or $\alpha_v \beta_5$ integrins on the cell surface, which provides them with an efficient cell internalization mechanism [157]. RGD binds up to 10 integrins present on cell surfaces and has been used to improve the cellular uptake of nonviral gene vectors by linking them to the carriers [158–161]. When the adenovirus binds to the extracellular domain of the integrins, it stimulates conformational changes in the structure of the integrins and activation of downstream signaling molecules that ultimately leads to endocytosis of the virus [162–164]. Thus, attachment of an RGD group would be expected to enhance receptor-mediated endocytosis of siRNA delivery vehicles in cells using a similar mechanism. For example, a "sterically stabilized nanoparticle" was developed to deliver unmodified siRNAs to neuroblastoma N2 A tumors in nude mice [99]. The particles contained PEI, PEI+PEG, or PEI+PEG plus an Arg-Gly-Asp (RGD) peptide to promote vascular targeting. SiRNA complexed with the targeting cationic polymer provided protection to the siRNA from serum based degradation and provided improved biodistribution kinetics *in vivo*. Control siRNAs or siRNAs without the delivery vehicle did not accumulate in the lung, liver, or tumors and were predominantly degraded or excreted. Conjugation of the RGD to the delivery vehicle resulted in greater and more selective accumulation in the tumors than complexes without the ligand. An anti-*VEGF R2* siRNA injected in mice with N2A resulted in greater than 90% suppression of tumor growth in comparison with vehicle-only or control siRNA-treated mice. Further improvements of this system may enhance the antitumor activity further [165].

6.4.3 Folate

Malignant tissues, such as the ovarian, nasopharyngeal, cervical, and chorionic carcinomas, express high levels of folate receptors that are accessible via the bloodstream [166]. Folate receptors are also present in a number of normal tissues including the placenta, kidney, fallopian tube, and choroidal plexus, where expression is restricted to the luminal surface of epithelial cells and is thus not accessible via the bloodstream [167, 168]. Folic acid is a water-soluble B vitamin that has a high affinity for the folate receptor even after chemical modification. Folate receptor targeting has been evaluated for enhancing tumor cell-selective delivery of a wide variety of therapeutic agents including radiopharmaceuticals [169], chemotherapeutics [170], anti-sense oligodeoxyribonucleotides [171], prodrug-converting enzymes [171], antibodies [172], gene transfer vectors [173–175], nanoparticles [176], and liposomal drug carriers [174]. For siRNA delivery, a target-specific delivery system of green fluorescent protein (GFP) specific siRNA was developed using folate-modified cationic PEI linked to PEG (PEI-PEG-FOL). Folate overexpressing KB cells expressing GFP were treated with various formulations of siRNA/PEI-PEG-FOL complexes to inhibit expression of GFP. SiRNA/PEI-PEG-FOL complexes markedly reduced GFP expression of KB cells in comparison with siRNA/PEI complexes without folate modification. This same complex showed significantly lower inhibition of GFP expression when tested in A549 cells, which express lower levels of folate receptors [177, 178]. Folate targeted uptake of siRNA has also been utilized in a nasopharyngeal cancer model that is a low level differentiated upper respiratory tract cancer that has high expression of human folate receptors. Folate was conjugated to adenosine 5′-monophosphate (AMP) using 1,6 hexadiamine linkages. The folate-AMP conjugate was incorporated into the 5′ end of bacteriophage phi29 motor pRNA. When this system was used to deliver a siRNA that suppresses an antiapoptosis factor to nasopharyngeal epidermal carcinoma cells, it did not stimulate antigenic responses but was significantly more effective at suppressing the target gene in comparison with the same formulation without a folate ligand [179].

6.4.4 Tat Peptides

HIV-1 Tat peptide binds strongly to glycosaminoglycan-specific structures of heparin sulfate and cell surface heparin sulfates [180]. As a result, Tat modification can enhanced cell uptake [181] and may have potential for enhancing the delivery of siRNAs. In a positive example of the utility of TAT peptides, Dowdy and colleagues have reported on the development of an efficient siRNA delivery approach that uses a peptide transduction domain–dsRNA-binding domain (PTD–DRBD) fusion protein. The DRBD component of the delivery system binds to siRNAs efficiently. This neutralizes the siRNA's negative charge, which allows for more efficient cellular uptake. The PTD component contained TAT peptide sequences that promote cell penetration. The authors showed that the PTD–DRBD system could deliver siRNA that triggered quick RNAi in significant proportions of a number of primary and transformed cells. Cytotoxicity, off-target effects, and the triggering of immune responses were all limited relative to other delivery systems [182]. The same group subsequently used the PTD–DRBD to deliver siRNA via direct intratumor injection in mouse brain to treat an *in vivo* glioblastoma tumor model [183]. However, it should be noted that some studies that have used Tat ligands reported negative results. In this study, a G5 PAMAM dendrimer was reacted with various linkers to conjugate the Tat peptide. The G5 dendrimer-Tat conjugate was complexed with antisense and siRNA oligonucleotides that target the gene *MDR1*. Both antisense and siRNA readily formed complexes with the G5 dendrimer-Tat conjugate and primarily localized in intracellular vesicles when incubated with NIH 3T3 MDR cells. Dendrimer–oligonucleotide complexes were somewhat effective for delivering the antisense oligonucleotides but were less effective for delivery of the siRNA. In this study, conjugation of a dendrimer with the Tat cell penetrating peptide failed to improve effectiveness of the dendrimers alone [184].

6.4.5 Fab-Antibody Targeting Ligands

Antibodies have high specificity and a variety of well-characterized reagents are available that recognize many different cell surface markers. One recent study reported use of this approach to target a cell surface marker to deliver unmodified siRNAs in mice by IV administration [125]. In these experiments, a Fab fragment (F105) specific for the HIV envelope glycoprotein gp160 was linked to protamine (F105-P), a cationic delivery vehicle discussed in Section Dimethylaminoethyl Methacrylate-Propylacrylic Acid. The ratio of siRNA to F10P-5 was 6:1 and the complex effectively delivered siRNA to all cells tested that expressed the HIV *env* gene, including T-cells, which are typically very difficult to transfect. The complex did not stimulate an immune response in B16 melanoma cells *in vitro*; further studies evaluating immune responses *in vivo* are necessary to validate these results. SiRNAs were injected IV or by direct intratumor injection, with or without the F105-P ligand, in mice bearing B16 melanoma tumors. Both intratumor and IV administration of a siRNA cocktail specific for *c-myc*, *MDM2*, and *VEGF* with F105-P delivery significantly reduced tumor size, whereas naked siRNAs or control treatments had no effect.

6.4.6 Other Cell Targeting Ligands

Antibodies, folate, transferrin, Tat, and RGD peptides represent only a fraction of the cell targeting ligands that have the potential to enhance siRNA delivery. For example, the DNA-packaging motor of bacteriophage phi29 has been conjugated to siRNAs and shown to facilitate cell entry [185]. Modified virus envelopes can be adapted to deliver nucleic acids to cells. Fusogenic influenza virus envelopes were used to deliver fluorescent dye-labeled siRNAs by IP injection in mice [186], hemagglutinating virus of Japan (HVJ) envelopes were used to deliver siRNAs via direct intratumor injection in mice [187], and SV40 pseudovirions are being tested as a delivery vehicle [188]. These delivery tools and other potential ligands such as mannose and aptamers [151] will need careful evaluation for efficacy and potential antigenicity if they are to be considered for therapeutic applications.

6.5   RATIONALE DESIGN OF MODULAR MULTICOMPONENT siRNA DELIVERY SYSTEMS

The most promising commercial systems in development synergistically combine the advantages of a cationic polymer, pegylation and a cell targeting ligand. For example, Intradigm is developing the PEI-PEG-RGD delivery system (Figure 6.6), which was described in Section 6.4.2. This rationally designed delivery system has multiple functionalities. The disulfide stabilized RGD peptide can target integrin expression, which is upregulated at sites of neovasculaturization(such as tumors). The PEG component decreases toxicity and ensures that the particles formed are sterically stabilized with the RGD sequences exposed on the surface. Finally, the cationic PEI complexes and condenses the siRNA providing it with protection against enzymatic degradation. Syntheses of delivery systems of this kind are relatively straightforward. In the PEI-PEG-RGD system, a 10 mer RGD sequence is oxidized to form an intramolecular disulfide bridge. This is reacted with NHS-PEG-VS to form RGD-PEG-VS, which is then purified by HPLC. The RGD-PEG-VS is finally reacted with PEI, with conjugation levels of PEI amines to RGD-PEG averaging 7%, or 40 RGD-PEG molecules per 25 kDa PEI. One

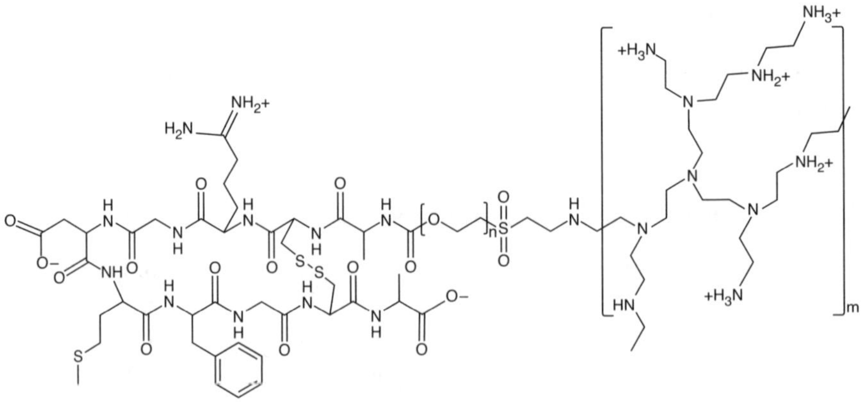

FIGURE 6.6   Structure of PEI-PEG-RGD polymer (adapted from [95]).

would anticipate that new versions of this chemistry that switch targeting ligands would be relatively straightforward, which is important for adapting this system to target other tissues [99]. This is illustrated in Section 4.3 with the description of a multicomponent PEI-PEG-folate siRNA delivery system.

In another example of industrial development of a rationally designed siRNA delivery vehicle, Calando Pharmaceuticals is developing cyclodextrin-containing polycations (CDP) with PEG and transferrin (Trf) cell targeting proteins and a siRNA delivery vehicle for oncology indications. Cyclodextrin was chosen because of its low toxicity profiles. Modification of the cyclodextrin with cationic amine functionalities allows it to condense siRNA into colloidal nanoparticles protecting it from enzymatic degradation. The PEG component, similar to the Intradigm PEI-PEG-RGD system, provides stabilization of the nanoparticles in the presence of biological fluids (serum) and is incorporated by inclusion complex formation between the terminal adamantine and the cyclodextrins. Some PEG units also have transferrin attached, which acts as a targeting ligand to tumor cells that overexpress the cell-surface transferrin receptor, as discussed in Section 6.4.1. Without the transferrin ligand, these nanoparticles could still provide tumor localization but the nanoparticles are not internalized by the tumor cells with the same high efficiency [155]. Using optimized manufacturing and formulations methods, the CDP vehicle forms particles with sizes ranging from 60 to 150 nm, molecular weights from approximately 7×10^7 to 1×10^9 g mol^{-1} and zeta potentials from 10 to 30 mV. A single 70 nm particle contains approximately 2000 siRNA molecules, 4000 adamantine-PEG molecules, 10,000 CDP polymer chains, and 100 adamantine-PEG-transferrin molecules. This represents a ratio of siRNA to targeting ligand of 20:1 [189]. The advanced CDP polymer is fairly nontoxic and can be safely administered to nonhuman primates at high levels, with toxicity only appearing at the highest doses examined (27 mg/kg) [190]. This compound complexed with an anti-*RRM2* (ribonucleotide reductase, subunit M2) siRNA was taken into Phase 1 clinical trial by Calando Pharmaceuticals in 2009; results of this trial have not yet been released.

6.6 CONCLUSIONS

RNAi-based therapeutics is undergoing active development by many pharmaceutical and biotechnology companies. RNAi has proven to be an extremely potent and versatile tool to specifically reduce expression of targeted genes. Widespread adoption of RNAi using synthetic siRNAs as an *in vivo* research tool will accelerate, as more effective mammalian delivery tools become commercially available. Although some laboratories have reported success using *in vivo* administration of "naked" siRNAs, a greater number of investigators reported that using some kind of delivery system improved results. Careful formulation, choice of delivery vehicle and cell targeting ligand strategies will be critical for successful *in vivo* application of siRNA.

REFERENCES

1. Fire, A., et al. (1998). Potent and specific genetic interference by double-stranded RNA in *Caenorhabditis elegans*. *Nature* **391**(6669): 806–11.
2. Zamore, P. D., et al. (2000). RNAi: double-stranded RNA directs the ATP-dependent cleavage of mRNA at 21 to 23 nucleotide intervals. *Cell* **101**(1): 25–33.
3. Elbashir, S. M., Lendeckel, W., and Tuschl, T. (2001). RNA interference is mediated by 21- and 22-nucleotide RNAs. *Genes Dev* **15**(2): 188–200.
4. Bernstein, E., et al. (2001). Role for a bidentate ribonuclease in the initiation step of RNA interference. *Nature* **409**(6818): 363–6.
5. Elbashir, S. M., et al. (2001). Duplexes of 21-nucleotide RNAs mediate RNA interference in cultured mammalian cells. *Nature* **411**(6836): 494–8.
6. Matranga, C., et al. (2005). Passenger-strand cleavage facilitates assembly of siRNA into ago2-containing RNAi enzyme complexes. *Cell* **123**(4): 607–20.
7. Rand, T. A., et al. (2005). Argonaute2 cleaves the anti-guide strand of siRNA during RISC activation. *Cell* **123**(4): 621–9.
8. Kim, D. H., et al. (2005). Synthetic dsRNA Dicer substrates enhance RNAi potency and efficacy. *Nat Biotechnol* **23**(2): 222–6.
9. Dykxhoorn, D. M. and Lieberman, J. (2005). The silent revolution: RNA interference as basic biology, research tool, and therapeutic. *Annu Rev Med* **56**: 401–23.
10. Leung, R. K. and Whittaker, P. A. (2005). RNA interference: from gene silencing to gene-specific therapeutics. *Pharmacol Ther* **107**(2): 222–39.
11. Tong, A. W., Zhang, Y. A., and Nemunaitis, J. (2005). Small interfering RNA for experimental cancer therapy. *Curr Opin Mol Ther* **7**(2): 114–24.
12. Fountaine, T. M., Wood, M. J., and Wade-Martins, R. (2005). Delivering RNA interference to the mammalian brain. *Curr Gene Ther* **5**(4): 399–410.
13. Carstea, E. D., et al. (2005). State-of-the-art modified RNAi compounds for therapeutics. *IDrugs* **8**(8): 642–7.
14. Uprichard, S. L. (2005). The therapeutic potential of RNA interference. *FEBS Lett* **579**(26): 5996–6007.
15. Lu, P. Y., Xie, F., and Woodle, M. C. (2005). In vivo application of RNA interference: from functional genomics to therapeutics. *Adv Genet* **54**: 117–42.
16. Cejka, D., Losert, D., and Wacheck, V. (2006). Short interfering RNA (siRNA): tool or therapeutic? *Clin Sci (Lond)* **110**(1): 47–58.

17. Campochiaro, P. A. (2005). Potential applications for RNAi to probe pathogenesis and develop new treatments for ocular disorders. *Gene Ther* **13**(6): 559–62.

18. Pai, S. I., et al. (2005). Prospects of RNA interference therapy for cancer. *Gene Ther* **13**(6): 464–77.

19. Behlke, M. A. (2006). Progress towards in vivo use of siRNAs. *Mol Ther* **13**(4): 644–70.

20. Behlke, M. A. (2008). Chemical modification of siRNAs for in vivo use. *Oligonucleotides* **18**(4): 305–20.

21. Morrissey, D. V., et al. (2005). Potent and persistent in vivo anti-HBV activity of chemically modified siRNAs. *Nat Biotechnol* **23**(8): 1002–7.

22. de Veer, M. J., Sledz, C. A., and Williams, B. R. (2005). Detection of foreign RNA: implications for RNAi. *Immunol Cell Biol* **83**(3): 224–8.

23. Robbins, M. A. and Rossi, J. J. (2005). Sensing the danger in RNA. *Nat Med* **11**(3): 250–1.

24. Karpala, A. J., Doran, T. J., and Bean, A. G. (2005). Immune responses to dsRNA: implications for gene silencing technologies. *Immunol Cell Biol* **83**(3): 211–6.

25. Stark, G. R., et al. (1998). How cells respond to interferons. *Annu Rev Biochem* **67**: 227–64.

26. Yoneyama, M., et al. (2004). The RNA helicase RIG-I has an essential function in double-stranded RNA-induced innate antiviral responses. *Nat Immunol* **5**(7): 730–7.

27. Marques, J. T. and Williams, B. R. (2005). Activation of the mammalian immune system by siRNAs. *Nat Biotechnol* **23**(11): 1399–405.

28. Mohmmed, A., et al. (2003). In vivo gene silencing in *Plasmodium berghei*—a mouse malaria model. *Biochem Biophys Res Commun* **309**(3): 506–11.

29. Filleur, S., et al. (2003). SiRNA-mediated inhibition of vascular endothelial growth factor severely limits tumor resistance to antiangiogenic thrombospondin-1 and slows tumor vascularization and growth. *Cancer Res* **63**(14): 3919–22.

30. Duxbury, M. S., et al. (2004). RNA interference targeting the M2 subunit of ribonucleotide reductase enhances pancreatic adenocarcinoma chemosensitivity to gemcitabine. *Oncogene* **23**(8): 1539–48.

31. Duxbury, M. S., et al. (2004). Systemic siRNA-mediated gene silencing: a new approach to targeted therapy of cancer. *Ann Surg* **240**(4): 667–74; discussion 675–6.

32. Liang, Z., et al. (2005). Silencing of CXCR4 blocks breast cancer metastasis. *Cancer Res* **65**(3): 967–71.

33. Putnam, D. and Doody, A. (2006). RNA-interference effectors and their delivery. *Crit Rev Ther Drug Carrier Syst* **23**(2): 137–64.

34. Golzio, M., et al. (2005). Inhibition of gene expression in mice muscle by in vivo electrically mediated siRNA delivery. *Gene Ther* **12**(3): 246–251.

35. Schiffelers, R. M., et al. (2005). Effects of treatment with small interfering RNA on joint inflammation in mice with collagen-induced arthritis. *Arthritis Rheum* **52**(4): 1314–8.

36. Inoue, A., et al. (2005). Electro-transfer of small interfering RNA ameliorated arthritis in rats. *Biochem Biophys Res Commun* **336**(3): 903–8.

37. Salem, A. K., Searson, P. C., and Leong, K. W. (2003). Multifunctional nanorods for gene delivery. *Nat Mater* **2**(10): 668–71.

38. Salem, A. K., et al. (2005). Multi-component nanorods for vaccination applications. *Nanotechnology* **16**(4): 484–7.

39. Kim, T. W., et al. (2005). Modification of professional antigen-presenting cells with small interfering RNA in vivo to enhance cancer vaccine potency. *Cancer Res* **65**(1): 309–16.

40. Kinoshita, M. and Hynynen, K. (2005). A novel method for the intracellular delivery of siRNA using microbubble-enhanced focused ultrasound. *Biochem Biophys Res Commun* **335**(2): 393–9.

41. Tsunoda, S., et al. (2005). Sonoporation using microbubble BR14 promotes pDNA/siRNA transduction to murine heart. *Biochem Biophys Res Commun* **336**(1): 118–27.

42. McCaffrey, A. P., et al. (2002). RNA interference in adult mice. *Nature* **418**(6893): 38–9.

43. Lewis, D. L., et al. (2002). Efficient delivery of siRNA for inhibition of gene expression in postnatal mice. *Nat Genet* **32**(1): 107–8.

44. Song, E., et al. (2003). RNA interference targeting Fas protects mice from fulminant hepatitis. *Nat Med* **9**(3): 347–51.

45. Hamar, P., et al. (2004). Small interfering RNA targeting Fas protects mice against renal ischemia-reperfusion injury. *Proc Natl Acad Sci USA* **101**(41): 14883–8.

46. Zender, L., et al. (2003). Caspase 8 small interfering RNA prevents acute liver failure in mice. *Proc Natl Acad Sci USA* **100**(13): 7797–802.

47. Contreras, J. L., et al. (2004). Caspase-8 and caspase-3 small interfering RNA decreases ischemia/reperfusion injury to the liver in mice. *Surgery* **136**(2): 390–400.

48. Giladi, H., et al. (2003). Small interfering RNA inhibits hepatitis B virus replication in mice. *Mol Ther* **8**(5): 769–76.

49. Morrissey, D. V., et al. (2005). Activity of stabilized short interfering RNA in a mouse model of hepatitis B virus replication. *Hepatology* **41**(6): 1349–56.

50. Hagstrom, J. E., et al. (2004). A facile nonviral method for delivering genes and siRNAs to skeletal muscle of mammalian limbs. *Mol Ther* **10**(2): 386–98.

51. Toumi, H., et al. (2006). Rapid intravascular injection into limb skeletal muscle: a damage assessment study. *Mol Ther* **13**(1): 229–36.

52. Keller, M. (2005). Lipidic carriers of RNA/DNA oligonucleotides and polynucleotides: what a difference a formulation makes! *J Control Release* **103**(3): 537–40.

53. Koltover, I., et al. (1998). An inverted hexagonal phase of cationic liposome-DNA complexes related to DNA release and delivery. *Science* **281**(5373): 78–81.

54. Verma, U. N., et al. (2003). Small interfering RNAs directed against beta-catenin inhibit the in vitro and in vivo growth of colon cancer cells. *Clin Cancer Res* **9**(4): 1291–300.

55. Flynn, M. A., et al. (2004). Efficient delivery of small interfering RNA for inhibition of IL-12p40 expression in vivo. *J Inflamm (Lond)* **1**(1): 4.

56. Yin, C., et al. (2005). Silencing heat shock factor 1 by small interfering RNA abrogates heat shock-induced cardioprotection against ischemia-reperfusion injury in mice. *J Mol Cell Cardiol* **39**(4): 681–9.

57. Hassani, Z., et al. (2005). Lipid-mediated siRNA delivery down-regulates exogenous gene expression in the mouse brain at picomolar levels. *J Gene Med* **7**(2): 198–207.

58. Luo, M. C., et al. (2005). An efficient intrathecal delivery of small interfering RNA to the spinal cord and peripheral neurons. *Mol Pain* **1**: 29.

59. Maeda, Y., et al. (2005). In vitro and in vivo suppression of GJB2 expression by RNA interference. *Hum Mol Genet* **14**(12): 1641–50.

60. Palliser, D., et al. (2006). An siRNA-based microbicide protects mice from lethal herpes simplex virus 2 infection. *Nature* **439**(7072): 89–95.

61. Spagnou, S., Miller, A. D., and Keller, M. (2004). Lipidic carriers of siRNA: differences in the formulation, cellular uptake, and delivery with plasmid DNA. *Biochemistry* **43**(42): 13348–56.

62. Meyerhoff, A. (1999). U.S. food and drug administration approval of AmBisome (liposomal amphotericin B) for treatment of visceral leishmaniasis. *Clin Infect Dis* **28**(1): 42–8; discussion 49–51.

63. Wang, S., et al. (1995). Delivery of antisense oligodeoxyribonucleotides against the human epidermal growth factor receptor into cultured KB cells with liposomes conjugated to folate via polyethylene glycol. *Proc Natl Acad Sci USA* **92**(8): 3318–22.

64. Dubey, P. K., et al. (2004). Liposomes modified with cyclic RGD peptide for tumor targeting. *J Drug Target* **12**(5): 257–64.

65. Oupicky, D., et al. (2002). Importance of lateral and steric stabilization of polyelectrolyte gene delivery vectors for extended systemic circulation. *Mol Ther* **5**(4): 463–72.

66. Moghimi, S. M. and Szebeni, J. (2003). Stealth liposomes and long circulating nanoparticles: critical issues in pharmacokinetics, opsonization and protein-binding properties. *Prog Lipid Res* **42**(6): 463–78.

67. Gao, D., et al. (2005). CD40 antisense oligonucleotide inhibition of trinitrobenzene sulphonic acid induced rat colitis. *Gut* **54**(1): 70–7.

68. Pal, A., et al. (2005). Systemic delivery of RafsiRNA using cationic cardiolipin liposomes silences Raf-1 expression and inhibits tumor growth in xenograft model of human prostate cancer. *Int J Oncol* **26**(4): 1087–91.

69. Chien, P. Y., et al. (2005). Novel cationic cardiolipin analogue-based liposome for efficient DNA and small interfering RNA delivery in vitro and in vivo. *Cancer Gene Ther* **12**(3): 321–8.

70. Tousignant, J. D., et al. (2000). Comprehensive analysis of the acute toxicities induced by systemic administration of cationic lipid:plasmid DNA complexes in mice. *Hum Gene Ther* **11**(18): 2493–513.

71. Semple, S. C., et al. (2001). Efficient encapsulation of antisense oligonu-cleotides in lipid vesicles using ionizable aminolipids: formation of novel small multilamellar vesicle structures. *Biochim Biophys Acta* **1510**(1–2): 152–66.

72. Dass, C. R. (2002). Cytotoxicity issues pertinent to lipoplex-mediated gene therapy in-vivo. *J Pharm Pharmacol* **54**(5): 593–601.

73. Audouy, S. A., et al. (2002). In vivo characteristics of cationic liposomes as delivery vectors for gene therapy. *Pharm Res* **19**(11): 1599–605.

74. Simberg, D., et al. (2004). DOTAP (and other cationic lipids): chemistry, bio-physics, and transfection. *Crit Rev Ther Drug Carrier Syst* **21**(4): 257–317.

75. Landen, C. N., Jr., et al. (2005). Therapeutic EphA2 gene targeting in vivo using neutral liposomal small interfering RNA delivery. *Cancer Res* **65**(15): 6910–8.

76. Leonetti, C., et al. (2001). Encapsulation of c-myc antisense oligodeoxynu-cleotides in lipid particles improves antitumoral efficacy in vivo in a human melanoma line. *Cancer Gene Ther* **8**(6): 459–68.

77. Heyes, J., et al. (2005). Cationic lipid saturation influences intracellular delivery of encapsulated nucleic acids. *J Control Release* **107**(2): 276–87.

78. Heyes, J., et al. (2006). Synthesis and characterization of novel poly(ethylene glycol)-lipid conjugates suitable for use in drug delivery. *J Control Release* **112**(2): 280–90.

79. Zimmermann, T. S., et al. (2006). RNAi-mediated gene silencing in non-human primates. *Nature* **441**(7089): 111–4.

80. Isacson, R., et al. (2003). Lack of efficacy of "naked" small interfering RNA applied directly to rat brain. *Acta Physiol Scand* **179**(2): 173–7.

81. Senn, C., et al. (2005). Central administration of small interfering RNAs in rats: a comparison with antisense oligonucleotides. *Eur J Pharmacol* **522**(1–3): 30–7.

82. Tompkins, S. M., et al. (2004). Protection against lethal influenza virus chal-lenge by RNA interference in vivo. *Proc Natl Acad Sci USA* **101**(23): 8682–6.

83. Bitko, V., et al. (2005). Inhibition of respiratory viruses by nasally administered siRNA. *Nat Med* **11**(1): 50–5.

84. Sioud, M. (2005). Induction of inflammatory cytokines and interferon responses by double-stranded and single-stranded siRNAs is sequence-dependent and requires endosomal localization. *J Mol Biol* **348**(5): 1079–90.

85. Heidel, J. D., et al. (2004). Lack of interferon response in animals to naked siRNAs. *Nat Biotechnol* **22**(12): 1579–82.

86. Sioud, M. and Sorensen, D. R. (2003). Cationic liposome-mediated delivery of siRNAs in adult mice. *Biochem Biophys Res Commun* **312**(4): 1220–5.

87. Ma, Z., et al. (2005). Cationic lipids enhance siRNA-mediated interferon response in mice. *Biochem Biophys Res Commun* **330**(3): 755–9.

88. Barreau, C., et al. (2006). Liposome-mediated RNA transfection should be used with caution. *Rna-a Publ Rna Soc* **12**(10): 1790–3.

89. Akinc, A., et al. (2008). A combinatorial library of lipid-like materials for delivery of RNAi therapeutics. *Nat Biotechnol* **26**(5): 561–9.

90. Wolfrum, C., et al. (2007). Mechanisms and optimization of in vivo delivery of lipophilic siRNAs. *Nat Biotechnol* **25**(10): 1149–57.

91. Love, K. T., et al. (2010). Lipid-like materials for low-dose, in vivo gene silencing. *Proc Natl Acad Sci USA* **107**(5): 1864–9.

92. Semple, S. C., et al. (2010). Rational design of cationic lipids for siRNA delivery. *Nat Biotechnol* **28**(2): 172–6.

93. Boussif, O., et al. (1995). A versatile vector for gene and oligonucleotide transfer into cells in culture and in vivo: polyethylenimine. *Proc Natl Acad Sci USA* **92**(16): 7297–301.

94. Akinc, A., et al. (2005). Exploring polyethylenimine-mediated DNA transfection and the proton sponge hypothesis. *J Gene Med* **7**(5): 657–63.

95. Chollet, P., et al. (2002). Side-effects of a systemic injection of linear polyethylenimine-DNA complexes. *J Gene Med* **4**(1): 84–91.

96. Godbey, W. T., Wu, K. K., and Mikos, A. G. (1999). Size matters: molecular weight affects the efficiency of poly(ethylenimine) as a gene delivery vehicle. *J Biomed Mater Res* **45**(3): 268–75.

97. Godbey, W. T., Wu, K. K., and Mikos, A. G. (2001). Poly(ethylenimine)-mediated gene delivery affects endothelial cell function and viability. *Biomaterials* **22**(5): 471–80.

98. Wightman, L., et al. (2001). Different behavior of branched and linear polyethylenimine for gene delivery in vitro and in vivo. *J Gene Med* **3**(4): 362–72.

99. Schiffelers, R. M., et al. (2004). Cancer siRNA therapy by tumor selective delivery with ligand-targeted sterically stabilized nanoparticle. *Nucleic Acids Res* **32**(19): e149.

100. Thomas, M., et al. (2005). Full deacylation of polyethylenimine dramatically boosts its gene delivery efficiency and specificity to mouse lung. *Proc Natl Acad Sci USA* **102**(16): 5679–84.

101. Hwa Kim, S., et al. (2005). Target-specific gene silencing by siRNA plasmid DNA complexed with folate-modified poly(ethylenimine). *J Control Release* **104**(1): 223–32.

102. Ge, Q., et al. (2004). Inhibition of influenza virus production in virus-infected mice by RNA interference. *Proc Natl Acad Sci USA* **101**(23): 8676–81.

103. Robbins, M., et al. (2008). Misinterpreting the therapeutic effects of small interfering RNA caused by immune stimulation. *Hum Gene Ther* **19**(10): 991–9.

104. Urban-Klein, B., et al. (2005). RNAi-mediated gene-targeting through systemic application of polyethylenimine (PEI)-complexed siRNA in vivo. *Gene Ther* **12**(5): 461–6.

105. Pun, S. H., et al. (2004). Cyclodextrin-modified polyethylenimine polymers for gene delivery. *Bioconjug Chem* **15**(4): 831–40.

106. Hwang, S. J., Bellocq, N. C., and Davis, M. E. (2001). Effects of structure of beta-cyclodextrin-containing polymers on gene delivery. *Bioconjug Chem* **12**(2): 280–90.

107. Davis, M. E., et al. (2004). Self-assembling nucleic acid delivery vehicles via linear, water-soluble, cyclodextrin-containing polymers. *Curr Med Chem* **11**(2): 179–97.

108. Putnam, D. (2006). Polymers for gene delivery across length scales. *Nat Mater* **5**(6): 439–51.

109. Omidi, Y., et al. (2005). Polypropylenimine dendrimer-induced gene expression changes: the effect of complexation with DNA, dendrimer generation and cell type. *J Drug Target* **13**(7): 431–43.

110. Tsutsumi, T., et al. (2006). Potential use of dendrimer/alpha-cyclodextrin conjugate as a novel carrier for small interfering RNA (siRNA). *J Incl Phenom Macro Chem* **56**(1–2): 81–4.

111. Convertine, A. J., et al. (2009). Development of a novel endosomolytic diblock copolymer for siRNA delivery. *J Control Release* **133**(3): 221–9.

112. Roy, K., et al. (1999). Oral gene delivery with chitosan–DNA nanoparticles generates immunologic protection in a murine model of peanut allergy. *Nat Med* **5**(4): 387–91.

113. Koping-Hoggard, M., et al. (2001). Chitosan as a nonviral gene delivery system. Structure-property relationships and characteristics compared with polyethylenimine in vitro and after lung administration in vivo. *Gene Ther* **8**(14): 1108–21.

114. Mao, H. Q., et al. (2001). Chitosan-DNA nanoparticles as gene carriers: synthesis, characterization and transfection efficiency. *J Control Release* **70**(3): 399–421.

115. Sato, T., Ishii, T., and Okahata, Y. (2001). In vitro gene delivery mediated by chitosan. Effect of pH, serum, and molecular mass of chitosan on the transfection efficiency. *Biomaterials* **22**(15): 2075–80.

116. Guliyeva, U., et al. (2006). Chitosan microparticles containing plasmid DNA as potential oral gene delivery system. *Eur J Pharm Biopharm* **62**(1): 17–25.

117. Zhang, W., et al. (2005). Inhibition of respiratory syncytial virus infection with intranasal siRNA nanoparticles targeting the viral NS1 gene. *Nat Med* **11**(1): 56–62.

118. Howard, K. A., et al. (2006). RNA interference in vitro and in vivo using a novel chitosan/siRNA nanoparticle system. *Mol Ther* **14**(4): 476–84.

119. Liu, X. D., et al. (2007). The influence of polymeric properties on chitosan/siRNA nanoparticle formulation and gene silencing. *Biomaterials* **28**(6): 1280–8.

120. MacLaughlin, F. C., et al. (1998). Chitosan and depolymerized chitosan oligomers as condensing carriers for in vivo plasmid delivery. *J Control Release* **56**(1–3): 259–72.

121. Li, X. W., et al. (2003). Sustained expression in mammalian cells with DNA complexed with chitosan nanoparticles. *Biochim et Biophys Acta-Gene Struct Expr* **1630**(1): 7–18.

122. Pille, J. Y., et al. (2006). Intravenous delivery of anti-RhoA small interfering RNA loaded in nanoparticles of chitosan in mice: safety and efficacy in xenografted aggressive breast cancer. *Hum Gene Ther* **17**(10): 1019–26.

123. Howard, K. A., et al. (2009). Chitosan/siRNA nanoparticle-mediated TNF-alpha knockdown in peritoneal macrophages for anti-inflammatory treatment in a murine arthritis model. *Mol Ther* **17**(1): 162–8.

124. Sorgi, F. L., Bhattacharya, S., and Huang, L. (1997). Protamine sulfate enhances lipid-mediated gene transfer. *Gene Ther* **4**(9): 961–8.

125. Song, E., et al. (2005). Antibody mediated in vivo delivery of small interfering RNAs via cell-surface receptors. *Nat Biotechnol* **23**(6): 709–17.

126. Svintradze, D. V. and Mrevlishvili, G. M. (2005). Fiber molecular model of atelocollagen-small interfering RNA (siRNA) complex. *Int J Biol Macromol* **37**(5): 283–6.

127. Takeshita, F., et al. (2005). Efficient delivery of small interfering RNA to bone-metastatic tumors by using atelocollagen in vivo. *Proc Natl Acad Sci USA* **102**(34): 12177–82.

128. Takei, Y., et al. (2004). A small interfering RNA targeting vascular endothelial growth factor as cancer therapeutics. *Cancer Res* **64**(10): 3365–70.

129. Banno, H., et al. (2006). Controlled release of small interfering RNA targeting midkine attenuates intimal hyperplasia in vein grafts. *J Vasc Surg* **44**(3): 633–41.

130. Bianco, A., et al. (2005). Biomedical applications of functionalised carbon nanotubes. *Chem Commun (Camb)* (5): 571–7.

131. Ajima, K., et al. (2005). Carbon nanohorns as anticancer drug carriers. *Mol Pharmacol* **2**(6): 475–80.

132. Sun, Y. P., et al. (2002). Functionalized carbon nanotubes: properties and applications. *Acc Chem Res* **35**(12): 1096–104.

133. Balasubramanian, K. and Burghard, M. (2005). Chemically functionalized carbon nanotubes. *Small* **1**(2): 180–92.

134. Jain, K. K. (2005). The role of nanobiotechnology in drug discovery. *Drug Discov Today* **10**(21): 1435–42.

135. Yang, R., et al. (2006). Single-walled carbon nanotubes-mediated in vivo and in vitro delivery of siRNA into antigen-presenting cells. *Gene Ther* **13**(24): 1714–23.

136. Bala, I., Hariharan, S., and Kumar, M. N. (2004). PLGA nanoparticles in drug delivery: the state of the art. *Crit Rev Ther Drug Carrier Syst* **21**(5): 387–422.

137. Panyam, J. and Labhasetwar, V. (2003). Biodegradable nanoparticles for drug and gene delivery to cells and tissue. *Adv Drug Deliv Rev* **55**(3): 329–47.

138. Shive, M. S. and Anderson, J. M. (1997). Biodegradation and biocompatibility of PLA and PLGA microspheres. *Adv Drug Deliv Rev* **28**(1): 5–24.

139. Kim, D., et al. (2005). Interaction of PLGA nanoparticles with human blood constituents. *Colloids Surf B Biointerfaces* **40**(2): 83–91.

140. Wang, D., et al. (1999). Encapsulation of plasmid DNA in biodegradable poly(D, L-lactic-co-glycolic acid) microspheres as a novel approach for immunogene delivery. *J Control Release* **57**(1): 9–18.

141. Capan, Y., et al. (1999). Preparation and characterization of poly (D,L-lactide-co-glycolide) microspheres for controlled release of poly(L-lysine) complexed plasmid DNA. *Pharm Res* **16**(4): 509–13.

142. Walter, E., et al. (2001). Hydrophilic poly(DL-lactide-co-glycolide) microspheres for the delivery of DNA to human-derived macrophages and dendritic cells. *J Control Release* **76**(1–2): 149–68.

143. Yuan, X. D., et al. (2006). siRNA drug delivery by biodegradable polymeric nanoparticles. *J Nanoscience Nanotechnology* **6**(9–10): 2821–8.

144. Fu, K., et al. (2000). Visual evidence of acidic environment within degrading poly(lactic-co-glycolic acid) (PLGA) microspheres. *Pharm Res* **17**(1): 100–6.

145. Schwendeman, S. P. (2002). Recent advances in the stabilization of proteins encapsulated in injectable PLGA delivery systems. *Crit Rev Ther Drug Carrier Syst* **19**(1): 73–98.

146. Walter, E., et al. (1999). Microencapsulation of DNA using poly(DL-lactide-co-glycolide): stability issues and release characteristics. *J Control Release* **61**(3): 361–74.

147. Luo, D., et al. (1999). Controlled DNA delivery systems. *Pharm Res* **16**(8): 1300–8.

148. Woodrow, K. A., et al. (2009). Intravaginal gene silencing using biodegradable polymer nanoparticles densely loaded with small-interfering RNA. *Nat Mater* **8**(6): 526–33.

149. Brannon-Peppas, L. and Blanchette, J. O. (2004). Nanoparticle and targeted systems for cancer therapy. *Adv Drug Deliv Rev* **56**(11): 1649–59.

150. Walker, G. F., et al. (2005). Toward synthetic viruses: endosomal pH-triggered deshielding of targeted polyplexes greatly enhances gene transfer in vitro and in vivo. *Mol Ther* **11**(3): 418–25.

151. Dassie, J. P., et al. (2009). Systemic administration of optimized aptamer-siRNA chimeras promotes regression of PSMA-expressing tumors. *Nat Biotechnol* **27**(9): 839–U95.

152. Manoharan, M. (2002). Oligonucleotide conjugates as potential antisense drugs with improved uptake, biodistribution, targeted delivery, and mechanism of action. *Antisense Nucleic Acid Drug Dev* **12**(2): 103–28.

153. Weissleder, R., et al. (2005). Cell-specific targeting of nanoparticles by multivalent attachment of small molecules. *Nat Biotechnol* **23**(11): 1418–23.

154. Kircheis, R., et al. (2002). Tumor-targeted gene delivery: an attractive strategy to use highly active effector molecules in cancer treatment. *Gene Ther* **9**(11): 731–5.

155. Hu-Lieskovan, S., et al. (2005). Sequence-specific knockdown of EWS-FLI1 by targeted, nonviral delivery of small interfering RNA inhibits tumor growth in a murine model of metastatic Ewing's sarcoma. *Cancer Res* **65**(19): 8984–92.

156. Ogris, M., et al. (2003). Tumor-targeted gene therapy: strategies for the preparation of ligand-polyethylene glycol-polyethylenimine/DNA complexes. *J Control Release* **91**(1–2): 173–81.

157. Medina-Kauwe, L. K. (2003). Endocytosis of adenovirus and adenovirus capsid proteins. *Adv Drug Deliv Rev* **55**(11): 1485–96.

158. Wittekindt, C., et al. (2004). Integrin specificity of the cyclic Arg-Gly-Asp motif and its role in integrin-targeted gene transfer. *Biotechnol Appl Biochem* **40**: 281–90.

159. Ruoslahti, E. (1996). RGD and other recognition sequences for integrins. *Annu Rev Cell Dev Biol* **12**: 697–715.

160. Harvie, P., et al. (2003). Targeting of lipid-protamine-DNA (LPD) lipopolyplexes using RGD motifs. *J Liposome Res* **13**(3–4): 231–47.

161. Colin, M., et al. (1998). Liposomes enhance delivery and expression of an RGD-oligolysine gene transfer vector in human tracheal cells. *Gene Ther* **5**(11): 1488–98.

162. Wickham, T. J., et al. (1993). Integrin-alpha-V-beta-3 and integrin-alpha-V-beta-5 promote adenovirus internalization but not virus attachment. *Cell* **73**(2): 309–19.

163. Li, E., et al. (1998). Adenovirus cell entry requires the Rho family of small GTPases. *Mol Biol Cell* **9**: 344A–344A.

164. Arnaout, M. A., Goodman, S. L., and Xiong, J. P. (2002). Coming to grips with integrin binding to ligands. *Curr Opin Cell Biol* **14**(5): 641–51.

165. Schiffelers, R. M., et al. (2005). Transporting silence: design of carriers for siRNA to angiogenic endothelium. *J Control Release* **109**(1–3): 5–14.

166. Wu, M., Gunning, W., and Ratnam, M. (1999). Expression of folate receptor type alpha in relation to cell type, malignancy, and differentiation in ovary, uterus, and cervix. *Cancer Epidemiol Biomarkers Prev* **8**(9): 775–82.

167. Weitman, S. D., et al. (1992). Distribution of the folate receptor Gp38 in normal and malignant-cell lines and tissues. *Cancer Res* **52**(12): 3396–401.

168. Weitman, S. D., et al. (1992). Cellular-localization of the folate receptor—potential role in drug toxicity and folate homeostasis. *Cancer Res.* **52**(23): 6708–11.

169. Guo, W., et al. (1999). Mechanisms of methotrexate resistance in osteosarcoma. *Clin Cancer Res* **5**(3): 621–7.

170. Leamon, C. P., Pastan, I., and Low, P. S. (1993). Cytotoxicity of folate-pseudomonas exotoxin conjugates toward tumor-cells—contribution of translocation domain. *J Biol Chem* **268**(33): 24847–54.

171. Lu, J. Y., et al. (1999). Folate-targeted enzyme prodrug cancer therapy utilizing penicillin-V amidase and a doxorubicin prodrug. *J Drug Target* **7**(1): 43–53.

172. Kranz, D. M., et al. (1995). Conjugates of folate and anti-T-cell-receptor antibodies specifically target folate-receptor-positive tumor-cells for lysis. *Proc Natl Acad Sci USA* **92**(20): 9057–61.

173. Lee, R. J. and Guo, W. (1999). Targeted gene delivery via the folate receptor. *Abstr Pap Am Chem Soc* **217**: U557–U557.

174. Lee, R. J. and Huang, L. (1996). Folate-targeted, anionic liposome-entrapped polylysine-condensed DNA for tumor cell-specific gene transfer. *J Biol Chem* **271**(14): 8481–7.

175. Lee, R. J., Wang, S., and Low, P. S. (1996). Measurement of endosome pH following folate receptor-mediated endocytosis. *Biochim Biophys Acta-Mol Cell Res* **1312**(3): 237–42.

176. Oyewumi, M. O. and Mumper, R. J. (2003). Influence of formulation parameters on gadolinium entrapment and tumor cell uptake using folate-coated nanoparticles. *Int J Pharm* **251**(1–2): 85–97.

177. Kim, S. H., et al. (2005). Target-specific gene silencing by siRNA plasmid DNA complexed with folate-modified poly(ethylenimine). *J Control Release* **104**(1): 223–32.

178. Kim, S. H., et al. (2006). Comparative evaluation of target-specific GFP gene silencing efficiencies for antisense ODN, synthetic siRNA, and siRNA plasmid complexed with PEI-PEG-FOL conjugate. *Bioconjug Chem* **17**(1): 241–4.

179. Guo, S., Huang, F., and Guo, P. (2006). Construction of folate-conjugated pRNA of bacteriophage phi29 DNA packaging motor for delivery of chimeric siRNA to nasopharyngeal carcinoma cells. *Gene Ther* **13**(10): 814–20.

180. Ishihara, Y., et al. (2004). HER2/neu-derived peptides recognized by both cellular and humoral immune systems in HLA-A2(+) cancer patients. *Int J Oncol* **24**(4): 967–75.

181. Suk, J. S., et al. (2006). Gene delivery to differentiated neurotypic cells with RGD and HIV Tat peptide functionalized polymeric nanoparticles. *Biomaterials* **27**(29): 5143–50.

182. Eguchi, A., et al. (2009). Efficient siRNA delivery into primary cells by a peptide transduction domain-dsRNA binding domain fusion protein. *Nat Biotechnol* **27**(6): 567–71.

183. Michiue, H., et al. (2009). Induction of in vivo synthetic lethal RNAi responses to treat glioblastoma. *Cancer Biol Ther* **8**(23): 2306–13.

184. Kang, H. M., et al. (2005). Tat-conjugated PAMAM dendrimers as delivery agents for antisense and siRNA oligonucleotides. *Pharm Res* **22**(12): 2099–106.

185. Guo, S., et al. (2005). Specific delivery of therapeutic RNAs to cancer cells via the dimerization mechanism of phi29 motor pRNA. *Hum Gene Ther* **16**(9): 1097–109.

186. de Jonge, J., et al. (2005). Reconstituted influenza virus envelopes as an efficient carrier system for cellular delivery of small-interfering RNAs. *Gene Ther* **13**(5): 400–11.

187. Ito, M., et al. (2005). Rad51 siRNA delivered by HVJ envelope vector enhances the anti-cancer effect of cisplatin. *J Gene Med* **7**(8): 1044–52.

188. Kimchi-Sarfaty, C., et al. (2005). Efficient delivery of RNA interference effectors via in vitro-packaged SV40 pseudovirions. *Hum Gene Ther* **16**(9): 1110–5.

189. Bartlett, D. W. and Davis, M. E. (2007). Physicochemical and biological characterization of targeted, nucleic acid-containing nanoparticles. *Bioconjug Chem* **18**(2): 456–68.

190. Heidel, J. D., et al. (2007). Administration in non-human primates of escalating intravenous doses of targeted nanoparticles containing ribonucleotide reductase subunit M2 siRNA. *Proc Natl Acad Sci USA* **104**(14): 5715–21.

CHAPTER 7

INTERFERON, CYTOKINE INDUCTION, AND OTHER POTENTIAL *IN VIVO* TOXICITIES

ADAM JUDGE, MARJORIE ROBBINS, and IAN MACLACHLAN

7.1 INTRODUCTION

The promise of molecular therapy will be realized in the development of nucleic acid-based drugs that act through their intended mechanism, while at the same time, causing a minimum of undesired side effects. A potential hurdle to be overcome is that many types of nucleic acid, including both single-stranded (ss) and double-stranded (ds) DNA and RNA species, are potent activators of the mammalian innate immune system [1–6]. Canonical small interfering RNA (siRNA) duplexes can also be included in the long list of immunostimulatory nucleic acids [7, 8].

Synthetically manufactured siRNA duplexes can induce high levels of inflammatory cytokines and type I interferons (IFNs), in particular interferon-alpha (IFN-α), following systemic administration in mammals [7]. Effective intracellular delivery of siRNA to human peripheral blood mononuclear cells also induces significant cytokine release, including high level IFN-α production from plasmacytoid dendritic cells (pDCs). These immune responses are greatly potentiated by the use of delivery vehicles that facilitate cellular uptake [7, 9]. Although the immunomodulatory effects of nucleic acids may be harnessed therapeutically, for example, in oncology and allergy applications [10, 11], in many cases immune activation represents a significant undesirable side effect. This is due to the toxicities associated with excessive cytokine release and associated inflammatory syndromes. The potential for nucleic acid-based drugs to be rendered immunogenic is also a cause for concern since

RNA Interference: Application to Drug Discovery and Challenges to Pharmaceutical Development, Edited by Paul H. Johnson
Copyright © 2011 John Wiley & Sons, Inc.

the establishment of an antibody response may severely compromise both its safety and efficacy. Historically, concerns around immunogenicity have hampered the development of other drug classes including protein-based therapeutics such as monoclonal Ab's. Clearly, there are significant implications both for the development of siRNA as a safe and effective therapeutic and in the interpretation of gene silencing effects elicited by siRNA in an immunological setting. This chapter provides the background information required to anticipate, manage, and abrogate the immunological effects of siRNA containing drugs and will assist the reader in the successful *in vivo* application of siRNA.

7.1.1 Basic Concepts in Immunology

Although central to our understanding of health and disease, immunology has garnered a reputation as one of the less tractable fields of study available to students of the biological sciences. In part, this is due to the numerous components of the immune system that interact in a seemingly endless array of pathways designed to protect the self from nonself. Although a review of immunology is beyond the scope of this chapter, a degree of familiarity is required to appreciate its relevance to siRNA and the appropriate design of RNAi experiments.

The immune system can be regarded as having two branches known as the innate and adaptive systems. The innate response is that which acts immediately to protect the host from potentially pathogenic infectious agents or other foreign bodies. Immune cells express proteins called pattern recognition receptors (PRRs) that have evolved to recognize molecular features common to many pathogens. These features, known as pathogen-associated molecular patterns (PAMPs), comprise a wide variety of highly conserved bacterial, fungal, and viral elements that serve as hallmarks of microbial infection when they are engaged by PRRs. Therefore, the specific recognition of microbial elements by PRRs represents one of the mechanisms used by the immune system to distinguish self from nonself. Cells respond to PAMPs by triggering a series of autocrine and paracrine signals that coordinate the host organism's immune response to the foreign threat. PRRs of the innate immune system are encoded in the germ line and expressed in a variety of specialized immune cells as well as other cell types. Many of the components of the innate immune system, including PRR, evolved early and can be found in invertebrates as well as vertebrates [12]. In the case of nucleic acids, receptors have evolved in mammals that recognize the ssRNA and the dsRNA of viruses, unmethylated CpG motifs of nonvertebrate DNA and other nucleic acid structures not typically present in mammalian cells. This has driven many pathogens to coevolve countermeasures that aim to prevent their recognition by the host innate immune response.

One family of PRR, the Toll-like receptors (TLRs), consists of up to 15 family members in mammals, with 10 known TLRs in humans, and 12 in mice. TLRs function as homo or heterodimers with each family member having different ligand specificity. They are oriented such that they have an N-terminal ligand-binding domain and a C-terminal cytoplasmic domain that transmits activation signals to the cell. TLR signaling results in cellular responses that include enhanced phagocytosis of invading bacterial pathogens, induction of apoptosis in response to certain viral pathogens, or activation of immune cells such that they produce IFNs, cytokines, and other inflammatory mediators. Other classes of PRRs include the RNA helicases RIG-I and MDA-5 and the dsRNA-binding protein kinase (PKR), an IFN-inducible serine–threonine kinase [13]. These cytoplasmic receptors are expressed in a wide variety of cell types and detect RNA species characteristic of intracellular viral infections, triggering IFN release and a generalized antiviral response inside the cell.

The innate immune response protects healthy individuals from most threats, detecting, reacting to and clearing pathogens within minutes or hours. The innate response also serves to orchestrate the slower developing adaptive immune response that may be required if the invading pathogen becomes established. Unlike the germ line encoded PRRs of the innate response, the adaptive response relies on the recognition of specific pathogen components (antigens) by receptors that are generated through the complex rearrangement of genes during T-cell and B-cell development. This process of gene rearrangement generates B-cell (antibody) and T-cell receptor repertoires capable of recognizing literally millions of distinct antigens or epitopes. Successful activation of the adaptive immune response results in the foundation of antigen-specific effector cell populations that can target specific pathogens through the secretion of antibodies and T-cell-directed killing. The adaptive response also establishes memory B and T cells that, in conjunction with long-lived antibody responses, confer long-term protection from subsequent reinfection; that which we call "immunity."

The adaptive immune system relies on the innate immune system to provide many of its cues. In this way, the two systems are linked. From the drug development perspective this can be both a blessing and a curse. In certain applications, such as infectious disease and oncology, activation of the innate immune system can potentiate an adaptive response resulting in successful immunization against infection or the establishment of long-term antitumor immunity. However, the activation of uncontrolled or misdirected innate responses can lead to undesired dose-limiting toxicities and inflammation as well as potentiating antibody responses against the drug carrier or the drug itself.

With this in mind, it is important to consider the particular immunological context in which a drug will be utilized. Since pathogens have evolved an array of entry routes to infect their hosts, the innate immune system has evolved so that most tissues contain the requisite immune cells required to mount a response to local invasion. As such, each of the common routes of drug administration results in exposure of the drug to cells of the immune system. Naïve and activated immune cells, together with antigens entering the body migrate through the peripheral tissues via the blood and lymphatic system into specialized lymphoid tissues where immune responses develop. These so-called secondary lymphoid tissues, including the spleen, lymph nodes, tonsils, adenoids and Peyer's patches of the gut, contain both resident and recirculating immune cells and are ideally located to receive incoming antigens from the skin, mucosae, and blood (Figure 7.1). There are a small number of tissues within the body that are considered to be immune privileged, a status that is thought to protect these sites from the damaging effects of an immune

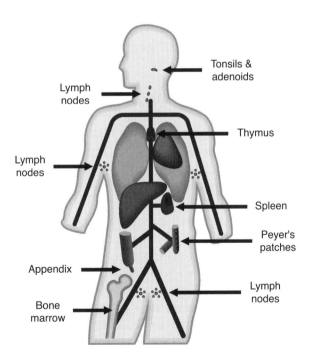

FIGURE 7.1 Lymphoid tissues in the Body. Naïve and activated immune cells circulate through the lymphatic and blood systems of the body via the secondary lymphoid tissues such as the spleen, tonsils, adenoids, thymus, and Peyer's patches. Immune cells are available to interact with immunostimulatory siRNA delivered via various routes of administration and thereby initiate both innate and adaptive immune responses.

response. Immune privilege is established by a number of mechanisms including reduced accessibility to immune effector cells and active inhibition of immune cell function by local immunosuppressive factors. These tissues include the brain, separated from the rest of the body by the blood brain barrier, and the vitreous humor compartment of the eye. Although it is conceivable that the direct administration of drugs into these immune-privileged sites may be less encumbered by immunological considerations, the diseased state can compromise immune privilege due to local inflammation, vascular permeability, and the recruitment of immune effector cells. The choroidal neovascularization underlying certain eye diseases, including those being currently targeted by siRNA-based therapeutics, is one example where this may occur. In any case, the development of nucleic acid-based drugs, including those using siRNA, requires careful consideration of the potential for immune-mediated complications. In order to better understand this potential, some understanding of the mechanism of nucleic acid-mediated immune stimulation is required.

7.2 MECHANISMS OF NUCLEIC ACID-MEDIATED IMMUNE STIMULATION

Innate immune responses can be triggered through a variety of TLR-dependent and TLR-independent mechanisms according to the nature of the pathogen-derived signal and the type of PRR that they engage. One arm of the TLR-independent response comprises a disparate series of cytoplasmic nucleic acid sensing proteins, including PKR, retinoic acid-inducible gene 1 (RIG-1), melanoma differentiation-associated gene 5 (MDA-5), and likely other yet unidentified proteins that are activated by RNA species containing viral signatures. The TLR-dependent arm of the innate immune response is founded on a number of TLR family members, each one having a specialized function in recognizing particular pathogen-associated molecules. These include bacterial cell wall components, lipopolysaccharides (LPS), flagellae, and nucleic acids derived from bacteria and viruses. An important feature of all PRRs is that the ability to engage their target ligands is dictated by the cellular location of the receptor. For example, TLRs that have evolved to sense external features of bacteria such as LPS and flagellin are typically expressed on the outer cell membrane, where they can engage bacteria that are outside of the cell. In contrast, the nucleic acid sensing TLRs are typically located inside the cell and engage nucleic acids released from invading pathogens, as they are degraded within the endosomal/lysosomal compartment. Similarly, the TLR-independent PRRs that detect viral RNA are ideally situated within the cell's cytoplasm to monitor for viral infection and replication. This compartmentalization of receptors provides an additional mechanism by which the host immune response is able to distinguish between self and nonself. This is particularly important in the case of the nucleic acid sensing TLRs where their endosomal location helps to prevent exposure to endogenous nucleic acids from healthy cells. As we describe in this chapter, siRNAs have the capacity to activate both TLR-dependent and -independent immune responses based on two fundamental principles: (1) siRNA can possess the same molecular signatures as viral RNA and (2) siRNA transfection into cells exposes this exogenous RNA to the nucleic acid sensing receptors of the innate immune system. We will begin our discussion by describing the role of the TLR family in nucleic acid recognition.

7.2.1 Toll-Like Receptors

TLRs derive their name from Toll, a transmembrane receptor first described for its role in establishing the dorsal-ventral pattern of differentiation in the developing *Drosophila* embryo [14]. This protein was later discovered to play a role in the *Drosophila* innate immune system, responding to extracellular stimuli by inducing gene expression in an NF-κB-dependent manner [15]. Subsequently, a whole family of human TLRs was identified having significant homology to *Drosophila* Toll [16–18], a finding that has lead to significant advances in our understanding of the innate immune system in mammals.

Of the 10 or more known members of the mammalian TLR family, 4 are involved in the recognition of nucleic acids. TLR3, TLR7, and TLR8 recognize RNA-based ligands and are primarily located within the endosomal compartment of immune cells, although TLR3 may also be found at the cell surface of certain cell types (Figures 7.2 and 7.3). TLR9 is located in the endoplasmic reticulum of resting cells and also translocates into the endosomal/lysosomal compartment upon cellular activation where it can engage exogenous DNA that has been taken up by the cell [19–21]. Functional signaling through these nucleic acid sensing TLRs appears to require endosomal maturation associated with the concomitant acidification of this cellular compartment [22, 23]. This process can be inhibited by chloroquine, a compound that prevents acidification in cellular vacuoles such as endosomes, lysosomes, and Golgi. Therefore, TLR-dependent immune activation by nucleic acids is characterized as being highly sensitive to inhibition by chloroquine or related compounds (e.g., [5, 7, 24]). Of the four TLRs involved in the recognition of nucleic acids, TLR7 and TLR8 are the most relevant when considering the immunobiology of siRNA. However, closely related TLR9 is more highly characterized, so we will begin our discussion there.

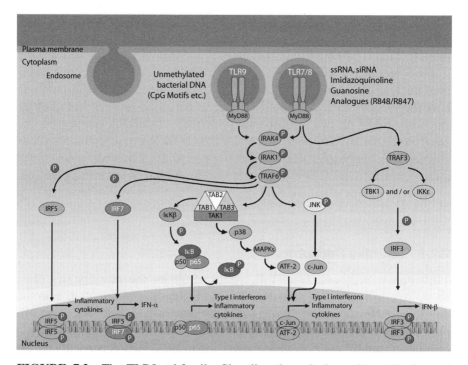

FIGURE 7.2 The TLR9 subfamily. Signaling through the endosomally located TLR7, TLR8, and TLR9 occurs through the adaptor protein MyD88. Activated MyD88 forms a complex with IRAK-1, IRAK-4, and TRAF6, resulting in the activation and nuclear translocation of NF-κB and activation of ATF2-c-Jun transcription factor through MAPKs. NF-κB and ATF-2-c-Jun activity are responsible for expression of inflammatory cytokines. The MyD88-IRAK1, IRAK4, TRAF6 complex also activates the transcription factor IRF-7 resulting in the transcription of IFNα subtypes. MyD88 also directly interacts with TRAF3, facilitating the production of IFN β via activation of IRF3. (For a color version of this figure, see plate 6.)

TLR9 Invertebrate DNA, including bacterial DNA, has stimulatory effects on mammalian immune cells due to the presence of unmethylated CpG dinucleotides [25]. This mammalian response to invertebrate and bacterial DNA is mediated by TLR9 [26]. The molecular basis for how TLR9 distinguishes self from nonself DNA is centered on the fact that mammalian (host) DNA contains very few unmethylated CpG dinucleotides. The frequency of CpG dinucleotides in mammalian genomic DNA is only a quarter of that predicted by random distribution [27]. Furthermore, the majority of these CpG dinucleotides in mammalian DNA are methylated posttranscription by DNA methyltransferase enzymes, converting the 5′-cytosine base to 5-methyl-cytosine (5 mC), a configuration no longer recognized by TLR9.

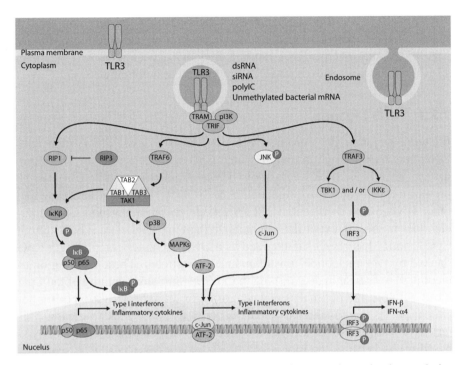

FIGURE 7.3   TLR3. Binding of dsRNA to TLR3 causes its activation and signaling through the adaptor protein TRIF. Upon activation, TRIF forms a complex with TRAF3 and TBK1 leading to IRF3 and IRF7 activation and the downstream production of Type I IFNs. TLR3 signaling through TRIF also activates RIP1 and TRAF6, leading to the downstream activation of NF-κB, ATF, and c-Jun transcription factors and induction of inflammatory cytokines such as IL-6 and TNF-α. (For a color version of this figure, see plate 7.)

It is interesting to note the prevailing theory that CpG methylation itself has driven CpG suppression in the mammalian genome due to the high frequency of spontaneous deamination that converts 5 mC to thymidine. The resulting point mutations have long been associated with a number of diseases [28]. However, if the consequence of CpG methylation is an unacceptably high mutation rate, why have mammals not abandoned the practice? Part of the answer may lie in the role of methylated CpG motifs in differentiating self from nonself DNA.

TLR9 mRNA is found in lymphoid tissues including the spleen, lymph nodes, bone marrow, and peripheral blood leukocytes. In humans, TLR9 is functionally expressed in B cells and pDCs, making these immune cell types directly responsive to CpG containing DNA [20]. In addition to B cells and pDCs, mice express TLR9 in monocytes and myeloid dendritic cells (mDCs).

As with all TLRs, the TLR9 protein has N-terminal leucine-rich repeats (LRRs) that are thought to mediate ligand recognition and binding specificity [29, 30]. A putative CpG DNA-binding domain has been identified in human TLR9 with homology to other DNA-binding protein domains [31].

7.2.2 TLR9 Ligands

Bacterial genomic and plasmid DNA, invertebrate DNA, and certain viral DNA genomes are rich in unmethylated CpG sequences and are, therefore, natural ligands for TLR9 activation. These stimulatory motifs can also be present in synthetic DNA oligonucleotides (ODNs) including antisense and other DNA-based therapeutics. TLR9 recognizes unmethylated CpG dinucleotides in the context of their immediate flanking sequences. The resulting CpG "motif" has been characterized as a DNA hexamer comprising a CpG flanked by two nucleotides upstream and downstream. These flanking dinucleotides are critical in determining the TLR9 stimulatory activity of the CpG motif. Of note, the optimal sequence motifs for immune activation differ between species due to inherent genetic differences in the TLR9 receptor. This has significant consequences for the preclinical development of CpG DNA-based drugs because the biological effects of a given CpG DNA sequence can differ markedly between mice, large animal models, and ultimately humans [11].

Since the discovery that the fundamental characteristics of CpG DNA motifs can be captured in simple ssDNA ODNs, a large body of research has been devoted to understanding the immunological mechanisms surrounding TLR9-mediated immune activation and how to exploit these effects for therapeutic purpose (reviewed in [11, 20]). Synthetic CpG ODNs can be designed either to trigger TLR9 responses or to inhibit TLR9-mediated immune activation through some form of receptor antagonism [32]. Immunostimulatory CpG ODN may be categorized as belonging to one of three classes [33]; type A ODNs contain a stretch of guanosines at their 3'end in addition to the CpG motif. This stretch of guanosines facilitates tetramer formation or oligomerization, leading to the formation of nanoparticles that are thought to be necessary for the TLR9-mediated IFN-induction in pDCs [34]. Type B ODNs lack the contiguous guanosines found in type A ODNs and are unable to form higher order structures. Type B ODNs strongly activate B cells to produce inflammatory cytokines such as interleukin-6 (IL-6) and tumor necrosis factor-alpha (TNF-α) but induce much lower levels of IFN-α than type A ODNs. Type C ODNs contain palindromic sequences that may facilitate the formation of dimers and/or hairpins and combine the immune effects of type A and B ODNs to induce production of IFN-α in pDCs as well as production of inflammatory cytokines in B cells [35]. Despite these various classes, all of the immunostimulatory effects of CpG ODNs are attributable to TLR9 engagement as the CpG DNA is trafficked through the endosomal compartment. The importance of intracellular trafficking is illustrated by the different activities of type A and B ODNs. Type A ODNs are retained in the endosome longer than type B ODNs, which are quickly trafficked to the lysosome [36]. Formulation of type B ODN as DOTAP lipoplexes facilitates their intracellular delivery and confers longer endosomal retention times, increasing their IFN-inducing capacity [36]. As we describe later in this chapter, the use of delivery vehicles greatly potentiates the immunostimulatory effects of synthetic siRNA, most likely through facilitating engagement of TLR7 and TLR8 that also reside in the endosomal compartment.

Synthetic CpG ODNs often contain a phosphorothioate (PS) backbone to enhance their resistance to nucleases and to facilitate their uptake by cells both *in vitro* and *in vivo*. CpG ODNs containing a PS backbone are typically more efficient at activating B cells and relatively less efficient at activating IFN-α production from pDCs when compared with a native phosphodiester (PO) backbone [11]. This difference in IFN-α induction could be due to an altered secondary structure that results from the incorporation of PS linkages in the ODN. PS ODNs are also more promiscuous than their PO counterparts, exhibiting CpG-independent binding to TLR2 and TLR9, although activation only occurs via TLR9 [31]. CpG ODNs can be encapsulated in various delivery vehicles, including liposomes, to protect them from nuclease-mediated degradation and to improve their drug-like properties. This bypasses the immediate requirement for PS chemistries to stabilize the naked ODN molecules. These formulations potentiate intracellular delivery and typically increase the immune stimulatory effects of the CpG DNA. When formulated into liposomes, the native PO chemistry is often more effective than the PS backbone at inducing cytokine production, suggesting that the natural PO backbone acts as a more effective ligand for TLR9-mediated immune recognition [37].

TLR7 and TLR8   TLR7 and TLR8 are highly homologous to TLR9 and together form the "TLR9 subfamily" of nucleic acid sensing TLRs (reviewed in [19, 38]). As would be expected for such closely related molecules, members of the TLR9 subfamily share many structural and functional characteristics including their cellular expression pattern, intracellular localization, common downstream signaling pathways, and the consequent biological effects of receptor activation. The primary difference lies in their respective ligands; whereas TLR9 recognizes DNA, TLR7 and TLR8 are both activated by RNA species that are taken up into the endosomal compartment. For the purposes of this chapter, it is important to highlight here that TLR7/8 ligands can include siRNAs and their constituent RNA ODNs.

As with TLR9, TLR7 is constitutively expressed by pDCs and B cells and can be upregulated in certain other immune cell types upon activation. Although TLR8 is phylogenetically close to TLR7 and is activated by structurally similar ligands, their cellular expression patterns are distinct with TLR8 being constitutively expressed by mDC and monocytes in humans. These differences in expression pattern likely account for the bias toward predominantly pDC-derived IFN-α (TLR7) or mDC-derived proinflammatory cytokines (TLR8) in response to TLR7 or TLR8 activation [39]. Murine TLR8 does not respond to conventional TLR7/8 ligands, and until recently [40], has been considered to be nonfunctional in mice. This is an important consideration when comparing RNA-mediated immune activation in murine and human model systems.

TLR7 and TLR8 Ligands *Nucleoside analogs*: The functionality of TLR7 and TLR8 was first revealed when they were identified as the cognate receptors for a class of synthetic nucleoside analogs that exert therapeutic antiviral effects via immune stimulation [41, 42]. TLR7 is directly activated by small molecule synthetic guanosine analogs, such as loxoribine, and imidazoquinoline amines, such as imiquimod and resiquimod (R-848), that resemble adenine. Some of these TLR7 ligands, for example, R-848, also activate human TLR8 suggesting a degree of redundancy between these receptors. However, differences in cellular expression and cytokine induction profiles illustrate that these receptors play distinct biological roles and likely act in concert to facilitate fine-tuning of the immune response [39, 42]. In this regard, continued work developing small molecule "immune response modifiers" has identified a number of synthetic compounds that preferentially activate either TLR7 or TLR8 in human systems, thereby allowing the interplay between these two closely related receptors to be more closely examined [39].

ssRNA: It was not until 2004 when three independent groups identified ssRNA as the natural ligand for TLR7 and TLR8 that their predicted role in antiviral defense became more fully appreciated [4, 5, 43]. TLR7 has been shown to recognize ssRNA viruses (such as vesicular stomatitis virus or influenza), as well as polyuridine and synthetic ssRNA rich in guanosine and uridine (such as RNA40, derived from a GU-rich segment of HIV RNA) [4, 5, 43]. In humans, TLR8 recognizes similar U-rich or GU-rich ssRNA and is also likely activated by RNA viruses [4]. More recently, it has been suggested that RNA ligands for TLR7 are defined simply by the presence of a ribose sugar backbone and multiple uridine groups in close proximity [44]. In this respect, the sequence specificity for TLR7 binding to RNA is considerably less strict than the corresponding interaction between TLR9 and defined CpG motifs within a DNA sequence. However, despite the apparent lack of a defined motif, it is clear that TLR7 is differentially activated according to the nucleotide sequence of the RNA. As such, the immunological effects of RNA ODNs can range from being highly potent immune activators equivalent to defined CpG ODNs to having no apparent immunostimulatory capacity. The importance of these sequence related effects on TLR7 activation become apparent when we consider how different siRNA duplexes can activate the innate immune response.

siRNA: Synthetic or *in vitro* transcribed siRNAs and short hairpin RNAs (shRNAs) are immunostimulatory when delivered into immune cells, triggering IFN-α production from pDCs and inflammatory cytokine production from mDCs [7, 8, 45]. The magnitude of this innate immune response is governed by the siRNA sequence, and in mice, this response to siRNA is primarily mediated via TLR7 activation [7, 8]. The striking similarities between immune responses to siRNA in mouse and human systems (e.g., IFN-α induction from pDC, chloroquine sensitivity, and RNA sequence specificity) imply that siRNA activates TLR7 in human immune cells and is also likely to be a ligand for human TLR8 [7].

A formal demonstration that siRNA directly activates human TLR7 and TLR8 has proven somewhat difficult. In the widely utilized HEK293 model cell lines that stably express human TLRs, TLR7 expressing cells are responsive to small molecule agonists yet the same cells appear unresponsive to either immunostimulatory siRNAs or ssRNAs such as RNA40 [4, 7]. Some reports have found that TLR8 but not TLR7-HEK293 cells are activated by immunostimulatory ssRNA [4, 46] although we have been unable to elicit specific responses to siRNA in either cell line ([7] and A. Judge and M. Robbins, 2007, unpublished observations). These discrepancies may simply reflect the fact that forced expression of TLRs in this model system does not fully recapitulate the natural biology of TLR7/8 expression in immune cells. An alternative explanation is that some other cofactor that is lacking in HEK293 cells is required for the recognition of RNA ligands by TLR7 and TLR8. Recent data describing a coreceptor in TLR9-mediated IFN induction via type A ODN provides one such example of a cofactor that modulates intracellular TLR signaling [47].

As we shall describe in detail in the following sections, TLR7/8-mediated recognition of siRNA can be inhibited by chemical modification. This can be achieved by introducing 2'-O-methyl (2'OMe)-modified nucleotides into the RNA sequence, thereby preventing TLR7/8 activation and profoundly inhibiting immune stimulation. Although in some ways analogous to the inhibition of TLR9 signaling by direct methylation of CpG motifs, 2'OMe-nucleotides reflect methylation of the ribose sugar backbone and appear to require no sequence or positional context to inhibit RNA from activating TLR7/8. As an extension to these studies, we have found that 2'OMe-modified

RNA acts as an antagonist to TLR7-mediated immune activation by both ssRNA and small molecule TLR7 agonists [48].

TLR3 TLR-3 has a unique gene structure among the TLRs and belongs to its own subfamily distinct from the TLR9 subfamily of nucleic acid sensing receptors [38]. At the cellular level, TLR3 expression in humans is largely restricted to mature mDCs [49], while in mice, TLR3 is found in a wider variety of cell types [50]. It can also be expressed in a number of cell lines including endothelial, epithelial, and fibroblast lines. TLR3 is considered to be a sensor of viral infection and is activated within the endosomal compartment of immune cells by long dsRNA [6]. Not only is TLR3 evolutionarily distinct from the TLR9 subfamily, its engagement by dsRNA activates distinct intracellular signaling pathways. TLR3 signaling is potentiated by the pattern recognition protein CD14, a coreceptor that is required for full responses to dsRNA in mice [51]. CD14 also potentiates LPS recognition and signaling through TLR4. Since dsRNA can activate multiple signaling pathways within the same cell, including TLR3 as well as alternate cytoplasmic receptors such as PKR, it is often difficult to dissect which of these pathways may be responsible for the observed immunostimulatory effects of dsRNA. Rather than acting in isolation, it is becoming apparent that there is significant interplay between TLR3, PKR, and likely other dsRNA sensing receptors that act in concert to provide an antiviral defense mechanism. This has led to significant complexity in the literature describing the immunological effects of dsRNA.

TLR3 Ligands Alexopoulou et al. identified dsRNA as a TLR3 agonist by examining the response of TLR3 knockout mice to exogenous nucleic acids [6]. These studies demonstrated that responses to polyinosinic:polycytidylic acid (polyI:C), a synthetic analog of long dsRNA, were substantially reduced in TLR3-deficient cells. Similar immunodeficiencies were also observed in response to viral genomic dsRNA, suggesting that this viral nucleic acid likely reflects the natural ligand for TLR3. Activation of TLR3 is sensitive to the length of dsRNA. Short polyI:C duplexes up to 40 base pairs fail to activate TLR3 expressing HEK293 cells (HEK-TLR3), suggesting that shorter dsRNA are ineffective at signaling through TLR3 [52]. However, short (20 nucleotide) stretches of complimentary duplex within a long polyI or polyC ssRNA can activate TLR3 [52], suggesting that secondary structures within long ssRNA may also act as TLR3 ligands. Support for this comes from the observation that long mRNAs [53] and poly-inosinic acid [54] that can form four-stranded structures [55] have also been reported as ligands for TLR3. The preference of TLR3 for inosine may reflect a recognition mechanism for exogenous viral and cellular RNAs that contain hypermutations of adenosine to inosine mediated by adenosine deaminases (ADARs) [52].

It has been reported that siRNA can activate cellular responses through TLR3 [56]. This is an attractive hypothesis simply because siRNA is indeed a dsRNA molecule. Experimental evidence for siRNA as a TLR3 ligand comes from the observation that high concentrations of lipid-transfected 21-mer siRNA can induce IFN-β in HEK-TLR3 cells [56]. However, there is some dispute regarding the precise mechanism underlying these observations and whether or not TLR3 plays any significant role in siRNA-mediated activation of the innate immune response [7, 8, 57]. For example, several of the siRNAs tested in the HEK-TLR3 model were generated using *in vitro* transcription [56], a method now known to generate RNA capable of activating IFN responses through the cytoplasmic RNA receptor RIG-1 [58, 59]. In addition, RIG-1 can be activated by synthetic 21-mer siRNAs if the siRNA is not of sufficient purity or quality [59]. We have observed that stably transfected cell lines such as HEK-TLR3 cells may be primed for activation via RIG-1 (M. Robbins, unpublished observations), a finding supported by Schlee et al. who conclude that HEK-TLR3 cells have provided no evidence of a direct interaction between siRNA and TLR3 [57]. Therefore, it remains to be seen whether canonical siRNAs are a ligand for TLR3, particularly in primary cells and at doses relevant to RNAi. However, reports utilizing primary immune cell cultures and TLR7-deficient mice to define the siRNA-mediated cytokine response clearly indicate that these are primarily driven by TLR7/8 activation and not via TLR3 [7, 8].

TLR Signaling   The TLR9 subfamily that includes TLR7 and TLR8 signal exclusively through an adaptor protein called MyD88 [29, 60, 61]. These TLR signaling pathways are summarized in Figure 7.2. MyD88 contains a C-terminal domain with considerable homology to both TLRs and the IL-1 receptor, a so-called cytoplasmic Toll/interleukin-1R (TIR) domain. MyD88 also contains a region of significant homology to the N-terminal region of TNF-R1 and Fas, a so-called death domain. MyD88 associates with the TIR domains of TLR7, -8, and -9 [29], and upon activation, forms a signaling complex with the intermediate molecules, IRAK-1, IRAK-4, and TRAF6. This initiates signaling events that result in the translocation of NF-κB to the nucleus and activation of transcription factors, including IRF5 and IRF7 that are responsible for upregulating expression of IFN-α and inflammatory cytokines [60, 61]. This process occurs rapidly in immune cells that are directly responsive to TLR9 family ligands, such as pDC and B cells, due to their constitutive expression of the TLRs together with key signaling components including IRF7. The outcome of TLR9 engagement has been shown to depend on the spatiotemporal regulation of the MyD88-IRF7 pathway [36, 62]. Production of inflammatory cytokines, such as TNF-α, appears to be promoted when TLR9 engagement and signaling occur in the lysosomal compartment, whereas production of IFN-α occurs when the signals are propagated within early endosomes. The balance between these two responses is dictated by the rate of trafficking through the endo/lysosomal compartment that is influenced by the structure of the nucleic acid and its mechanism of uptake. This dichotomy also likely exists for TLR7 signaling [62] and has implications for understanding the impact of different delivery systems on the nature of the immune response to siRNA.

TLR3 signaling proceeds through an entirely different pathway to that of the TLR9 subfamily. Unlike the other nucleic acid sensing TLRs that use MyD88 as an adaptor protein, TLR3 signals through the TRIF adaptor protein [63]. This pathway is summarized in Figure 7.3. TRIF signals for the downstream production of IFN-β and IFN-α4 via TANK-binding kinase-1 (TBK1), which mediates activation of the transcription factor IRF3 [64,65]. A positive feedback mechanism occurs in TLR3 signaling in which the production of IFN-β and IFN-α4 signals back to the cell causing the upregulation of IRF7 and other IFN-inducible genes. This leads to the production of additional IFN-α subtypes and amplification of the response [61]. TLR3 activation through TRIF also activates RIP1 and TRAF6, leading to the downstream activation of NF-κB, ATF, and c-Jun transcription factors and the induction of inflammatory cytokines such as IL-6 and TNF-α [61]. TBK1 activation is sufficient for TLR3-mediated IRF3 dimerization and nuclear translocation but the induction of gene transcription also requires PI3 kinase activity [66]. This "two-step" activation of TLR3 signaling appears to be unique among the TLRs.

TLR-Independent Mechanisms   In addition to the TLR systems described above, mammalian cells have evolved a number of TLR-independent mechanisms to recognize cytoplasmic RNA species that are hallmarks of viral infection and replication. Cellular responses to cytoplasmic RNA can be induced via PKR, RIG-1, and MDA-5 proteins. These pathways are summarized in Figure 7.4. Recently, cytoplasmic recognition of microbial RNA and nucleoside analogs has also been shown for Nalp3, a member of the NOD-LRR protein family [67].

RIG-1 and MDA-5   RIG-1 is a cytoplasmic RNA helicase that has recently been shown to play an important role in antiviral defense [68–70]. For example, RIG-1 expression was found to be essential for IFN production in conventional DCs and fibroblasts following infection by particular RNA viruses [69]. RIG-1 acts as a sensor of viral RNA through its binding and activation by dsRNA and ssRNA containing uncapped 5′triphosphates that are characteristic of certain viral RNA [59, 68, 71, 72]. As we describe in more detail later in this chapter, these physical characteristics of RIG-1

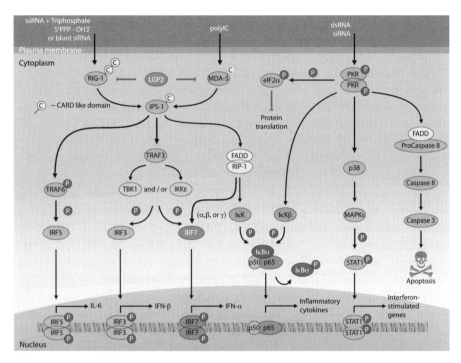

FIGURE 7.4   The cytoplasmic RNA receptors RIG-1, MDA5, and PKR. Upon binding to dsRNA or ssRNA-triphosphate, the cytoplasmic proteins RIG-1 and MDA-5 signal through the IFNβ promoter stimulator 1 (IPS-1) protein adaptor. The closely related protein LGP2 acts as an inhibitor of RIG-1 and MDA-5 signaling. IPS-1 signals through TRAF6 for the activation of IRF5 and inflammatory cytokine production. IPS-1 also activates TRAF3 leading to IRF3 and IRF7 phosphorylation and ultimately to type I IFN production. FADD is required for IPS-1-mediated production of IRF-7 and IFN induction. Binding of dsRNA to PKR causes its dimerization and transphosphorylation. PKR activation leads to the phosphorylation of proteins such as eIF2α and IκB, causing a general inhibition of translation and nuclear translocation of the NF-κB transcription factor, respectively. FADD is required for PKR-mediated apoptosis through caspase-8 and caspase-3. Phosphorylated PKR leads to activation of p38 MAPK and STAT1 culminating in the transcription of interferon-stimulated genes (ISGs). (For a color version of this figure, see plate 8.)

ligands are also found in certain siRNA constructs including blunt-ended and *in vitro* transcribed siRNA. Therefore, there is strong evidence that some siRNA species can activate TLR-independent cellular responses via the RIG-1 pathway and that this may be the prevalent mechanism for siRNA-mediated IFN induction from nonimmune cells.

RIG-1 is a DexD/H-box-containing RNA helicase that encodes two caspase recruitment domains (CARD) at its N terminus. Upon dsRNA binding at the C-terminal helicase domain, RIG-1 signals for the activation of IRF3 and NF-κB, leading to the production of IFN-β and inflammatory mediators, respectively [73,74]. RIG-1 signaling is transmitted through an adaptor protein variously named IFN-β promoter stimulator 1 (IPS-1; [75]), mitochondrial antiviral signaling ([76], virus-induced signaling adaptor [77], or Cardif [78] The adaptor FADD (Figure 7.4) is also required for dsRNA signaling via RIG-1, functioning downstream of the IPS-1 adaptor and upstream of IRF-7 for the production of type I IFN [79].

Two other DexD/H-box-containing RNA helicases, MDA-5 and LGP2, are closely related to RIG-1 [73]. MDA-5 contains RNA helicase and CARD domains and also signals through IPS-1/FADD, IRF3, and NF-κB to mediate the production of IFN-β [73]. LGP2 differs from RIG-1 and MDA-5 in that it contains an RNA helicase domain but does not have a CARD domain. Therefore, it is unable to engage the adaptor proteins utilized by RIG-1 and MDA-5. For this reason, LGP2 acts as a dominant-negative regulator of RIG-1 and MDA-5 signaling by sequestering dsRNA [73]. RIG-1, MDA-5, and LGP2 are all IFN-inducible genes, and therefore, their expression is rapidly upregulated in an autocrine or paracrine manner following initiation of an IFN response.

PKR PKR is an IFN-inducible serine–threonine kinase expressed in most mammalian cells, and until the identification of TLRs and the cytoplasmic RNA helicases, it was long considered to be the primary sensor of viral dsRNA (Figure 7.4) [13, 80]. PKR is present in cells in an inactive form but is activated in association with long dsRNA binding at its N terminus, causing homodimer formation and autophosphorylation on serine/threonine residues. dsRNA-activated PKR catalyzes the phosphorylation of proteins such as eIF2α and IκB, leading to the general inhibition of translation [13,81]. Several earlier studies ascribed the upregulation of IFN-inducible genes by siRNA in cell lines to a PKR-mediated effect (e.g., [82]). However, given our current understanding, it is now thought that RIG-1 activation likely accounts for many of these observations [58,71]. Therefore, it is unclear whether siRNA can induce functional activation of the PKR response. PKR can interact with dsRNA as short as 11 bp independent of nucleotide sequence although more than 30 bp of contiguous dsRNA is thought to be required for PKR activation [83]. Recently, higher sensitivity kinase assays have facilitated the observation that synthetic siRNA, either blunt or 21-mer duplex containing canonical 3′overhangs, can activate PKR to some degree [59, 84, 85]. However, it is not clear from these *in vitro* studies whether NF-kB activation or translation inhibition are induced by this level of PKR signaling.

7.3   FACTORS INFLUENCING IMMUNE STIMULATION

Unlike invertebrate systems, the introduction of long dsRNA into mammalian cells typically leads to the global degradation of mRNA, inhibition of protein synthesis, and activation of the IFN system. These processes reflect activation of the cells' autonomous antiviral response [86] that is based on the recognition of cytoplasmic dsRNA as a signature of viral infection. As described above, these intracellular events are mediated by the activation of dsRNA-binding receptors such as PKR [87] and the RNA helicases RIG-1 and MDA-5 [68–70]. One consequence of this near ubiquitous defense mechanism is that it precludes the use of long dsRNA Dicer substrates to study RNAi in mammalian cell lines due to the myriad of off-target effects associated with activation of the innate antiviral response. However, this barrier was overcome by the identification of siRNAs as the active Dicer product and the demonstration that these short 21-mer duplexes can mediate RNAi in mammalian cell lines without apparently activating the IFN response associated with transfection of longer dsRNA [88]. The seminal work describing RNAi in mammalian cells inadvertently helped foster the then widely held belief that siRNA molecules, in general, are immunologically inert. This is despite several later reports showing that even in certain *in vitro* culture systems, chemically synthesized and virally transcribed siRNA are capable of activating components of the IFN system [58, 82]. Given the early focus on whether or not siRNA could induce an IFN response, it is remarkable that the potential for siRNA to activate mammalian immune cells possessing multiple nucleic acid sensing receptors in addition to PKR has, until recently, been largely ignored. This is particularly surprising when one considers that a few years earlier, studies on the off-target effects associated with antisense ODNs, considered a novel class of gene silencing agent at the time, helped define immunostimulatory CpG motifs in DNA [20]. An understanding of these immunological side effects subsequently led to the reevaluation of antisense experiments and the mechanism of action underlying various "antisense" drugs.

   In many ways mirroring the early history of antisense technology, we and several other groups have shown recently that siRNA has the inherent capacity to activate potent immune responses *in vivo* or when transfected into responsive cell types *in vitro*. Immune stimulation and the induction of IFNs by siRNA provides not only the potential for strong nonspecific effects with respect to target gene expression and function, but the ensuing inflammatory response can also result in significant toxicities when siRNA are administered *in vivo*. In this section, we outline some of the factors that may influence the immunostimulatory properties of siRNA and highlight the need for these to be taken into consideration when designing and interpreting results from siRNA experiments.

7.3.1 The Influence of Cell Type

Unlike PKR, which is nearly ubiquitous in its expression, TLRs and the RNA helicase's show different expression patterns depending on cell type. This heterogeneity in receptor expression has been a contributing factor in the numerous conflicting reports on the immunobiology of siRNA. It is now clear that there are specialized cells of the mammalian innate immune system that are highly responsive to stimulation by siRNA. Uptake of synthetic siRNA duplexes or hairpin RNA into primary human or murine blood cell cultures elicits the secretion of IFN-α and inflammatory cytokines at levels comparable to those induced by immunostimulatory CpG ODN. Not surprisingly, this robust *in vitro* response is recapitulated when formulated siRNA are administered to mice, bringing about the characteristic activation of the innate immune response. Immune cell sensitivity to siRNA is primarily dictated by their pattern of TLR expression, in particular, the functional expression of TLR7 and/or TLR8. pDCs that constitutively express TLR7 in both mice and humans are directly activated by siRNA to secrete high levels of IFN-α [7,8]. In contrast, human myeloid lineage cells including monocytes and mDC preferentially express TLR8 and respond to stimulatory siRNA by secreting inflammatory cytokines such as IL-6 and TNF rather than IFN-α [7, 39]. siRNA can also activate a variety of primary dendritic cell and macrophage cultures, mouse splenocytes, as well as certain macrophage-like cell lines.

Recent work has focused on the ability of siRNA to induce innate cytokine responses, however, cells of the adaptive immune system can also be directly activated by TLR ligands. B cells that are responsible for antibody production have a similar TLR expression profile as pDC, constitutively expressing both TLR7 and TLR9. Accordingly, they are activated by similar TLR ligands including stimulatory RNA. B-cell responsiveness to RNA has been highlighted by studies of autoimmune diseases such as systemic lupus erythematosus (SLE) in which TLR7 has been found to play a major role in the activation of autoreactive B cells [89–93]. The production of both pathogenic autoantibodies and type I IFNs that are hallmarks of SLE pathogenesis [94] can be driven by RNA associated autoantigens and immune complexes through TLR7 activation [89, 90, 95]. Similarly, we have found that loading immunostimulatory siRNA into liposomes can render an otherwise inert delivery vehicle immunogenic. This is evidenced by the induction of antibody responses against certain vehicle components and is driven by the activation of B cells that have taken up the stimulatory siRNA. Similar reports have recently been published in primates where the administration of a cyclodextrin-formulated siRNA resulted in an antibody response against a targeting ligand incorporated into the delivery vehicle [96]. This provides another example of the potential pitfalls associated with the *in vivo* use of immunostimulatory nucleic acids.

Although work to date indicates that the TLR-mediated response to siRNA *in vivo* is dominated by immune cell activation, the expression of TLRs is not entirely restricted to cells of the immune system. Fibroblasts, epithelial cells, endothelial cells, and hepatocytes, for example, can express functional TLRs that are upregulated by inflammatory stimuli and IFNs. It is possible that following siRNA administration, additional cell types may be stimulated through TLR engagement.

Nonhematological cell lines do not typically express TLR7/8, and therefore, do not manifest the robust innate immune response to siRNA that is readily observed both *in vivo* and in primary blood cell cultures. However, unlike nucleic acid sensing TLR, cytoplasmic RNA receptors are expressed in a wider variety of mammalian cell types, providing the cells with an autonomous antiviral defense mechanism. Numerous, often conflicting, reports have questioned whether or not siRNA can stimulate IFN responses in cell lines through these alternate RNA receptor pathways. Recent *in vitro* studies, however, have now started to delineate more clearly the cell types and conditions under which this is likely to occur. As described in this chapter, structural features of certain transcribed and synthetic siRNA have now been shown to activate the RIG-1 pathway. Accordingly, cell lines that naturally express high levels of RIG-1, such as the lung fibroblast MRC-5, or glioblastoma T98G, mount strong IFN responses when transfected with blunt-ended siRNA [59]. In our experience, blunt-ended siRNA can also induce IFN responses, albeit weaker, in a number of other commonly used human cell lines of diverse lineage, with the magnitude of the response presumably dictated by the differential expression levels of RIG-1 or equivalent RNA receptors. It should be noted that cell culture conditions can also directly affect the sensitivity of cells to siRNA-mediated activation. For example, PKR, RIG-1, and a number of TLRs including TLR3 and TLR7 are themselves induced by IFNs, while critical components of these signaling pathways can also be upregulated by other physiological factors such as cellular stress. Therefore, the potential exists for many cell types to be primed, either intentionally or inadvertently, to respond to siRNA, depending on the experimental conditions. In addition, the ability of siRNA to activate an immune response is influenced by a number of other factors including the siRNA sequence, the chemical structure, and the mode of intracellular delivery, all of which must be taken into account. Each of these is discussed in more detail below.

7.3.2 Delivery Vehicles

Many nucleic acid-based drugs, including synthetic siRNA and plasmid DNA, require enablement via some method of intracellular delivery. This is due to the poor cellular uptake of the naked nucleic acid molecules. For this reason, the use of delivery vehicles to enable synthetic siRNA uptake and presentation to the cytoplasmic RNAi machinery is seen as essential by researchers conducting both *in vitro* and *in vivo* studies. The most widely used vehicles for this purpose are based around positively charged (cationic) agents that complex with, or encapsulate, the negatively charged nucleic acid. These include cationic lipid formulations, for example, lipofectamine, and cationic polymers such as polyethylenimine (PEI), both of which form positively charged complexes with siRNA and facilitate intracellular delivery through electrostatic interactions with the membrane of the target cell. One important feature of these delivery vehicles is that they are typically taken up into cells by endocytosis and are concentrated in the endosomal compartment prior to releasing siRNA into the cytoplasm. An inadvertent consequence of this process is the efficient delivery of siRNA into the very cellular compartments where the RNA sensing PRRs are localized. It is worth noting that immunologists have exploited this feature of cationic lipids and polycations to potentiate the immunostimulatory effects of RNA and DNA for many years. Therefore, it should come as no surprise that similar effects are also observed with siRNA.

Naked siRNA molecules do not typically activate an immune response from blood cells either *in vitro* or *in vivo* [7, 97]. The relationship between siRNA delivery and immune stimulation reflects a number of factors: (1) the relative efficiency of intracellular uptake, (2) enhanced bioavailability and exposure to innate immune cells *in vivo*, (3) protection of the siRNA from rapid nuclease degradation, and (4) altered physical characteristics of the siRNA complex resulting in more efficient engagement of immune receptors. The nature of the delivery vehicle utilized in a given experiment can have a dramatic effect on both the quality and magnitude of the immune response to siRNA. For example, our group has shown that human blood cells stimulated with siRNA encapsulated in stable nucleic acid lipid particles (SNALP) or complexed with PEI induce a response that is dominated by IFN-α secretion. In contrast, lipofectamine and polylysine that form larger, more heterogeneous complexes with siRNA tend to elicit a predominantly inflammatory cytokine biased response from the same human blood cell population [7]. We have found that a number of parameters affect how delivery vehicles potentiate immune stimulation by a particular siRNA duplex. These include the chemical composition of the delivery vehicle as well as physical properties such as the size and charge ratio of the formulated material. *In vivo*, additional variables also need to be considered including the pharmacokinetics and biodistribution of the formulated siRNA as well as the route of administration. We have noted that differences in these parameters can result in the magnitude of the immune response changing by greater than 100-fold. In our experience to date, however, we have found that siRNA duplexes with inherent immunostimulatory activity will invariably activate some measure of immune stimulation when tested appropriately in responsive immune cell types, irrespective of the delivery system employed. These include the typical commercial transfection reagents as well as our own proprietary lipid delivery technologies (SNALP).

7.3.3 siRNA Sequence and Purity

The initial reports describing ssRNA as the natural ligands for TLR7 and TLR8 demonstrated that RNA activates these receptors in a sequence dependent manner [4, 5]. In particular, uridine (U) or guanosine/uridine (GU) rich RNA sequences are particularly effective in activating TLR7/8-mediated cytokine responses in human and murine systems. Perhaps not surprisingly, similar rules seem to apply to synthetic siRNA duplexes and their constitutive ssRNA ODNs [7, 8, 45]. As such, individual siRNA duplexes vary considerably in their capacity to activate the innate immune response due to inherent differences in their nucleotide sequence. Unlike the defined CpG motifs within DNA that characterize TLR9 agonists, the precise nature of the RNA motifs recognized by TLR7/8 remain obscure. We originally described siRNA duplexes with GU-rich sequences as being highly immunostimulatory and identified 5'-UGU-3' motifs within particular siRNA that apparently confer this activity [7]. Substitution of the uridine groups in this motif significantly reduced immunostimulatory capacity of the duplex whereas introduction of the 5'-UGU-3' motif into an siRNA duplex had the predicted effect of increasing cytokine induction. By avoiding GU-rich sequences, we have shown that it is possible to select functional siRNA duplexes with inherently low immunostimulatory capacity [7]. It is clear, however, from our own work and others that the 5'-UGU-3' motif is not the only RNA sequence recognized by TLR7/8 [5, 7, 8, 44, 45]. This is illustrated by the fact that the large majority of unmodified siRNA sequences demonstrate at least some level of immunostimulatory activity, suggesting that TLR7/8 likely recognizes a simple pattern of ribonucleotides occurring at high frequency in conventionally designed synthetic siRNA. This hypothesis has recently been validated by Diebold et al. [44], who demonstrated that the presence of uridine and a ribose sugar backbone (two hallmarks that define RNA from DNA) are both necessary and sufficient for TLR7 recognition and that short ssRNA only require several uridines in close proximity to one and other to render the ODNs TLR7 agonists. These findings go some way to refining the basic concept of what may be regarded as the stimulatory "motifs" within RNA and are consistent with our own observations relating to siRNA duplexes. As discussed later in this chapter, the fact that siRNA duplexes have inherently different capacities to activate a TLR-mediated immune response based on their unique RNA sequence has significant consequences in the development of siRNA technologies. It also highlights the critical requirement for the use of appropriate controls that allow genuine RNAi effects to be distinguished from nonspecific effects induced by active and control siRNA sequences that have distinct immunostimulatory profiles.

Although ssRNA has been defined as a natural ligand for TLR7/8, it is clear that the immune stimulatory activity of synthetic siRNA duplexes is not due to contaminating single-stranded ODNs [7, 8]. This was important to demonstrate given the fact that the annealing of siRNA duplexes is not a completely efficient process and results in synthetic siRNA preparations containing low levels of unincorporated ssRNA. The implication is that immune activation by siRNA cannot be overcome by improved manufacture or downstream purification of the duplexes. In support of this, PAGE-purified siRNA (>95% duplex) and nonpurified siRNA preparations (75–80% duplex) induce cytokine responses of equal magnitude [7]. In our work developing siRNA for therapeutic use, we have also found that HPLC-purified synthetic siRNA duplexes of a purity equivalent to material qualified for use in human clinical trials induce IFN-α and inflammatory cytokine responses that are equivalent to those of crude siRNA preparations. Although duplexed siRNA clearly activates TLR7/8, it is not known at present if this response reflects TLR engagement of the intact duplex itself within the endosome or whether degradation or denaturation of the duplex to ssRNA is required.

7.3.4 Structural and Physical Characteristics of siRNA

Unlike TLR7/8, the recognition of RNA by the cytoplasmic receptors RIG-1, MDA-5, and PKR is considered to be sequence independent. However, these nucleic acid sensing receptors have evolved to recognize certain other physical and structural characteristics of RNA. Here, we shall briefly discuss several of these features that relate to current siRNA design strategies.

Following the initial discovery that 21-mer siRNA can initiate RNAi in mammalian cells without activation of the PKR-mediated IFN response [88, 98], several studies have subsequently reported that IFN induction from cell lines may still occur under certain experimental conditions [58, 82, 99]. Kim et al. [58] demonstrated that phage polymerase transcribed siRNA-activated IFN responses when transfected into nonhematopoietic cell lines due to the presence of uncapped 5′-triphosphate groups that are a feature of these transcribed RNA. This observation likely explains earlier reports of IFN induction in RNAi experiments that utilized transcribed siRNA [82]. The molecular mechanism underlying these effects has now been elucidated. It appears that RNA containing uncapped 5′ triphosphate groups binds to, and activates RIG-1 resulting in potent IFN responses from RIG-1 expressing cells [71, 72]. Therefore, uncapped 5' triphosphate groups on RNA represent a pathogen-associated molecular pattern that helps distinguish virally derived from self RNA. For siRNA constructs synthesized using phage polymerase, the induction of an IFN response through RIG-1 activation needs to be considered, even when working in cell lines that do not express TLR7/8. In this regard, Kim et al. [58] provide a methodology for engineering T7 siRNA synthesis in order to remove the initiating 5' triphosphate, and therefore, alleviate IFN induction by this class of siRNA.

Further studies have highlighted additional structural features of chemically synthesized siRNA that can also activate the RIG-1-mediated IFN pathway in cell lines [59]. Asymmetrical siRNA that contain a standard 3' overhang at one end and a blunt 5'-antisense end have become more widely used in an attempt to improve RNAi potency [100, 101]. Marques et al. [59] have subsequently demonstrated that blunt-ended RNA, including siRNA, can also bind to and activates RIG-1. Again, this effect appears to be independent of the RNA sequence but is enhanced as the length of the blunt-ended siRNA is increased from 21 to 27 base pairs and is reduced if the blunt end is converted to an overhang. This study also reported the interesting observation that certain batches of conventional 21-mer siRNA with 3' overhangs could activate IFN responses equivalent to those induced by blunt-ended or 5'-triphosphate siRNA. This appears to be associated with siRNA batches of poor quality or purity that presumably contain uncharacterized RNA products capable of activating RIG-1 or one of the other cytoplasmic RNA receptors. Such variability between siRNA batches and the differences in RNA quality between suppliers means that it is up to individual researchers to determine whether or not their particular siRNA preparations are capable of activating an IFN response, even when working *in vitro* with cell lines. Unfortunately, it would appear insufficient to rely solely on the generalized principles described in the literature to make this assessment.

It should be appreciated that a given siRNA duplex may contain multiple structural, physical, and sequence-related features that are recognized by the various immune receptors. As such, a particular siRNA may be able to simultaneously activate both TLR and non-TLR pathways depending on its sequence and structural characteristics, and the cell types that are transfected. For example, an unmodified, blunt-ended siRNA such as the 21/23-mer ApoB1 duplex can be a potent activator of both TLR7/8 as it traffics through the endosomal compartment [102] and RIG-1 when it is released into the cell cytoplasm ([59] and A. Judge and M. Robbins, 2007, unpublished observation). Each pathway results in the induction of type I IFNs and may contribute to the toxic and off-target effects observed with these unmodified siRNA. Therefore, it is important that the ability of a chosen siRNA to activate any one of multiple pathways is taken into consideration.

7.3.5 Chemical Modification Strategies

Stabilization of synthetic siRNA against rapid nuclease degradation is often regarded as a prerequisite for *in vivo* and therapeutic applications. This is achieved using stabilization chemistries that were previously developed for ribozymes or antisense oligonucleotide drugs [103]. These include chemical modifications to the $2'$-OH group in the ribose sugar backbone, such as $2'$-O-methyl ($2'$OMe) and $2'$-fluoro ($2'$F) substitutions, that are introduced into the RNA as $2'$-modified nucleotides during RNA synthesis. A number of reports have shown that siRNA containing $2'$OMe, $2'$F, $2'$-deoxy ($2'$H), or "locked nucleic acid" (LNA) modifications may retain functional RNAi activity, indicating that these chemistries can be compatible with the RNAi machinery [8, 104–109]. However, these modifications to siRNA appear to be tolerated only in certain ill-defined positional or sequence-related contexts as, in many cases, their introduction can have a negative impact on RNAi activity [8, 104, 106, 107, 109].

The use of appropriate delivery vehicles that confer nuclease protection to the encapsulated or complexed siRNA bypasses the absolute requirement for stabilization chemistries to be applied to siRNA for either *in vitro* or *in vivo* use. However, work in developing siRNA as potential therapeutic agents has revealed that these same chemistries, in particular the use of $2'$OMe nucleotides, can also prevent recognition of the siRNA by the innate immune system [102, 110]. This has the striking result of rendering appropriately designed siRNA immunologically inert, without any need to modify the basic RNA sequence that confers RNAi activity.

One chemical modification strategy to generate siRNA suitable for use as naked molecules involves the systematic substitution of all ribonucleotides with $2'$F, $2'$OMe, or $2'$-deoxy nucleotides based on the pattern of purines and pyrimidines in the given sequence (Figure 7.5) [107, 111, 112]. We have found that these siRNA molecules (so-called as they contain no native ribose sugar) exhibit only minimal immunostimulatory activity compared with the native siRNA sequence when administered to mice in lipidic formulations [112]. This is perhaps unsurprising given the fact that the ribose sugar is a definitive characteristic of RNA, and therefore, likely plays an integral role in the recognition of RNA by nucleic acid sensing receptors. This has recently been directly demonstrated in the case of TLR7-mediated recognition of RNA [44]. From the initial studies in which multiple stabilization chemistries were simultaneously substituted into the siRNA duplex, it was not possible to determine which chemical modifications in particular were responsible for abrogating immune stimulation. It should also be noted that the application of this chemical modification strategy to unmodified active siRNA sequences frequently causes significant inhibition of RNAi activity [107] and calls for

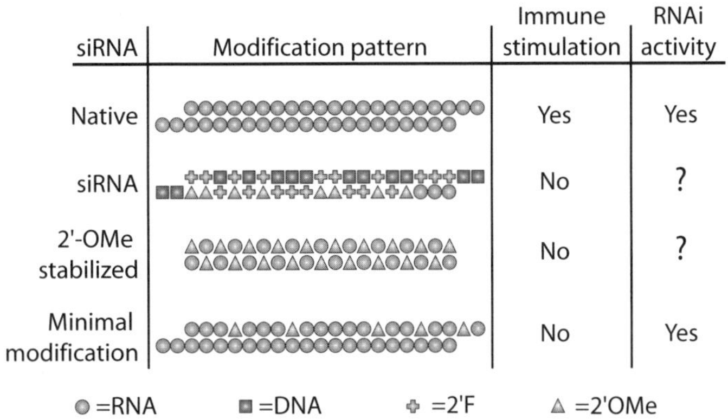

siRNA	Modification pattern	Immune stimulation	RNAi activity
Native		Yes	Yes
siRNA		No	?
2'-OMe stabilized		No	?
Minimal modification		No	Yes

◎ =RNA   ▣ =DNA   ✛ =2'F   △ =2'OMe

FIGURE 7.5 Chemical modification of siRNA. Chemical modifications have been applied to siRNA in an effort to either confer stability from nuclease-mediated degradation or abrogate the inherent immunostimulatory properties of canonical siRNA duplexes. Various approaches are discussed in the text.

a stochastic screening approach to select modified duplexes that retain gene silencing activity.

We have found that the selective incorporation of as few as two 2'OMe guanosine or uridine residues in the sense strand of highly immunostimulatory siRNA molecules is sufficient to abrogate siRNA-mediated IFN and inflammatory cytokine induction in human PBMC and in mice *in vivo* (Figure 7.5) [102]. This most likely reflects profound inhibition of the TLR7/8-mediated pathway that dominates the response to siRNA in immunological settings. Strikingly, the degree of 2'OMe modification required to exert this profound anti-inflammatory effect on the RNA represents ~5% of the native 2'-OH positions in the siRNA duplex and no other stabilization chemistries are required. This can be achieved using either 2'OMe-uridine, -guanosine, or -adenosine residues in any combination (surprisingly, the incorporation of 2'OMe cytidines by themselves has significantly less effect in dampening immune stimulation [46, 102]). Coupled with a suitable delivery vehicle, these minimally modified siRNAs are able to mediate potent RNAi effects *in vitro* and *in vivo* without induction of a detectable cytokine response [102].

Researchers who utilize synthetic siRNA in their studies can readily adopt this simple approach to siRNA design, as 2'OMe nucleotides are a standard chemistry offered by many of the RNA suppliers at minimal additional cost over conventional ribonucleotides. The incorporation of 2'OMe nucleotides, however, can impact the gene silencing activity of a given siRNA sequence [102,104,106]. Therefore, testing of the modified duplex should be conducted alongside the native duplex to confirm RNAi potency has been retained. We have found that 2'OMe modification of less than 20% of the total nucleotides is generally well tolerated ([102] and A. Judge and M. Robbins, 2007, unpublished observations). Since our original description of this chemical modification strategy [102], two studies examining the mechanism of RNAi have shown that the sense strand of an siRNA duplex is typically cleaved as a precursor to efficient assembly of the RISC complex [113,114]. This process follows the same rules established for the siRNA-guided cleavage of a target mRNA, resulting in RISC-directed cleavage between positions 9 and 10 of the sense strand. Leuschner et al. showed that chemical modification of the nucleotide at position 9 of the sense strand (or introduction of a PS linker between nucleotides 9 and 10) could inhibit sense strand cleavage and subsequently reduce the efficiency of RISC assembly and RNAi activity [114]. In line with these results, we have found that the introduction of 2'OMe nucleotides at position 9 in the sense strand can reduce RNAi activity, even in the absence of any chemical modifications to the antisense strand of the siRNA duplex (A. Judge, 2007, unpublished observations). Although this negative effect is not absolute and does not appear to affect all duplexes, the chemical modification of this particular sense strand nucleotide is best avoided when designing siRNA to have minimal immunostimulatory activity.

It has been suggested that human TLR may be preferentially activated by pathogen-derived RNA based on their lack of modified nucleosides that typically occur at much higher frequency in most mammalian RNA [46]. The introduction of a variety of naturally occurring modified nucleosides, including 2'OMe nucleosides, into RNA was shown to inhibit TLR activation and immune stimulation [46]. Findings with 2'OMe-modified siRNA are consistent with this report, particularly with respect to the low degree of modification required to abrogate RNA-mediated immune stimulation and the differential effects of modifying uridine versus cytidine residues on the activation of primary immune cells. This suggests that 2'OMe-modified siRNA may avoid recognition by the innate immune system due to an evolutionary mechanism by which immune receptors distinguish pathogen-derived RNA from self RNA. Whether or not the immune system has evolved to distinguish self from nonself RNA by such a mechanism remains an open question.

Chemical modification of siRNA can also block their interaction with RIG-1 in the cell cytoplasm, and therefore, inhibit IFN responses that are induced via this pathway. As we have described in this chapter, blunt-ended duplex RNA are able to bind to and activate RIG-1 in a variety of cell lines. In the original description of this phenomenon by Marques et al. [59], the authors also illustrated a simple way of preventing this immune recognition by the incorporation of two DNA nucleotides into the blunt end of the siRNA. This is anticipated to have minimal impact on the RNAi activity of the duplex and appears to be adequate to significantly reduce RIG-1-mediated IFN responses in sensitive cell lines [59]. We have confirmed these observations in our own unpublished studies; however, these DNA-modified blunt-ended siRNAs are still fully capable of eliciting potent inflammatory responses through TLR7/8-mediated immune stimulation. Initial reports describing RIG-1 activation by 5'-triphosphate RNA indicated that global substitution of uridines with 2'OMe–uridine in these transcribed RNA profoundly inhibited IFN induction in monocyte cultures [71]. This implies that 2'OMe nucleotides are also able to inhibit the recognition of stimulatory RNA by RIG-1. We have found that minimal 2'OMe modification to blunt-ended siRNA not only inhibits TLR7/8-mediated immune activation but also completely abrogates the IFN response in RIG-1 sensitive cell lines such as T98G and MRC5 (A. Judge and M. Robbins, in preparation). Therefore. it would appear that the use of 2'OMe-modified siRNA is able to circumvent both the TLR-dependent and -independent mechanisms primarily responsible for initiating immune responses against siRNA duplexes.

It is unclear at present how the introduction of 2'OMe nucleotides into siRNA prevents recognition of the duplex RNA by the immune system. The exact nature of the physical interaction between TLR7/8 and RNA is not known. This is also true for other defined TLR7 and TLR8 ligands such as the commonly used guanosine analogues [115]. Therefore, further work is required to confirm the precise mechanism of siRNA-mediated TLR activation before the molecular basis underlying the inhibitory effects of 2'OMe modification can be fully elucidated. However, it is interesting to note that 2'OMe RNA is also able to inhibit immune stimulation by small molecule TLR7 agonists, suggesting that its inhibitory effects reflect some form of TLR7 antagonism [48].

A number of other stabilization chemistries are routinely used in synthetic siRNA design that may also influence immune recognition and RNAi. LNAs that contain a 2'-O, 4'-C methylene bridge in the sugar ring have been shown to partially reduce the immunostimulatory activity of an siRNA [8], while siRNAs containing inverted deoxy a basic end caps retain immunostimulatory activity [112]. No evidence of a transinhibitory effect similar to that observed with 2'OMe modifications (whereby 2'OMe-modified RNA annealed to unmodified immunostimulatory RNA generates a nonimmunostimulatory duplex [48, 102]) has been observed with LNA-modified duplexes. As we have described, a complex combination of 2'F, 2'H, and 2'OMe chemistries can generate a fully modified siRNA duplex with minimal immunostimulatory activity [112]. The introduction of 2'F-modified nucleotides into RNA has been reported to reduce immune stimulation [110] although we have found that the inhibitory effects of this chemistry appear to depend on the siRNA sequence and/or the position and extent of the modified nucleotides. As such, the use of 2'-F and 2'-H chemistries alone tends to have unpredictable effects on the immunostimulatory activity of the modified siRNA (A. Judge and I. MacLachlan, 2007, unpublished observations). Taken as a whole, these observations suggest that immune stimulation by siRNA is particularly sensitive to inhibition by 2'OMe modifications versus other, well characterized, stabilization chemistries.

7.3.6   Detection of the Immune Response to siRNA

The immune response to siRNA is characterized by the induction of type I IFN and/or inflammatory cytokine responses from both *in vitro* cell cultures and in animal studies. As we have described in this section, the nature and extent of this response is dictated by a multitude of variables that differ with each experimental model and methodology employed to affect RNA interference. Therefore, it is essential that researchers conduct the appropriate studies that are able to monitor for the induction of an immune response in their particular experimental setting. We shall describe here the basic parameters that need to be considered when designing such experiments.

7.3.7   Testing for Appropriate Cytokines

As the nature of the cytokine response to siRNA can differ according to cell type, delivery vehicle, route of administration, and so on, the absence of immune stimulation cannot be concluded from testing for the presence or absence of a single cytokine. Antibodies and enzyme linked immunosorbent assay (ELISA) kits are widely available for the determination of IFN-α, IFN-β, and a whole variety of inflammatory cytokines. For *in vivo* studies, we recommend testing for both IFN-α and suitable inflammatory cytokines (including IL-6 and TNF-α) in the plasma of treated animals to monitor for systemic activation of the innate immune response. A similar panel of cytokines can also be used to test for stimulation of primary immune cell cultures *in vitro*. For cell lines, the detection of IFN-β, IL-6, or the chemokine IL-8 in the supernatant of treated cells can be used as a measure of siRNA-mediated activation through the RIG-1/MDA-5/PKR pathways. However, the secretion of these cytokines in response to activation is cell-line dependent and cannot be used in isolation to determine whether these cytoplasmic RNA receptor pathways have been engaged.

7.3.8   Timing

Measurement of the immune response at an appropriate time after siRNA treatment is critical in order to make a valid assessment. Systemic administration of immunostimulatory siRNA formulations to mice can lead to detectable elevations in serum cytokines within 1–2 h, with the timing dependent on the type of delivery vehicle and the cytokine being assessed. However, it is important to note that elevations in serum cytokines are transient and typically resolve within 12–24 h after initial treatment. This is true even for highly stimulatory siRNA that can induce nanograms per milliliter amounts of cytokines in the blood. By way of example, intravenous administration of lipidic (SNALP) siRNA formulations leads to elevations in serum IL-6 by 2 h, with a peak between 4 and 6 h and resolution by 16 h after a single treatment. IFNα follows a similar pattern but with a 2-h delay in peak serum levels. However, it should be emphasized that these timeframes are entirely dependent on the nature of the delivery vehicle. Therefore, it is important that researchers define this parameter within their own models and select an appropriate time point that is able to capture this aspect of the innate immune response. The assessment of cytokine responses from *in vitro* cell cultures is less time sensitive since the secreted cytokines tend to accumulate in the tissue culture supernatant. Therefore, the measurement of cytokines at a single time point 16–24 h after siRNA treatment is often adequate for detection of a response. However, this does not reflect the dynamics of the cytokine response per se; researchers who choose to monitor cytokine induction through mRNA analysis also need to define the most appropriate time point for sample collection (e.g., [59]).

7.3.9 Sensitivity

Although the measurement of secreted cytokines is both an efficient and meaningful readout of innate immune stimulation, it is not necessarily the most sensitive method to assess the response. Therefore, great care should be taken when interpreting negative cytokine data; the absence of proof is not the proof of absence. Within our laboratory, we have utilized IFN-inducible IFIT1 (p56) mRNA, the most strongly induced mRNA in response to type I IFN [116] or dsRNA [117], as a more sensitive measure of immune stimulation than plasma cytokines. We have measured strong IFIT1 mRNA induction in both liver and spleen of siRNA-treated mice in the absence of any detectable plasma IFN-α protein or related immunotoxicity (A. Judge and M. Robbins manuscript submitted). This likely reflects low level, local IFN induction that does not manifest as a systemic cytokine response. Alternatively, direct induction of IFIT1 via activation of IRF3 in the absence of type I IFN protein has also been reported to occur [117]. Although the immunostimulatory activity that can be detected by IFIT1 mRNA analysis is not sufficient to cause overt symptoms of toxicity in mice, it is clearly associated with off-target effects in gene expression patterns. It will be up to individual researchers to demonstrate whether or not such low-grade responses to siRNA are of sufficient magnitude to mediate nonspecific antiviral or antitumoral effects in preclinical models.

7.3.10 Testing for Vehicle Immunogenicity

When developing siRNA formulations as therapeutic agents, the potential for antibody responses to the carrier must be monitored. Immunostimulatory siRNA can render delivery vehicles immunogenic, even in the absence of what may be regarded as conventional antigens such as peptides or proteins in the formulation. In our own work, we have found that robust antibody responses can develop against polyethylene glycol (PEG), one of the least likely components of a formulation to be considered immunogenic [118]. Therefore, researchers should test for the development of antibodies against each component of their preferred delivery vehicle, as the siRNA formulations are advanced through preclinical studies. Typically, this can initially be assessed in mouse models following single or repeat dosing regimens. Appropriate time points range from days or weeks after administration depending on the antibody isotype (e.g., IgM or IgG) and whether a long-lived response has been established. We have described a sensitive method for the detection of serum antibodies against PEG [118] that is based on a modified ELISA originally developed for the detection of anticholesterol antibodies [119]. This method should be readily adaptable for the detection of antibodies against the lipids of particular interest to individual researchers. ELISA methods to detect antipeptide antibodies are well described in the literature and immunology textbooks.

7.4 IMPLICATIONS FOR PHARMACEUTICAL PRODUCT DEVELOPMENT

7.4.1 False Positive Efficacy

When reviewing the list of features advertised for the forthcoming wave of siRNA-based therapeutics one cannot help but be attracted by the possibility of developing drugs with little or no side effects, their selectivity conferred simply by choosing the appropriate siRNA sequence with activity against one, and only one, target transcript. However, the reality is that much of the discussion of the therapeutic potential of RNAi has been concerned with so-called off target effects. With respect to siRNA, off target effects are generally described as any effect other than the RNAi-mediated downregulation of expression of the intended target transcript. Although much has been said about the potential for RNAi-mediated downregulation of unintended, "off-target" transcripts, an equally if not more important class of off-target effects are those that are mediated by the induction of the innate immune response to siRNA.

Although it is now well known that synthetically manufactured siRNA duplexes can induce high levels of inflammatory cytokines and type I IFNs following systemic administration in mammals [7], very little of the literature is devoted to determining the extent to which these effects may contribute to the "efficacy" associated with the use of siRNA. siRNA have been reported as efficacious in several *in vivo* virus infection models, including influenza A [120, 121], herpes simplex virus (HSV) [122], respiratory syncitial virus (RSV) [123], parainfluenza (PIV) [123], and hepatitis B virus (HBV) [112] infections in mice, ebola virus infection in guinea pigs [124], and severe acute respiratory syndrome in both monkeys and mice [125]. Activation of innate immunity and production of cytokines such as type I IFN are known to inhibit viral infection. For example, polyI:C in complex with poly-L-lysine and methylcellulose (polyICLC), either alone or encapsulated in liposomes, protect mice from otherwise lethal influenza A infection [126]. In spite of the obvious interplay between immune stimulation and antiviral activity, at the time of this writing, only one published study has compared chemically modified with unmodified (immunostimulatory) siRNA [112] and found that nonspecific reduction of HBV titer *does* occur *in vivo* when using unmodified, immunostimulatory control siRNA. Chemical modification of both control and active siRNA in a manner that abrogates the siRNA's immunostimulatory activity prevents the nonspecific efficacy associated with the control while maintaining specific antiviral efficacy of the active siRNA [112]. This serves to highlight not only the potential contribution of immune stimulation to antiviral efficacy but also one of the strategies by which one may abrogate the effect.

The potential for immune stimulation to manifest as nonspecific "efficacy" is not confined to antiviral applications. In oncology, an area of intense interest to investigators working in RNAi, the immunostimulatory effects of nucleic acids have been intentionally harnessed for therapeutic benefit [11, 127, 128]. Furthermore, several IFNs are approved for use as drugs in humans and IFN-α in particular is used to treat many types of cancer. In spite of the well-known antitumor effects associated with stimulation of the innate immune system, reports that describe the extent to which siRNA-mediated immune stimulation contributes to antitumor efficacy are in the minority [129]. One mechanism by which IFN may contribute to antitumor effects involves the antiangiogenic activity of IFNs α and β [130]. IFN inhibits the ability of endothelial cells to form new blood capillaries, with IFN-α acting specifically to suppress vascular endothelial growth factor (VEGF) expression at the mRNA level [131, 132]. This highlights another area where the interpretation of preclinical results may be confounded by the immunostimulatory activity of active siRNA. The VEGF pathway is an attractive target for other applications, in addition to oncology. Macular degeneration, an eye disease characterized by dysregulated macular capillary growth, has been targeted using siRNA directed against VEGF. Given that unintended immune stimulation and concomitant IFN production has the potential to downregulate both VEGF protein and mRNA, confirmation that VEGF knockdown is mediated by RNAi and not via an IFN response induced by the active siRNA is fundamental to the interpretation of experiments targeting VEGF.

The use of appropriate controls should facilitate the straightforward interpretation of siRNA studies. However, there is currently little consensus as to what constitutes the "best" control for a given siRNA when considering immune-mediated effects. Noncoding siRNA or siRNA targeting genes that are not present in the mammalian genome, such as green fluorescent protein (GFP) or firefly luciferase (Luc), were once considered adequate controls. However, it is curious that a common EGFP siRNA selected for use as a negative control by several groups working on antiviral applications of RNAi [120, 121, 133–135] is an inherently nonimmunostimulatory sequence, while the active antiviral siRNAs used by these same groups are immunostimulatory when evaluated on either human PBMCs, murine bone marrow derived Flt3 L DCs, or *in vivo* in mice (M. Robbins, in preparation). This observation has prompted a retrospective analysis of previously reported *in vivo* influenza RNAi experiments [120]. When previously published antiviral efficacy studies are repeated using chemically modified, nonstimulatory active siRNA or alternately, immunostimulatory negative controls, the results clearly suggest that a differential induction of IFN between control and active siRNAs has affected the results and interpretation of a number of published *in vivo* knockdown studies (M. Robbins, in preparation). Since the inherent immunostimulatory activity of siRNA is sequence dependent, a certain amount of screening may be required to ensure that negative control siRNA are as immunostimulatory as their active counterparts (e.g., [124]). A preferred approach would be to utilize chemically modified siRNA with minimal residual immunostimulatory activity for both active and control duplexes and to confirm this within the context of the disease model in question. This may help avoid the misinterpretation of preclinical results.

7.4.2 Acute Toxicities

siRNA-based drugs have three classes of dose-limiting toxicities. In the first case, siRNA may be toxic as a result of exaggerated pharmacology, a direct consequence of the intentional knockdown of the siRNA target transcript. For example, antineoplastic siRNA that act to induce apoptosis in proliferating cells may be cytotoxic when delivered to normal, healthy cells. It is only recently that this type of toxicity has been a relevant concern when working with nucleic acid-based drugs. In some ways, the ability to elicit "too much" of a specific effect when using siRNA is a reflection of the potency of the RNAi mechanism and may bode well for the development of effective siRNA-based drugs. Another type of toxicity relates to the chemical nature of the siRNA and its associated delivery system. Certain nucleotide chemistries, including backbone modifications commonly used to confer stability to the siRNA duplex, have their own toxicological considerations [136] that are described in considerable detail elsewhere in this volume. As novel chemical entities, the increasingly wide variety of delivery vehicles and siRNA-conjugates under development also require formal evaluation. The use of delivery vehicles can alter the toxicity profile of a drug due to altered pharmacokinetics and biodistribution. In the case of liver targeting formulations, for example, elevations in serum transaminase levels can be a sensitive indicator of liver damage associated with an excessive chemical load into hepatocytes. The third type of toxicity is directly related to the subject of this chapter and is caused by the unintended activation of the innate immune response by immunostimulatory siRNA.

The recognition of canonical siRNA duplexes as a foreign entity by the mammalian TLR system acts as a trigger for the rapid release of inflammatory mediators as part of the host's natural defense against pathogens. The use of delivery systems to confer the required drug-like properties to siRNA promotes the immune response [7, 8], while "naked" siRNAs, in the absence of an siRNA delivery system, are not immunostimulatory [97]. TLR7 and TLR8 expression allow innate immune cells to respond directly to siRNA. pDC respond by producing large amounts of IFN-α that directly activates a generalized antiviral state in the body and causes the maturation of antigen presenting cells that can initiate potent T-cell responses [137]. Soluble factors that are released by pDC in this initial phase of the reaction, including IFN-α, also recruit and activate other immune cells to amplify the inflammatory response. This is brought about in part by the upregulation of TLR7 on monocytes, macrophages, NK cells, and neutrophils, enabling these cells to respond to siRNA [138, 139]. IFN-α signaling can also induce upregulation of the enzymes cyclooxygenase-2 (COX-2) [140] and nitric oxide synthase (iNOS) [141] resulting in the biosynthesis of eicosanoids and nitric oxide, respectively. In this manner, immunostimulatory siRNA can trigger an inflammatory cascade culminating in the high-level production of an array of cytokines plus other vasoactive and inflammatory mediators. In our experience, these inflammatory reactions can also exacerbate any underlying chemical toxicities associated with the siRNA or delivery vehicle.

Although beneficial in host defense, overstimulation of TLR-mediated pathways is pathological. Treatment of humans with the TLR ligands LPS (TLR4) [142, 143] or Poly I:C (TLR3) [144] results in an inflammatory response syndrome characterized by flu-like symptoms, fever, chills, rigors, and hypotension. Onset of symptoms typically occurs within hours of administration, distinguishing them from immediate hypersensitivity or infusion reactions. This response can be replicated in a number of animal models including rodents, although the doses required to induce symptoms can vary over orders of magnitude according to the species. Reasons for this remain unclear although it may reflect interspecies differences in either TLR signaling or differential sensitivity to the ensuing inflammatory response. Although the clinical syndrome induced by these agents is multifactorial, reflecting the complexity of the inflammatory cascade, many of the symptoms can be directly attributable to the action of cytokines. Evidence to support this comes from the clinical experience with recombinant cytokines as therapeutics, such as IFN-α, interleukin-1β (IL-1β), and TNF-α, where dose-limiting toxicities typically include fever, chills, rigors, and hypotension.

The experimental data from preclinical studies and the current understanding of the biology of these responses suggest the following mechanism of toxicity associated with systemic administration of immunostimulatory RNA (Figure 7.6). Similar pathways are also likely to be activated by local routes of administration, manifesting as inflammatory reactions at the site of injection:

1. Endocytosis of siRNA carriers (either lipidic or polycationic systems) by pDC in the blood or lymphoid tissues causes cell activation via TLR-mediated recognition of RNA. This results in the secretion of IFN-α and other cytokines including IL-6.

2. IFN-α acts on surrounding monocytes and macrophages, making them responsive to the stimulatory effects of RNA and inducing high-level production of inflammatory cytokines, including IL-6, IL-1β, and TNF-α, together with proinflammatory chemokines.

3. Cytokines released into the blood cause activation of vascular endothelial cells resulting in upregulation of adhesion molecules, IL-6, and other inflammatory mediators. Margination and pavementing of blood cells ensue, manifesting as transient lymphopenia, and thrombocytopenia.

4. Activation of cells by siRNA, either directly or via the action of cytokines, can upregulate COX-2 and NOS enzyme pathways resulting in eicosanoid (prostaglandins, etc.) and nitric oxide production. These mediators contribute to the symptoms of toxicity, including pain.

5. Systemic release of IFN-α, IL-6, and IL-1β induce symptoms of fever, rigors, and chills. These cytokines also act directly on the liver to induce the so-called acute phase reaction that elevates a range of serum protein components associated with host defense such as complement, pentraxins, and coagulation factors.

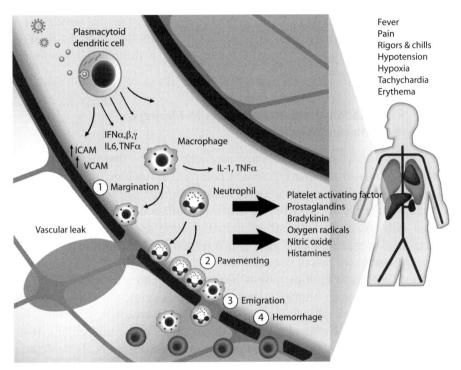

FIGURE 7.6 Downstream effects of innate immune stimulation. IFNα produced by pDC acts on surrounding monocytes and macrophages, causing the production of high levels of inflammatory cytokines including IL-6, IL-1β, and TNF-α. Systemic release of IFNα, IL-6, and IL-1β induce symptoms of fever, rigors, and chills. Cytokines released into the blood cause activation of vascular endothelial cells, resulting in a cascade of effects on blood cells characterized by (1) margination, (2) pavementing, (3) emigration, and (4) hemorrhage that exacerbate lymphopenia and thrombocytopenia. Activation of cells by siRNA, either directly or via the action of cytokines, can upregulate COX-2 and nitric oxide synthase enzyme pathways, resulting in eicosanoid (prostaglandins, etc.) and nitric oxide production contributing to the symptoms of toxicity, including pain. Effects of IL-1β and TNF-α on vascular endothelium result in the development of hypotension.

6. Effects of IL-1β, TNF-α, and other vasoactive molecules increase vascular permeability resulting in the development of hypotension. Emigration and hemorrhage exacerbate the preexisting lymphopenia and thrombocytopenia.

7. In the most severe cases, dysregulation of the protective negative feedback mechanisms allow continued amplification of the systemic inflammatory response, worsening hypotension, vascular leak, and intravascular coagulation that ultimately leads to multiorgan failure.

Although this pathway of events is modeled upon the characterized responses to TLR ligands, such as plasmid DNA, LPS and PolyI:C, there is good reason to believe that significant activation of the innate immune response by siRNA would manifest similarly.

7.4.3 Pharmacological Intervention to Manage Immune-Mediated Toxicities

Based on the mechanism of immune-mediated toxicity, there is a strong incentive to consider the management or complete abrogation of the toxicities associated with the administration of immunostimulatory RNA. Since these toxicities appear to result from an excessive inflammatory response, medication with an appropriate anti-inflammatory drug prior to treatment might be expected to avoid the induction of this response. Glucocorticoids, such as dexamethasone, are potent steroidal anti-inflammatory drugs that exert their inhibitory effects at multiple points in the inflammatory cascade. Based on prior experience with immunostimulatory nucleic acids, the immunostimulatory properties of siRNA may be expected to be exquisitely sensitive to inhibition by glucocorticoids. This is due to their known molecular effects on key components of the signaling pathways employed by TLRs, including TLR7 and TLR8, to induce cell activation [145]. In particular, glucocorticoids inhibit the actions of the transcription factors NF-κB and AP-1 and suppress the MAP kinase signaling cascade. These are the pathways utilized by TLR to activate an array of genes encoding cytokines and other inflammatory proteins. Therefore, it is expected that glucocorticoids could act to suppress cytokine release by inhibiting the initial trigger for the inflammatory response mediated by TLR recognition. In this respect, previous preclinical studies have demonstrated that pretreatment with dexamethasone in mice substantially inhibits the inflammatory cytokine response induced by plasmid DNA-lipid complexes [146]. In human studies, it has also been shown that glucocorticoid administration is a potent suppressor of the IFN-α response elicited from blood-derived pDC stimulated with lipid encapsulated plasmid DNA (A. Judge and I. MacLachlan, 2007, unpublished observations). Other beneficial actions of glucocorticoids that may ameliorate the inflammatory response to siRNA include the inhibition of COX-2 and iNOS consequently blocking both eicosanoid and nitric oxide biosynthesis. Both of these proinflammatory pathways can be upregulated, either directly or indirectly through cytokines such as IFN-α, produced in response to siRNA.

Glucocorticoids may also have a beneficial effect in symptom management in the event of cytokine release following siRNA administration in patients. This is due to their ability to block cytokine signaling through inhibition of the principal cytokine receptor signaling pathways [145, 147]. This could help manage the direct pyrogenic and hypotensive effects of cytokines such as IFN-α, IL-6, and IL-1. With symptom management in mind, it is also conceivable that premedication of patients with acetaminophen could be beneficial due to the known antipyretic effects and control of other flu-like symptoms triggered by prostaglandin biosynthesis. In this regard, it is important to consider that acetaminophen is oxidized to the reactive intermediate N-acetyl-p-benzoquinone imine (NAPQI), which reacts with sulfur-containing compounds. Reaction between metabolically activated acetaminophen and PS ODNs results in the formation of higher molecular weight products with NAPQI bound to the sulfur atoms in the PS backbone [148]. Although this interaction has been characterized as nontoxic and nonmutagenic, the extent to which it may interfere with the ability of PS-containing siRNA to mediate RNAi is not known. In the interim, other NSAIDS, such as ASA, may offer more suitable alternatives for premedicating patients.

7.4.4 Abrogation of Immune Stimulation via Chemical Modification of siRNA

A far more preferable alternative to managing the toxicities associated with the use of immunostimulatory siRNA is to avoid inducing them altogether. On the basis of the finding that immune activation by siRNA is sequence dependent, it is possible to design active siRNA with negligible immunostimulatory activity by selecting sequences that lack immunostimulatory sequence motifs [7]. Although this strategy has proven successful, it significantly limits the number of novel siRNA sequences that can be designed against a given target and requires a certain degree of screening due to the relatively ill-defined nature of immunostimulatory RNA sequence motifs. A more robust approach is to abrogate siRNA-mediated immune stimulation by selective incorporation of 2′OMe or other modified nucleotides in the siRNA duplex [102]. Since effective abrogation of the immune response may require only one of the RNA strands to be selectively modified, chemical modifications can be restricted to the sense strand of the duplex, therefore minimizing the potential for attenuating the potency of the siRNA. This method allows for rapid design and synthesis of nonimmunostimulatory siRNA on the basis of native sequences with proven RNAi activity. By combining selectively modified siRNA with an effective systemic delivery vehicle, potent silencing of endogenous gene targets can be achieved *in vivo* at therapeutically viable doses without the deleterious side effects associated with systemic activation of the innate immune response [102]. Highly active siRNA containing more extensive chemical modifications can also be generated if nuclease resistance of the naked duplex remains a requirement (e.g., [100, 104, 111]). Many of the published patterns of chemical modification employ 2′OMe nucleotides, either alone or in combination with other stabilization chemistries [100,104], and are, therefore, also predicted to avoid immune activation. As described earlier, we have confirmed that the extensively modified siRNA molecules, which contain less than 8% native ribonucleotides (and include 2'OMe pyrimidines in the antisense strand), do not activate an immune response [112].

As the 2'-OH in the ribose backbone is a distinguishing feature of RNA, it may be anticipated that extensive chemical substitutions at this position may be required to disrupt recognition of the modified nucleic acid by an RNA-binding receptor. However, 2'OMe-modified siRNA can be rendered nonimmunostimulatory by modification of less than 5% of their native ribonucleotides. O-methyl groups are considered to be a relatively bulky chemistry at the 2' position that sit within the minor groove of an RNA duplex without significantly distorting its A-form helical structure [107,149]. This may be sufficient to disrupt interactions between the RNA duplex and its putative immune receptors (TLRs) or accessory molecules.

7.4.5 Multiple Dosing and Toxicities Associated with Drug Immunogenicity

This chapter has, thus, far focused on the immunological considerations accompanying the single administration of an siRNA-based drug. In practice, siRNA drugs will likely be used in a manner analogous to their small molecule counterparts, including reliance on multiple dosing regimens that have an increased potential for the development of adaptive immune responses.

Activation of the innate immune response sensitizes the adaptive arm of the immune system. Normally, the benefits of this include successful immunization against infection and the establishment of long-term immunity. However, in the drug development context, the activation of innate immune responses can lead to adaptive responses against the drug carrier or the drug itself. The potential for a drug or its excipient to be immunogenic is a serious concern, since the establishment of an antibody response can severely compromise both the safety and efficacy of a drug. Evidence suggests that this can be a concern for the development of nucleic acid-based drugs as well. Synthetic siRNAs that induce potent immune stimulation *in vivo* can drive the production of a strong anti-PEG antibody response when the siRNAs are encapsulated in PEGylated liposomes ([118] and A. Judge, M. Robbins, and I. MacLachlan, in preparation). The immune response against PEGylated liposomes is surprisingly robust, generating both IgM and IgG isotypes directed against PEG following a single intravenous administration. The presence of serum antibodies results in accelerated blood clearance, a loss of disease site targeting and acute hypersensitive reactions upon subsequent readministration of PEGylated liposomes in mice. PEG is generally regarded as nonimmunogenic and empty liposomes appear to be immunologically inert; however, the encapsulation of immunostimulatory payloads such as nucleic acids that act as potent adjuvants render the drug vehicle immunogenic. In this example, the immunostimulatory activity of siRNA is thought to potentiate antibody responses against the PEG-lipids both by direct B-cell stimulation through TLR7 [150] and through the concurrent induction of cytokines that support activated B-cell growth and differentiation [151].

The immunogenicity of PEGylated liposomes containing siRNA can be greatly reduced by using alternative PEG-lipids with shorter alkyl chains. This modification has been shown to facilitate the exchange of the PEG-lipid from the liposomal bilayer, thereby allowing the PEG-lipid to dissociate more rapidly from the particle when administered *in vivo* [152]. By substantially reducing the antibody response to PEG, these modified liposomes can be safely readministered intravenously to mice while maintaining the effective delivery of the immunostimulatory payload to distal sites. Administration of modified liposomes is still associated with substantial cytokine induction, indicating that the reduced immunogenicity is not due to abrogation of the immunostimulatory activity of the payload. Instead, these findings suggest that the robust Ab response to PEG requires the close physical association of the weak PEG-lipid antigen with the immunostimulatory payload.

The ability to abrogate the immunogenicity of PEGylated liposomes by simple modification of their lipid composition without significantly compromising *in vivo* performance has implications for their design and clinical development. It is expected that attachment of targeting ligands to delivery systems carrying stimulatory nucleic acids may well exacerbate the problem of drug vehicle immunogenicity. Perhaps not surprisingly, unmodified, immunostimulatory siRNA delivered in human transferrin-conjugated-PEG-modified cyclodextrin-based carriers have been shown to elicit an adaptive response resulting in the production of antihuman transferrin antibodies in nonhuman primates [96]. It remains to be seen if active targeting technologies can be made to be compatible with the delivery of immunostimulatory siRNA.

Perhaps the most alarming aspect of the adaptive response to carriers containing immunostimulatory siRNA is the anaphylactic response that can result upon subsequent administration of the drug. These hypersensitive or "infusion-type" reactions develop within minutes of drug administration and are distinct from the acute inflammatory toxicities that manifest upon first challenge with an immunostimulatory siRNA. Antibodies can mediate hypersensitive reactions through a variety of mechanisms following drug administration. Classical allergic reactions can occur when antibody (typically IgE)–antigen binding triggers the release of histamine and other vasoactive molecules from mast cells and basophils. Alternatively, IgM and certain IgG

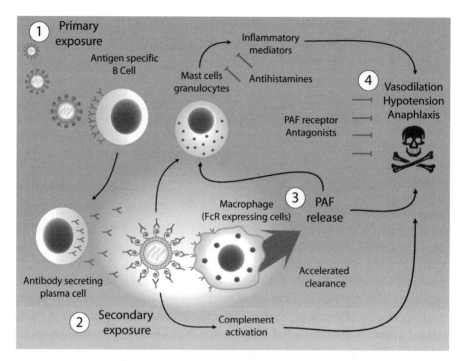

FIGURE 7.7 Mechanism of PAF-mediated anaphylaxis. In the mouse, a primary mechanism of Ab-mediated anaphylaxis involves platelet activating factor (PAF). This reaction can be initiated by the formation of IgG containing immune complexes in the blood that trigger excess PAF release from Fcγ receptor expressing cells. Antibody responses against an siRNA conjugate or delivery vehicle may be established following primary administration due to the immunostimulatory activity of the siRNA molecule.

subclasses can activate the complement cascade after binding their cognate antigens. Complement activation rapidly leads to the generation of so-called anaphylatoxins such as C3a and C5a that act directly on vascular endothelium and smooth muscle cells as well as triggering degranulation of mast cells and basophils to bring about the anaphylactic response. In the mouse, an additional mechanism of antibody-mediated anaphylaxis involves platelet-activating factor (PAF) [153] (Figure 7.7). This reaction can be initiated by the formation of IgG-containing immune complexes in the blood that trigger excess PAF release from Fcγ receptor expressing cells [153]. This mechanism is responsible for the anaphylactic reaction to PEGylated liposomes carrying pDNA in mice [118]. Prophylactic treatment of mice with PAF antagonists CV6209 or CV3988 fully inhibits the anaphylactic reaction to PEGylated liposomes at challenge doses that otherwise proved fatal in presensitized control mice. This suggests that the hypersensitive and acute toxicities following repeat administration of PEGylated liposomes are due to the systemic release of PAF, triggered by the formation of immune complexes between anti-PEG Ab and the drug carrier. In this model, levels of complement activation or histamine release detected in anaphylactic mice are insignificant, and hypersensitivity is not associated with excessive systemic cytokine release at the time of the second dose.

The induction of an adaptive response may actually be a more sensitive indicator of immune stimulation than conventional cytokine analysis. Substitution of 2'OMe uridines into the sense strand of an siRNA abrogates cytokine induction *in vivo* and *in vitro* [102]. However, despite a lack of measurable cytokine production, certain of these minimally 2'OMe-modified siRNA are still able to promote antibody responses against PEG in the delivery vehicle (A. Judge, 2007, unpublished observations). This adaptive immune response becomes more evident in multidosing regimes and most likely reflects residual immunostimulatory activity associated with the minimally modified siRNA. We have discovered that *in vivo* IFIT1 mRNA analysis may be a more sensitive indicator of siRNA-mediated immune stimulation than systemic cytokine production and therefore a more accurate predictor of this type of adaptive response. Complete elimination of IFIT1 mRNA induction by siRNA can be readily achieved by the incorporation of 2'OMe residues into both strands of the siRNA. This still requires less than 20% of the total nucleotides in the duplex to be 2'OMe modified and results in an siRNA molecule with no residual immunostimulatory activity. Importantly, we have found that this minimal alteration to the siRNA also acts to completely abrogate any antibody response against the lipid vehicle, resulting in a drug formulation that is nonimmunogenic. These findings suggest that in some cases both strands of an siRNA may need to be chemically modified in order to eliminate residual levels of immune stimulation and to prevent siRNA delivery vehicles from being rendered immunogenic.

7.4.6 Species Differences

At the time of this writing, siRNA-based therapeutics have yet to be systemically administered to humans. Therefore, no direct clinical precedent exists with which to compare the toxicities observed in preclinical studies to those in humans. In our experience, preclinical toxicology in mice has proven to be nonpredictive for the severe immunotoxicities observed in human subjects after the intravenous administration of immunostimulatory plasmid DNA (A. Judge and I. MacLachlan, 2007, unpublished observations). However, the discovery that these symptoms of toxicity in humans correlated with significant increases in blood cytokines and that the response to the DNA-based drug could be replicated *in vitro* using TLR9 expressing human blood cells, provides us a better understanding with which to extrapolate the effects of immune stimulation by siRNA-based drugs in preclinical models.

Although rat and mouse models successfully reproduce several aspects of the cytokine response and associated toxicities identified in human subjects receiving lipid-encapsulated plasmid DNA, neither model replicates the full extent of the toxicities observed in humans (most notably the development of hypotension), or predict that immunotoxicities would manifest at the low doses that they do in humans (less than 0.003 mg plasmid DNA per kilogram body weight). By our understanding, no pre-clinical model has been described for a DNA-based therapeutic that is predictive of the human response to low dose, systemic administration of immunostimulatory DNA. However, the pre-clinical toxicities associated with DNA-based drugs are typically ascribed to TLR9-mediated immune stimulation and this can be partly modeled in a human system using primary immune cell cultures containing TLR9 expressing pDC. Therefore, it is proposed that the etiology of the toxicities observed in preclinical models and in humans is fundamentally similar; the difference between species lies in the degree of sensitivity to the DNA and its immunostimulatory effects. In this respect, we see no reason to believe that the clinical effects of a TLR7/8-mediated immune response to an siRNA-based drug will be fundamentally different.

Critical differences in the sensitivity of human subjects to the toxic effects of immune stimulation compared with preclinical animal models have recently been highlighted in an ill-fated phase I study of a CD28 agonist mAb designed to activate T-cell responses. Life-threatening shock-like symptoms developed rapidly in a number of healthy volunteers following first administration of the immunostimulatory monoclonal antibodies. These symptoms were subsequently attributed to "on-target" effects of the CD28 agonist causing excessive cytokine release, leading to a severe shock-like syndrome [154]. Most strikingly, these effects occurred at very low dose and were apparently unpredicted by the extensive preclinical testing leading up to this first in human trial.

It is tempting to speculate that nonhuman primate models may be more predictive of the human response to nucleic acid-based drugs. Several nonhuman primate studies have examined the toxicity of DNA formulations injected systemically. In each case, the DNA was presumed or known to contain immunostimulatory CpG sequence motifs. Treatment of cynomolgus monkeys with a single administration of plasmid DNA in artificial viral envelope liposomes at a dose of ~0.2 mg DNA/kg induced no abnormalities in general condition or histopathology in the animals [155]. Another study, also in cynomolgus monkeys, reported that a dose of 18 mg/kg of plasmid DNA condensed with polyvinylpyrrolidone could be repeatedly administered via subcutaneous injection without ill effect [156]. Naked plasmid DNA has been administered intra-arterially to rhesus macaques at high doses (1–2 mg DNA/kg) with only minor changes in blood chemistry and no effect on WBC counts [157]. Immunostimulatory DNA ODNs encapsulated within PEGylated liposomes have been tested for toxicity in telemetered cynomolgus monkeys. Intravenous infusion at doses from 10 to 40 mg DNA/kg was accomplished without any clinical signs of an adverse event. No significant changes in mean arterial blood pressure, heart rate, or ECG readout were observed [158]. In our opinion, these studies suggest that nonhuman primate models may also be inadequate at predicting the consequences of TLR-mediated immune stimulation in humans.

The relative sensitivities of species to other stimulators of innate immunity via TLR pathways are considered idiosyncratic and notoriously difficult to predict. The most well defined of these is the response to LPS, also known as endotoxin. Humans and chimpanzees are exquisitely sensitive to the toxic effects of endotoxin, whereas baboons and other primates are highly resistant [159]. A spectrum of sensitivities within rodents is also seen. With respect to immunostimulatory nucleic acids, the dramatic differences between species in their sensitivity and response to plasmid DNA and other immunostimulatory nucleic acids may be due to several reasons:

1. It is well known that different species recognize and respond to different immunostimulatory motifs (sequences). Recognition of species-specific motifs is largely conferred by their respective TLR receptors.
2. There are significant differences between species in the pattern of TLR expression, resulting in different cell types being directly responsive to nucleic acid stimulation.
3. Species differ in their sensitivity to the toxic effects of the inflammatory cytokines released in response to immunostimulatory nucleic acids. This is illustrated by the clinical experience with systemic recombinant cytokine therapies. Several of these, such as TNF-α, are associated with unacceptable toxicities at low doses that were not predicted by preclinical studies.

Taken together, it is believed that the identification of a preclinical model for siRNA immunotoxicity that accurately replicates all of the clinical symptoms within an appropriate dose range would require a stochastic approach to screening species. To the best of our knowledge, no published studies have highlighted such a model. Available experimental evidence does not indicate that nonhuman primates would necessarily provide a predictive model of the toxicity of immunostimulatory siRNA anticipated in human subjects.

7.5 SUMMARY

The multitude of cell types and mechanisms through which siRNA can interact with the mammalian immune system means that the potential to activate off-target immune-mediated effects is a genuine concern for any researcher utilizing RNAi technologies. The extent to which these immunological pathways may be activated is dependent upon the sequence, structure, and quality of the siRNA together with the type of delivery system employed to transfect the siRNA into cells. Therefore, the onus falls on the individual researcher to determine whether or not a particular siRNA formulation activates an immune response within their experimental models. Appropriate study design is required to accurately make this assessment and needs to be conducted on each of the active and control siRNA sequences under consideration.

The implications of activating an immune response for siRNA-based therapeutics run significantly beyond the much discussed "off-target" effects on gene expression associated with the induction of an IFN response. Activation of TLR-mediated immune responses can lead to significant immunotoxicities caused by the release of proinflammatory cytokines and IFNs. These are of particular concern for systemic RNAi applications where dose-limiting immunotoxicities may manifest at subtherapeutic siRNA doses. Inflammatory responses are also a relevant concern for local routes of drug administration due to injection site reactions and the potential for these to spread systemically. Even in the absence of overt inflammatory reactions, low-grade stimulation of the immune system by siRNA significantly increases the likelihood of an antibody response developing against components of any siRNA delivery vehicle that is utilized *in vivo*. Antibody responses against the drug conjugate or carrier can severely impair multidose treatment regimes due to rapid drug clearance, loss of tissue targeting, and their potential to trigger hypersensitive reactions in patients when reexposed to the drug.

Clinical immunotoxicities are notoriously hard to predict using current preclinical models, particularly in the case of TLR-mediated immune reactions. This has been most clearly illustrated to us by our clinical experience with an immunostimulatory DNA formulation. In this case, single, systemic drug administration resulted in dose-limiting toxicities associated with excessive IFN-α and inflammatory cytokine release. Importantly, although the TLR9-mediated cytokine response was predicted by a number of preclinical models, none of these was able to predict the toxic effects such a response would have in human subjects. Therefore, the advancement of siRNA-based therapeutics into the clinic needs to proceed with caution and with a full understanding of the potential for the siRNA to activate innate immune responses in preclinical human and animal models.

Fortunately, relatively simple ways have been identified to engineer siRNA that avoid recognition by TLRs and other nucleic acid sensing receptors. In particular, this can be achieved by introducing chemically modified nucleotides into the siRNA duplex in a manner that does not significantly impact RNAi activity. These chemistries are commonly used in RNA synthesis and are readily available to researchers through conventional suppliers. The progress made in this aspect of siRNA design illustrates how chemical modification strategies can overcome many, if not all, of the problems surrounding the immunostimulatory capacity of siRNA. With appropriately designed siRNA coupled to increasingly effective delivery systems, time is fast approaching for the first successful demonstrations of systemic RNAi in human subjects.

REFERENCES

1. Yi, A. K., Chace, J. H., Cowdery, J. S., and Krieg, A. M. (1996). IFN-gamma promotes IL-6 and IgM secretion in response to CpG motifs in bacterial DNA and oligonucleotides. *J Immunol* **156**: 558–64.

2. Ballas, Z. K., Rasmussen, W. L., and Krieg, A. M. (1996). Induction of NK activity in murine and human cells by CpG motifs in oligonucleotides and bacterial DNA. *J Immunol* **157**: 1840–5.

3. Klinman, D. M., Yi, A. K., Beaucage, S. L., Conover, J., and Krieg, A. M. (1996). CpG motifs present in bacterial DNA rapidly induce lymphocytes to secrete interleukin 6, interleukin 12 and interferon gamma. *Proc Natl Acad Sci USA* **93**: 2879–33.

4. Heil, F., et al. (2004). Species-specific recognition of single-stranded RNA via toll-like receptor 7 and 8. *Science* **303**: 1526–9.

5. Diebold, S. S., Kaisho, T., Hemmi, H., Akira, S., and Reise Sousa, C. (2004). Innate antiviral responses by means of TLR7-mediated recognition of single-stranded RNA. *Science* **303**: 1529–31.

6. Alexopoulou, L., Czopik-Holt, A., Medzhitov, R., and Flavell, R. (2001). Recognition of double-stranded RNA and activation of NF-KB by toll-like receptor 3. *Nature* **413**: 732–8.

7. Judge, A., Sood, V., Shaw, J., Fang, D., McClintock, K., and MacLachlan, I. (2005). Sequence-dependent stimulation of the mammalian innate immune response by synthetic siRNA. *Nat Biotechnol* **23**(4): 457–62.

8. Hornung, V., et al. (2005). Sequence-specific potent induction of IFN-α by short interfering RNA in plasmacytoid dendritic cells through TLR7. *Nat Med* **11**(3): 263–70.

9. Gursel, I., Gursel, M., Ishii, K. J., and Klinman, D. M. (2001). Sterically stabilized cationic liposomes improve the uptake and immunostimulatory activity of CpG oligonucleotides. *J Immunol* **167**(6): 3324–8.

10. Klinman, D. M. (2004). Immuotherapeutic uses of CpG oligodeoxynucleotides. *Nat Rev Immunol* **4**: 249–58.

11. Krieg, A. M. (2006). Therapeutic potential of Toll-like receptor 9 activation. *Nat Rev Drug Discov* **5**(6): 471–84.

12. Roach, J. C., et al. (2005). The evolution of vertebrate Toll-like receptors. *Proc Natl Acad Sci USA* **102**(27): 9577–82.

13. Meurs, E., et al. (1990). Molecular cloning and characterization of the human double-stranded RNA-activated protein kinase induced by interferon. *Cell* **62**(2): 379–90.

14. Schneider, D. S., Hudson, K. L., Lin, T. Y., and Anderson, K. V. (1991). Dominant and recessive mutations define functional domains of Toll, a transmembrane protein required for dorsal-ventral polarity in the *Drosophila* embryo. *Genes Dev* **5**(5): 797–807.

15. Rosetto, M., Engstrom, Y., Baldari, C. T., Telford, J. L., and Hultmark, D. (1995). Signals from the IL-1 receptor homolog, Toll, can activate an immune response in a *Drosophila* hemocyte cell line. *Biochem Biophys Res Commun* **209**(1): 111–6.

16. Dushay, M. S. and Eldon, E. D. (1998). *Drosophila* immune responses as models for human immunity. *Am J Hum Genet* **62**(1): 10–4.

17. Rock, F. L., Hardiman, G., Timans, J. C., Kastelein, R. A., and Bazan, J. F. (1998). A family of human receptors structurally related to *Drosophila* Toll. *Proc Natl Acad Sci USA* **95**(2): 588–93.

18. Chuang, T. H. and Ulevitch, R. J. (2000). Cloning and characterization of a subfamily of human toll-like receptors: hTLR7, hTLR8 and hTLR9. *Eur Cytokine Netw* **11**(3): 372–8.

19. Wagner, H. (2004). The immunobiology of the TLR9 subfamily. *Trends Immunol* **25**(7): 381–6.

20. Krieg, A. M. (2002). CpG motifs in bacterial DNA and their immune effects. *Annu Rev Immunol* **20**: 709–60.

21. Latz, E., et al. (2004). TLR9 signals after translocating from the ER to CpG DNA in the lysosome. *Nat Immunol* **5**(2): 190–8.

22. Yi, A. K., Tuetken, R., Redford, T., Waldschmidt, M., Kirsch, J., and Krieg, A. M. (1998). CpG motifs in bacterial DNA activate leukocytes through the pH-dependent generation of reactive oxygen species. *J Immunol* **160**(10): 4755–61.

23. Hacker, et al. (1998). CpG-DNA-specific activation of antigen-presenting cells requires stress kinase activity and is preceded by non-specific endocytosis and endosomal maturation. *EMBO J* **17**(21): 6230–40.

24. Leadbetter, E. A., Rifkin, I. R., Hohlbaum, A. M., Beaudette, B. C., Shlomchik, M. J., and Marshak-Rothstein, A. (2002). Chromatin-IgG complexes activate B cells by dual engagement of IgM and Toll-like receptors. *Nature* **416**(6881): 603–7.

25. Krieg, A. M., et al. (1995). CpG motifs in bacterial DNA trigger direct B-cell activation. *Nature* **374**(6522): 546–9.

26. Hemmi, H., et al. (2000). A Toll-like receptor recognizes bacterial DNA. *Nature* **408**(6813): 740–5.

27. Bullock, E. and Elton, R. A. (1972). Dipeptide frequencies in proteins and the CpG deficiency in vertebrate DNA. *J Mol Evol* **1**(3): 315–25.

28. Cooper, D. N. and Krawczak, M. (1989). Cytosine methylation and the fate of CpG dinucleotides in vertebrate genomes. *Hum Genet* **83**(2): 181–8.

29. Takeda, K. and Akira, S. (2005). Toll-like receptors in innate immunity. *Int Immunol* **17**(1): 1–14.

30. Bell, J. K., Mullen, G. E., Leifer, C. A., Mazzoni, A., Davies, D. R., and Segal, D. M. (2003). Leucine-rich repeats and pathogen recognition in Toll-like receptors. *Trends Immunol* **24**(10): 528–33.

31. Rutz, M., et al. (2004). Toll-like receptor 9 binds single-stranded CpG-DNA in a sequence- and pH-dependent manner. *Eur J Immunol* **34**(9): 2541–50.

32. Krieg, A. M., et al. (1998). Sequence motifs in adenoviral DNA block immune activation by stimulatory CpG motifs. *Proc Natl Acad Sci USA* **95**: 12631–6.

33. Vollmer, J., et al. (2004). Oligodeoxynucleotides lacking CpG dinucleotides mediate Toll-like receptor 9 dependent T helper type 2 biased immune stimulation. *Immunology* **113**(2): 212–23.

34. Kerkmann, M., et al. (2005). Spontaneous formation of nucleic acid-based nanoparticles is responsible for high interferon-alpha induction by CpG-A in plasmacytoid dendritic cells. *J Biol Chem* **280**(9): 8086–93.

35. Jurk, M., et al. (2004). C-Class CpG ODN: sequence requirements and characterization of immunostimulatory activities on mRNA level. *Immunobiology* **209**(1–2): 141–54.

36. Honda, K., et al. (2005). Spatiotemporal regulation of MyD88-IRF-7 signalling for robust type-I interferon induction. *Nature* **434**(7036): 1035–40.

37. Mui, B., Raney, S. G., Semple, S. C., and Hope, M. J. (2001). Immune stimulation by a CpG-containing oligodeoxynucleotide is enhanced when encapsulated and delivered in lipid particles. *J Pharmacol Exp Ther* **298**(3): 1185–92.

38. Takeda, K., Kaisho, T., and Akira, S. (2003). Toll-like receptors. *Ann Rev Immunol* **21**: 335–76.

39. Gorden, K. B., et al. (2005). Synthetic TLR agonists reveal functional differences between human TLR7 and TLR8. *J Immunol* **174**(3): 1259–68.

40. Gorden, K. K., Qiu, X. X., Binsfeld, C. C., Vasilakos, J. P., and Alkan, S. S. (2006). Cutting edge: activation of murine TLR8 by a combination of imidazoquinoline immune response modifiers and PolyT oligodeoxynucleotides. *J Immunol* **177**(10): 6584–7.

41. Hemmi, H., et al. (2002). Small anti-viral compounds activate immune cells via the TLR7 MyD88-dependent signaling pathway. *Nat Immunol* **3**(2): 196–200.

42. Jurk, M., et al. (2002). Human TLR7 or TLR8 independently confer responsiveness to the antiviral compound R-848. *Nat Immunol* **3**(6): 499.

43. Lund, J. M., et al. (2004). Recognition of single-stranded RNA viruses by Toll-like receptor 7. *Proc Natl Acad Sci USA* **101**(15): 5598–603.

44. Diebold, S. S., Massacrier, C., Akira, S., Paturel, C., Morel, Y., and Reis e Sousa, C. (2006). Nucleic acid agonists for Toll-like receptor 7 are defined by the presence of uridine ribonucleotides. *Eur J Immunol* **36**(12): 3256–67.

45. Sioud, M. (2005). Induction of inflammatory cytokines and interferon responses by double-stranded and single-stranded siRNA is sequence dependent and requires endosomal localization. *J Mol Biol* **348**(5): 1079–90.

46. Karikó, K., Buckstein, M., Ni, H., and Weissman, D. (2005). Suppression of RNA recognition by Toll-like receptors: the impact of nucleoside modification and the evolutionary origin of RNA. *Immunity* **23**: 165–75.

47. Gursel, M., Gursel, I., Mostowski, H. S., and Klinman, D. M. (2006). CXCL16 influences the nature and specificity of CpG-induced immune activation. *J Immunol* **177**(3): 1575–80.

48. Robbins, M., Judge, A., Liang, L., McClintock, K., Yaworski, E., and Maclachlan, I. (2007). 2'-O-methyl-modified RNAs Act as TLR7 Antagonists. *Mol Ther* **15**(9):1663–1669.

49. Muzio, M., et al. (2000). Differential expression and regulation of toll-like receptors (TLR) in human leukocytes: selective expression of TLR3 in dendritic cells. *J Immunol* **164**(11): 5998–6004.

50. Applequist, S. E., Wallin, R. P., and Ljunggren, H. G. (2002). Variable expression of Toll-like receptor in murine innate and adaptive immune cell lines. *Int Immunol* **14**(9): 1065–74.

51. Lee, H. K., Dunzendorfer, S., Soldau, K., and Tobias, P. S. (2006). Double-stranded RNA-mediated TLR3 activation is enhanced by CD14. *Immunity* **24**(2): 153–63.

52. Okahira, S., Nishikawa, F., Nishikawa, S., Akazawa, T., Seya, T., and Matsumoto, M. (2005). Interferon-beta induction through toll-like receptor 3 depends on double-stranded RNA structure. *DNA Cell Biol* **24**(10): 614–23.

53. Kariko, K., Ni, H., Capodici, J., Lamphier, M., and Weissman, D. (2004). mRNA is an endogenous ligand for Toll-like receptor 3. *J Biol Chem* **279**(13): 12542–50.

54. Marshall-Clarke, S., Downes, J. E., Haga, I. R., Browie, A. G., Borrow, P., Pennock, J. L., Grencis, R. K., Rothwell, P. (2007) Polyinosinic acid is a ligand for toll-like receptor 3. *J Biol Chem.* **282**(34): 24759–66.

55. Arnott, S., Chandrasekaran, R., and Marttila, C. M. (1974). Structures for polyinosinic acid and polyguanylic acid. *Biochem J* **141**(2): 537–43.

56. Karikó, K., Bhuyan, P., Capodici, J., and Weissman, D. (2004). Small interfering RNAs mediate sequence-independent gene suppression and induce immune activation by signaling through Toll-like receptor-3. *J Immunol* **172**: 6545–9.

57. Schlee, M., Hornung, V., and Hartmann, G. (2006). siRNA and isRNA: two edges of one sword. *Mol Ther* **14**(4): 463–70.

58. Kim, D.-H., Longo, M., Han, Y., Lundberg, P., Cantin, E., and Rossi, J. J. (2004). Interferon induction by siRNAs and ssRNAs synthesized by phage polymerase. *Nat Biotechnol* **22**(3): 321–5.

59. Marques, J. T., et al. (2006). A structural basis for discriminating between self and nonself double-stranded RNAs in mammalian cells. *Nat Biotechnol* **24**(5): 559–65.

60. Akira, S. and Takeda, K. (2004). Toll-like receptor signalling. *Nat Rev Immunol* **4**: 499–511.

61. Kawai, T. and Akira, S. (2006). Innate immune recognition of viral infection. *Nat Immunol* **7**(2): 131–7.

62. Asselin-Paturel, C. and Trinchieri, G. (2005). Production of type I interferons: plasmacytoid dendritic cells and beyond. *J Exp Med* **202**(4): 461–5.

63. Yamamoto, M., et al. (2003). Role of adaptor TRIF in the MyD88-independent toll-like receptor signaling pathway. *Science* **301**(5633): 640–3.

64. Yamamoto, M., et al. (2002). Cutting edge: a novel Toll/IL-1 receptor domain-containing adapter that preferentially activates the IFN-beta promoter in the Toll-like receptor signaling. *J Immunol* **169**(12): 6668–72.

65. Peters, K. L., Smith, H. L., Stark, G. R., and Sen, G. C. (2002). IRF-3-dependent, NFkappa B- and JNK-independent activation of the 561 and IFN-beta genes in response to double-stranded RNA. *Proc Natl Acad Sci USA* **99**(9): 6322–7.

66. Sen, G. C. and Sarkar, S. N. (2005). Transcriptional signaling by double-stranded RNA: role of TLR3. *Cytokine Growth Factor Rev* **16**(1): 1–14.

67. Kanneganti, T. D., et al. (2006). Bacterial RNA and small antiviral compounds activate caspase-1 through cryopyrin/Nalp3. *Nature* **440**(7081): 233–6.

68. Yoneyama, M., et al. (2004). The RNA helicase RIG-1 has an essential function in double-stranded RNA induced innate antiviral responses. *Nat Immunol* **5**: 730–37.

69. Kato, H., et al. (2005). Cell type-specific involvement of RIG-I in antiviral response. *Immunity* **23**(1): 19–28.

70. Kato, H., et al. (2006). Differential roles of MDA5 and RIG-I helicases in the recognition of RNA viruses. *Nature* **441**(7089): 101–5.

71. Hornung, V., et al. (2006). 5′-Triphosphate RNA is the ligand for RIG-I. *Science* **314**(5801): 994–7.

72. Pichlmair, A., et al. (2006). RIG-I-mediated antiviral responses to single-stranded RNA bearing 5′-phosphates. *Science* **314**(5801): 997–1001.

73. Yoneyama, M., et al. (2005). Shared and unique functions of the DExD/H-box helicases RIG-I, MDA5, and LGP2 in antiviral innate immunity. *J Immunol* **175**(5): 2851–8.

74. Hiscott, J., Lin, R., Nakhaei, P., and Paz, S. (2006). MasterCARD: a priceless link to innate immunity. *Trends Mol Med* **12**(2): 53–6.

75. Kawai, T., et al. (2005). IPS-1, an adaptor triggering RIG-I- and Mda5-mediated type I interferon induction. *Nat Immunol* **6**(10): 981–8.

76. Seth, R. B., Sun, L., Ea, C. K., and Chen, Z. J. (2005). Identification and characterization of MAVS, a mitochondrial antiviral signaling protein that activates NF-kappaB and IRF 3. *Cell* **122**(5): 669–82.

77. Xu, L. G., Wang, Y. Y., Han, K. J., Li, L. Y., Zhai, Z., and Shu, H. B. (2005). VISA is an adapter protein required for virus-triggered IFN-beta signaling. *Mol Cell* **19**(6): 727–40.

78. Meylan, E., et al. (2005). Cardif is an adaptor protein in the RIG-I antiviral pathway and is targeted by hepatitis C virus. *Nature* **437**(7062): 1167–72.

79. Balachandran, S., Venkataraman, T., Fisher, P. B., and Barber, G. N. (2007). Fas-associated death domain-containing protein-mediated antiviral innate immune signaling involves the regulation of Irf7. *J Immunol* **178**(4): 2429–39.

80. Clemens, M. J. and Elia, A. (1997). The double-stranded RNA-dependent protein kinase PKR: structure and function. *J Interferon Cytokine Res* **17**(9): 503–24.

81. Williams, B. R. (2001). Signal integration via PKR. *Sci STKE* **2001**(89): RE2.

82. Sledz, C. A., Holko, M., de Veer, M. J., Silverman, R. H., and Williams, B. R. (2003). Activation of the interferon system by short-interfering RNAs. *Nat Cell Biol* **5**(9): 834–9.

83. Manche, L., Green, S. R., Schmedt, C., and Mathews, M. B. (1992). Interactions between double-stranded RNA regulators and the protein kinase DAI. *Mol Cell Biol* **12**(11): 5238–48.

84. Puthenveetil, S., Whitby, L., Ren, J., Kelnar, K., Krebs, J. F., and Beal, P. A. (2006). Controlling activation of the RNA-dependent protein kinase by siRNAs using site-specific chemical modification. *Nucleic Acids Res* **34**(17): 4900–11.

85. Zhang, Z., Weinschenk, T., Guo, K., and Schluesener, H. J. (2006). siRNA binding proteins of microglial cells: PKR is an unanticipated ligand. *J Cell Biochem* **97**(6): 1217–29.

86. Samuel, C. E. (2001). Antiviral actions of interferons. *Clin Microbiol Rev* **14**(4): 778–809.

87. Saunders, L. R. and Barber, G. N. (2003). The dsRNA binding protein family: critical roles, diverse cellular functions. *FASEB J.* **17**: 961–83.

88. Elbashir, S. M., Harborth, J., Lendeckel, W., Yalcin, A., Weber, K., and Tschi, T. (2001). Duplexes of 21-nucleotide RNAs mediate RNA interference in cultured mammalian cells. *Nature* **411**: 494–8.

89. Vollmer, J., et al. (2005). Immune stimulation mediated by autoantigen binding sites within small nuclear RNAs involves Toll-like receptors 7 and 8. *J Exp Med* **202**(11): 1575–85.

90. Lau, C. M., et al. (2005). RNA-associated autoantigens activate B cells by combined B cell antigen receptor/Toll-like receptor 7 engagement. *J Exp Med* **202**(9): 1171–7.

91. Pisitkun, P., Deane, J. A., Difilippantonio, M. J., Tarasenko, T., Satterthwaite, A. B., and Bolland, S. (2006). Autoreactive B cell responses to RNA-related antigens due to TLR7 gene duplication. *Science* **312**(5780): 1669–72.

92. Subramanian, S., et al. (2006). A TLR7 translocation accelerates systemic autoimmunity in murine lupus. *Proc Natl Acad Sci USA* **103**(26): 9970–5.

93. Christensen, S. R., Shupe, J., Nickerson, K., Kashgarian, M., Flavell, R. A., and Shlomchik, M. J. (2006). Toll-like receptor 7 and TLR9 dictate autoantibody specificity and have opposing inflammatory and regulatory roles in a murine model of lupus. *Immunity* **25**(3): 417–28.

94. Pascual, V., Farkas, L., and Banchereau, J. (2006). Systemic lupus erythematosus: all roads lead to type I interferons. *Curr Opin Immunol* **18**(6): 676–82.

95. Savarese, E., et al. (2006). U1 small nuclear ribonucleoprotein immune complexes induce type I interferon in plasmacytoid dendritic cells through TLR7. *Blood* **107**(8): 3229–34.

96. Heidel, J. D., et al. (2007). Administration in non-human primates of escalating intravenous doses of targeted nanoparticles containing ribonucleotide reductase subunit M2 siRNA. *Proc Natl Acad Sci USA* **104**(14): 5715–21.

97. Heidel, J. D., Hu, S., Liu, X. F., Triche, T. J., and Davis, M. E. (2004). Lack of interferon response in animals to naked siRNAs. *Nat Biotechnol* **22**: 1579–82.

98. Gitlin, L., Karelsky, S., and Andino, R. (2002). Short interfering RNA confers intracellular antiviral immunity in human cells. *Nature* **418**: 430–4.

99. Bridge, A. J., Pebernard, S., Ducraux, A., Nicoulaz, A.-L., and Iggo, R. D. (2003). Induction of an interferon response by RNAi vectors in mammalian cells. *Nat Genet* **34**(3): 263–4.

100. Soutschek, J., et al. (2004). Therapeutic silencing of an endogenous gene by systemic administration of modified siRNAs. *Nature* **432**: 173–8.

101. Kim, D. H., Behlke, M. A., Rose, S. D., Chang, M. S., Choi, S., and Rossi, J. J. (2005). Synthetic dsRNA Dicer substrates enhance RNAi potency and efficacy. *Nat Biotechnol* **23**(2): 222–6.

102. Judge, A. D., Bola, G., Lee, A. C. H., and MacLachlan, I. (2006). Design of noninflammatory synthetic siRNA mediating potent gene silencing in vivo. *Mol Ther* **13**(3): 494–505.

103. Manoharan, M. (2004). RNA interference and chemically modified small interfering RNAs. *Curr Opin Chem Biol* **8**: 570–9.

104. Czauderna, F., et al. (2003). Structural variations and stabilising modifications of synthetic siRNAs in mammalian cells. *Nucl Acids Res* **31**(11): 2705–16.

105. Allerson, C. R., et al. (2005). Fully 2′-modified oligonucleotide duplexes with improved in vitro potency and stability compared to unmodified small interfering RNA. *J Med Chem* **48**: 901–4.

106. Prakash, T., et al. (2005). Positional effect of chemical modifications on short interference RNA activity in mammalian cells. *J Med Chem* **48**: 4247–53.

107. Chiu, Y. and Rana, T. (2003). siRNA function in RNAi: a chemical modification analysis. *RNA* **9**: 1034–48.

108. Layzer, J., McCaffrey, A., Tanner, A., Huang, Z., Kay, M., and Sullenger, B. (2004). In vivo activity of nuclease resistant siRNAs. *RNA* **10**: 766–71.

109. Elmen, J., et al. (2005). Locked nucleic acid (LNA) mediated improvements in siRNA stability and functionality. *Nucleic Acids Res* **33**(1): 439–47.

110. Cekaite, L., Furset, G., Hovig, E., and Sioud, M. (2007). Gene expression analysis in blood cells in response to unmodified and 2'-modified siR-NAs reveals TLR-dependent and independent effects. *J Mol Biol* **365**(1): 90–108.

111. Morrissey, D. V., et al. (2005). Activity of stabilized short interfering RNA in a mouse model of hepatitis B virus infection. *Hepatology* **41**(6): 1349–56.

112. Morrissey, D. V., et al. (2005). Potent and persistent in vivo anti-HBV activity of chemically modified siRNA's. *Nat Biotechnol* **23**(8): 1002–7.

113. Matranga, C., Tomari, Y., Shin, C., Bartel, D. P., and Zamore, P. D. (2005). Passenger-strand cleavage facilitates assembly of siRNA into Ago2-containing RNAi enzyme complexes. *Cell* **123**(4): 607–20.

114. Leuschner, P. J., Ameres, S. L., Kueng, S., and Martinez, J. (2006). Cleavage of the siRNA passenger strand during RISC assembly in human cells. *EMBO Rep* **7**(3): 314–20.

115. Lee, J., et al. (2003). Molecular basis for the immunostimulatory activity of guanine nucleoside analogs: activation of Toll-like receptor 7. *Proc Natl Acad Sci USA* **100**(11): 6646–51.

116. Der, S. D., Zhou, A., Williams, B. R., and Silverman, R. H. (1998). Identification of genes differentially regulated by interferon alpha, beta, or gamma using oligonucleotide arrays. *Proc Natl Acad Sci USA* **95**(26): 15623–8.

117. Geiss, G., Jin, G., Guo, J., Bumgarner, R., Katze, M. G., and Sen, G. C. (2001). A comprehensive view of regulation of gene expression by double-stranded RNA-mediated cell signaling. *J Biol Chem* **276**(32): 30178–82.

118. Judge, A. D., McClintock, K., Shaw, J. R., and MacLachlan, I. (2006). Hypersensitivity and loss of disease site targeting caused by antibody responses to pegylated liposomes. *Mol Ther* **13**(2): 328–37.

119. Dijkstra, J., et al. (1996). Interaction of anti-cholesterol antibodies with human lipoproteins. *J Immunol* **157**: 2006–13.

120. Ge, Q., Filip, L., Bai, A., Nguyen, T., Eisen, H. N., and Chen, J. (2004). Inhibition of influenza virus production in virus-infected mice by RNA interference. *Proc Natl Acad Sci USA* **101**(23): 8676–81.

121. Tompkins, S. M., Lo, C. Y., Tumpey, T. M., and Epstein, S. L. (2004). Protection against lethal influenza virus challenge by RNA interference *in vivo*. *Proc Natl Acad Sci USA* **101**(23): 8682–6.

122. Palliser, D., et al. (2006). An siRNA-based microbicide protects mice from lethal herpes simplex virus 2 infection. *Nature* **439**(7072): 89–94.

123. Bitko, V., Musiyenko, A., Shulyayeva, O., and Barik, S. (2005). Inhibition of respiratory viruses by nasally administered siRNA. *Nat Med* **11**(1): 50–5.

124. Geisbert, T. W., et al. (2006). Postexposure protection of guinea pigs against a lethal ebola virus challenge by RNA interference. *J Infect Dis* **193**(12): 1650–7.

125. Li, B. J., et al. (2005). Using siRNA in prophylactic and therapeutic regimens against SARS coronavirus in Rhesus macaque. *Nat Med* **11**(9): 944–51.

126. Saravolac, E. G., et al. (2001). Immunoprophylactic strategies against respiratory influenza virus infection. *Vaccine* **19**(17-19): 2227–32.

127. Brannon-Peppas, L., Ghosn, B., Roy, K., and Cornetta, K. (2007). Encapsulation of nucleic acids and opportunities for cancer treatment. *Pharm Res* **24**(4): 618–27.

128. Foss, F. M. (2002). Immunologic mechanisms of antitumor activity. *Semin Oncol* **29**(3 Suppl 7): 5–11.

129. Behlke, M. A. (2006). Progress towards in vivo use of siRNAs. *Mol Ther* **13**(4): 644–70.

130. Folkman, J. and Ingber, D. (1992). Inhibition of angiogenesis. *Semin Cancer Biol* **3**(2): 89–96.

131. von Marschall, Z., et al. (2003). Effects of interferon alpha on vascular endothelial growth factor gene transcription and tumor angiogenesis. *J Natl Cancer Inst* **95**(6): 437–48.

132. Wu, W. Z., et al. (2005). Interferon alpha 2a down-regulates VEGF expression through PI3 kinase and MAP kinase signaling pathways. *J Cancer Res Clin Oncol* **131**(3): 169–78.

133. Novina, C. D., et al. (2002). siRNA-directed inhibition of HIV-1 infection. *Nat Med* **8**(7): 681–6.

134. Song, E., et al. (2003). Sustained small interfering RNA-mediated human immunodeficiency virus type 1 inhibition in primary macrophages. *J Virol* **77**(13): 7174–81.

135. Thomas, M., Lu, J. J., Ge, Q., Zhang, C., Chen, J., and Klibanov, A. M. (2005). Full deacylation of polyethylenimine dramatically boosts its gene delivery efficiency and specificity to mouse lung. *Proc Natl Acad Sci USA* **102**(16): 5679–84.

136. Zon, G. (1995). Antisense phosphorothioate oligodeoxynucleotides: introductory concepts and possible molecular mechanisms of toxicity. *Toxicol Lett* **82–83**: 419–24.

137. Ito, T., Amakawa, R., Inaba, M., Ikehara, S., Inaba, K., and Fukuhara, S. (2001). Differential regulation of human blood dendritic cell subsets by IFNs. *J Immunol* **166**(5): 2961–9.

138. Hornung, V., et al. (2002). Quantitative expression of Toll-like receptor 1–10 mRNA in cellular subsets of human peripheral blood mononuclear cells and sensitivity to CpG oligodeoxynucleotides. *J Immunol* **168**(9): 4531–7.

139. Kadowaki, N., et al. (2001). Subsets of human dendritic cell precursors express different toll-like receptors and respond to different microbial antigens. *J Exp Med* **194**(6): 863–9.

140. Yeo, S. J., Yoon, J. G., and Yi, A. K. (2003). Myeloid differentiation factor 88-dependent post- transcriptional regulation of cyclooxygenase-2 expression by CpG DNA—tumor necrosis factor-alpha receptor-associated factor 6, a diverging point in the Toll-like receptor 9- signaling. *J Biol Chem* **278**(42): 40590–600.

141. Sharara, A. I., Perkins, D. J., Misukonis, M. A., Chan, S. U., Dominitz, J. A., and Weinberg, J. B. (1997). Interferon (IFN)-alpha activation of human blood mononuclear cells in vitro and in vivo for nitric oxide synthase (NOS) type 2 mRNA and protein expression: possible relationship of induced NOS2 to the anti-hepatitis C effects of IFN-alpha in vivo. *J Exp Med* **186**(9): 1495–502.

142. Michie, H. R., et al. (1988). Detection of circulating tumor necrosis factor after endotoxin administration. *N Engl J Med* **318**(23): 1481–6.

143. Lynn, M., et al. (2003). Blocking of responses to endotoxin by E5564 in healthy volunteers with experimental endotoxemia. *J Infect Dis* **187**: 631–9.

144. Stevenson, H. C., Abrams, P. G., Schoenberger, C. S., Smalley, R. B., Herberman, R. B., and Foon, K. A. (1985). A phase I evaluation of poly(I,C)-LC in cancer patients. *J Biol Response Mod* **4**(6): 650–5.

145. Moynagh, P. N. (2003). Toll-like receptor signalling pathways as key targets for mediating the anti-inflammatory and immunosuppressive effects of glucocorticoids. *J Endocrinol* **179**(2): 139–44.

146. Tan, Y. D., Li, S., Pitt, B. R., and Huang, L. (1999). The inhibitory role of CpG immunostimulatory motifs in cationic lipid vector-mediated transgene expression in vivo. *Hum Gene Ther* **10**(13): 2153–61.

147. Bianchi, M., Meng, C., and Ivashkiv, L. B. (2000). Inhibition of IL-2-induced Jak-STAT signaling by glucocorticoids. *PNAS* **97**: 9573–8.

148. Copple, B. L., Gmeiner, W. M., and Iversen, P. L. (1995). Reaction between metabolically activated acetaminophen and phosphorothioate oligonucleotides. *Toxicol Appl Pharmacol* **133**(1): 53–63.

149. Cummins, L. L., et al. (1995). Characterization of fully 2′-modified oligoribonucleotide hetero- and homoduplex hybridization and nuclease sensitivity. *Nucl Acids Res* **23**(11): 2019–24.

150. Peng, S. (2005). Signaling in B cells via Toll-like receptors. *Curr Opin Immunol* **17**(3): 230–6.

151. Jego, G., Palucka, A. K., Blanck, J.-P., Chalouni, C., Pascual, V., and Banchereau, J. (2003). Plasmacytoid dendritic cells induce plasma cell differentiation through type I interferon and interleukin 6. *Immunity* **19**: 225–34.

152. Ambegia, E., Ansell, S., Cullis, P., Heyes, J., Palmer, L., and MacLachlan, I. (2005). Stabilized plasmid–lipid particles containing PEG-diacylglycerols exhibit extended circulation lifetimes and tumor selective gene expression. *Biochim Biophys Acta* **1669**(2): 155–63.

153. Strait, R., Morris, S., Yang, M., Qu, X.-W., and Finkelman, F. (2002). Pathways of anaphylaxis in the mouse. *J Allergy Clin Immunol* **109**: 658–68.

154. Suntharalingam, G., et al. (2006). Cytokine storm in a phase 1 trial of the anti-CD28 monoclonal antibody TGN1412. *N Engl J Med* **355**(10): 1018–28.

155. Tsuboniwa, N., et al. (2001). Safety evaluation of hemagglutinating virus of Japan-artificial viral envelope liposomes in nonhuman primates. *Hum Gene Ther* **12**(5): 469–87.

156. Quezada, A., et al. (2002). Safety toxicity study of plasmid-based IL-12 therapy in Cynomolgus monkeys. *J Pharm Pharmacol* **54**(2): 241–8.

157. Zhang, G. F., Budker, V., Williams, P., Subbotin, V., and Wolff, J. A. (2001). Efficient expression of naked DNA delivered intraarterially to limb muscles of nonhuman primates. *Hum Gene Ther* **12**(4): 427–38.

158. Webb, M. S., et al. (2001). Toxicity and toxicokinetics of a phosphorothioate oligonucleotide against the c-myc oncogene in cynomolgus monkeys. *Antisense Nucleic Acid Drug Dev* **11**(3): 155–63.

159. Smirnova, I., Poltorak, A., Chan, E. K. L., McBride, C., and Beutler, B. (2000). Phylogenetic variation and polymorphism at the Toll-like receptor 4 locus (TLR4). *Genome Biol* **1**(1): 1–10.

CHAPTER 8

APPLICATION OF RNA INTERFERENCE TO VIRAL DISEASES

RALPH A. TRIPP and STEPHEN MARK TOMPKINS

8.1 INTRODUCTION

RNA interference (RNAi) mediated by double-stranded short interfering RNAs (siRNAs) has been shown to have an important role in regulating gene expression in a sequence-specific manner. RNAi platforms to synthesize and deliver siRNAs are being widely adopted for research and therapeutic applications. Accumulating evidence demonstrating that siRNAs effectively silence or reduce expression of pathological proteins has driven therapeutic development of synthetic siRNAs as drug candidates to address viral diseases. A barrier in siRNA drug therapeutics is efficient siRNA delivery *in vivo*. This is due to the potential for enzymatic degradation before the siRNA reaches the target cells, the need to penetrate the target cell membrane to gain access to the RNA-induced silencing complex (RISC) in the cytoplasm, and the need to deliver an appropriate dose of siRNA required for gene silencing. Recent progress has been made protecting and targeting siRNAs for delivery, and evidence is emerging regarding their potential for robust virus gene silencing activity. This chapter focuses on synthetic siRNA drug development and therapeutic applications for respiratory syncytial virus (RSV) and influenza viruses.

8.2 RNAi PLATFORM TECHNOLOGY

RNAi is a conserved mechanism of gene silencing discovered in plant and mammalian cells [1–4]. RNAi is mediated by 19–23 nucleotide (nt) double-stranded RNA (dsRNA) molecules, or siRNA, which targets cognate RNA for

RNA Interference: Application to Drug Discovery and Challenges to Pharmaceutical Development, Edited by Paul H. Johnson
Copyright © 2011 John Wiley & Sons, Inc.

destruction with exquisite potency and selectivity causing posttranscriptional gene silencing [3–6]. There are two major platforms for delivering RNAi-inducing cargo into cells to regulate gene expression. One is delivery of synthetic siRNA molecules, naked or complexed with a carrier, and the other is delivery of plasmid or viral vector constructs that induce cells to express siRNA, or a short hairpin RNA (shRNA) [7–15]. This chapter focuses on delivery of synthetic siRNA molecules as an RNAi therapeutic application for silencing virus replication.

8.2.1 Synthetic siRNAs

Synthetic siRNA duplexes are composed of sense and antisense strands paired to have a 2-nt (UU) 3' overhang and to have a 23-nt sequence motif of AA(N19)TT (N, any nucleotide) [16–20]. Delivery of synthetic siRNAs incorporates the same pathways as naturally derived siRNAs; that is, within the cytoplasm, the duplexes become separated by the RISC [20–24]. Most commonly the antisense strand remains bound to the RISC and targets the RNA–RISC complex to mRNA within the cytoplasm having cognate nucleotide sequences, generally resulting in cleavage of mRNA and preventing protein expression [25, 26].

Pharmaceutical development of synthetic siRNA drug therapies for silencing virus replication has been limited. Alnylam Pharmaceuticals (Cambridge, MA) is presently performing clinical investigations of an siRNA drug for RSV infection [8, 27]. To date, their investigational new drug, ALN-RSV01, has been safe and well tolerated. The scope of siRNA drug therapies has been limited because questions remain regarding the siRNA pharmacokinetics, modalities for targeted delivery, and potential off-target or unintended effects of siRNA drugs. However, much has been learned in animal models regarding development and application of RNAi to viral diseases, particularly for RSV and influenza virus.

8.2.2 Strategies to Target Viruses

The decision to target a specific viral gene(s) to silence or reduce virus replication is dependent on factors that may include targeting a gene coding for viral receptors, targeting genes affecting the antiviral immune response, and/or targeting highly conserved genes required in the viral replication life cycle. The intended target sites should be blast-searched against genomic libraries to ensure that only the virus gene is targeted by the siRNA and not a host gene. It is important to compare potential target sites to the appropriate genome database to eliminate siRNA candidates with target sequences to other coding sequences [18, 19, 28, 29]. Since regions of mRNA may be structured or affected by regulatory proteins, several different siRNA target sites should be selected at different positions along the length of the gene sequence to ensure efficacy. It is also important to note that the siRNA specificity for the target region is critical as a single point mutation can be sufficient to abolish target mRNA degradation [30, 31].

There are several algorithms available to aid in defining suitable siRNA candidates. Most of these algorithms evaluate candidate siRNAs on the basis of binding affinity, GC content, and specific sequence motifs that are guided by considerations of siRNA duplexes composed of 21-nt sense and antisense strands paired to have a 2-nt (UU) 3′ overhang, target sites beginning with AA, and siRNAs having approximately 50% GC content [16–19]. It is critical that siRNA experiments include the appropriate control siRNA. A useful negative control for the siRNA is one with the same nucleotide composition (GC content) as the effector siRNA but which lacks sequence homology to the target.

Synthetic siRNA drugs are considered preferable for rapid but transient suppression of acute viral infections, whereas expression vectors may be more appropriate for sustained RNAi of chronic or persistent viruses. The delivery of the RNAi-inducing cargo to the appropriate cell type is critical to RNAi efficacy particularly for viruses that have specific cell tropism. For example, to silence RSV replication, RNAi therapeutics should target the ciliated epithelial cells in the respiratory tract [32, 33]. Other RNAi strategies for targeting viruses include (1) consideration of prophylactic or treatment applications, (2) the window available for RNAi therapeutics, as not all viruses replicate equivalently, (3) the lower dose limit of synthetic siRNA required to achieve efficacy, (4) the permissibility of the cell types for siRNA delivery, (5) unintended modulation of host gene expression, and (6) potential interactions with other endogenous pathways linked to gene regulation, for example, microRNA pathway.

8.2.3 Chemical Modifications

Synthetic siRNAs are generally unstable in serum as they are rapidly degraded by serum nucleases [34–37]. However, it has been shown that chemical modification to the sugars, backbone, or bases of siRNAs can substantially improve resistance without substantially modifying activity [35]. A common approach to stabilize synthetic siRNAs against nuclease degradation is by introducing a phosphorothioate backbone linkage at the 3′ end for exonuclease resistance, and 2′ modifications (2′-OMe) for endonuclease resistance [22, 38, 39]. It has been shown that 2′-OMe modifications may enhance both endonuclease stability and increase *in vitro* potency [35, 40, 41]; however, siRNA activity has been shown to depend on the position of the modification in the guide-strand sequence. Other approaches include 2′-O-allyl and 2′-deoxy-fluorouridine, which have been examined as a means to improve stability for the prospect of siRNA therapy. In addition, locked nucleic acids (LNAs) that use a methylene bridge connecting 2′ and 4′ carbons can substantially increase siRNA potency *in vitro* and *in vivo* with minimal toxicity [34]. This bridge locks the ribose ring in the 3′-*endo* conformation characteristic of RNA and introduces new features into the siRNA without affecting the overall helical structure required for activity. LNA is used to reduce off-target effects by either lowering incorporation of the siRNA sense strand and/or by reducing the ability of inappropriately loaded sense strand to cleave the target RNA.

8.2.4 Dicer Substrate siRNAs

Use of thermodynamic end stability rules and empiric design parameters [42–47] has provided a means to potentially make more potent siRNA reagents available for gene silencing by chemically synthesizing 27-mer RNA duplexes that are optimized for Dicer processing. The concept of delivering Dicer substrate siRNAs to cells builds on the natural pathway of RNAi findings and the notion that Dicer is not only important in endonuclease cleavage of long dsRNA into siRNAs, but is also involved with entry of the siRNA into RISC and participates in RISC assembly [25, 26, 42, 48, 49]. In this approach, Dicer substrate RNAs are synthesized as 27-mer RNA duplexes that are optimized for Dicer processing [42]. These duplexes when delivered to mammalian cells are cleaved by Dicer into active 21-mer siRNAs that associate with Dicer, TRBP, and Ago2 to form RISC. In RISC, the passenger (sense) strand is degraded or discarded, while the guide (antisense) strand directs the sequence specificity of gene silencing. It has been shown that 27-mer duplexes can be up to 100-fold more potent than traditional 21-mer duplexes [28]; however, not all 27-mer duplexes show increased potency [44]. The generation of Dicer substrate siRNAs for use in siRNA drug therapeutics for viruses has not been explored but is an emerging area of interest.

8.2.5 Endonuclease-Prepared siRNAs

A new approach in the development of synthetic siRNAs is to generate endonuclease-prepared siRNAs (esiRNA) for cell delivery. These esiRNAs are produced from 200 to 500 bp dsRNAs that are digested by either recombinant Dicer enzyme or bacterial RNase III [50–53]. The process produces a cocktail of siRNA molecules that potentially target a single gene. The esiRNAs have the advantage of multi-single site targeting, eliminating the need to test a large number of synthetic siRNAs. The procedures available for esiRNA purification generally produce small quantities of siRNAs for laboratory use;

thus, refinements of procedures are needed for larger scale *in vivo* studies. However, a new method of esiRNAs purification based on ion exchange chromatography and size exclusion chromatography has reported to yield high purity esiRNA that specifically suppress homologous gene expression without activating the interferon response—and with higher efficiency than chemically synthesized siRNAs [52]. There have been no reported studies using esiRNA to target viral genes; however, the ability to generate siRNA cocktails that may have comparable silencing efficacies to those of synthetic siRNAs makes these tools important to consider for RNAi silencing of virus replication. Also, esiRNAs may be quite useful in the development of cell microarrays, which offers high-throughput screening potential.

8.3 siRNA SCREENING

High-throughput screening of siRNAs remains a challenge due to the variability of cell culture needs and transfection efficiency. Efficient transfer of siRNAs into primary cells using commercially available lipid-based transfection reagents is generally restricted to a few cell types [13,54–59]. This can be a drawback as primary cells are often preferred for gene silencing experiments since they generally offer a more translatable model for corresponding *in vivo* studies than immortalized cells. Given this, several alternative approaches to lipid-mediated transfection of siRNAs have been examined including electroporation, which has been shown to provide improved transfection efficiencies in primary cell types [57, 60] (Table 8.1). An issue with electroporation is often loss of cell viability, thus the balance between this and transfection efficiencies must be considered, particularly for certain cell types.

Adherent transformed cell lines such Vero, A549, and HeLa offer a robust system to screen siRNAs, as they provide a cell monolayer that is useful for evaluating endpoints such as plaque formation that is often used to evaluate siRNA efficacy for virus studies. For many of these adherent cell types, transient transfection of siRNAs using lipid-based transfection reagents is highly efficient (>90%) and often does not have significant effects on cell viability [56,61]. It is important to note that siRNA transfection efficiencies are affected by the doubling time of the cell line and that this directly affects the duration of silencing. Studies to date suggest that siRNA efficacy in these cell types usually does not exceed 5–6 days [155].

An important consideration in screening siRNA candidates is the use of multiple siRNAs, or pools to target each gene. In this fashion, there is a higher probability of detecting gene silencing from many siRNA candidates. In general, 3–6 siRNAs are incorporated into pools. The pools of siRNAs can be initially screened for efficacy, and when found, the individual siRNAs of the

TABLE 8.1   siRNA Delivery Methods.

Transfection Method	Target(s)	Model	References
Cationic lipid-based agents	Host cell protein, virus, cancer	*In vitro, in vivo*	56, 61–72
DOTAP cationic liposomes	Host cell protein	*In vitro, in vivo*	73–76
Virosomes/VLPs	Cell delivery model	*In vitro*	77–130
Multivalent lipids/cholesterol	Cell delivery model	*In vitro*	76, 80, 81
Nanoparticles/ chitosan	Cell delivery model	*In vitro; in vivo*	82–99
Cell-penetrating peptides	Cancer cells	*In vitro*	100–102
SNALPs	Cell delivery model, virus, nonhuman primates	*In vitro; in vivo*	103–105
(PEI)-based polyplexes	Host cell protein, virus, cancer	*In vitro; in vivo*	106–116
Ligand/antibody directed	Host cell protein, virus, cancer	*In vitro; in vivo*	74, 101, 117–124
Photochemical internalization	Host cell protein	*In vitro*	125
Osmotic	Host cell protein	*In vitro*	126, 127
Atelocollagen	Host cell protein	*In vitro; in vivo*	128–132
Electroporation	Host cell protein, virus, cancer	*In vitro; in vivo*	57, 133–143
Hydrodynamic injection	Host cell protein, virus, cancer		(144–150)
Aptamer	Host cell protein	*In vitro; in vivo*	97, 121, 151–154
Baculoviral vectors	Host cell protein	*In vitro*	55

DOTAP, 1,2-dioleoyl-3-trimethylammonium-propane; VLPs, virus-like particles; SNALPs, stable nucleic acid lipid particles; PEI, polyethylenimine.

pool individually analyzed. The caveat is that this technique assumes that the silencing performance of the pool is at least as good as the individual siRNA. In some experiments, it has been shown that poorly performing siRNAs may compete with better ones and actually lower the efficacy of the pooled siRNAs [156]. However, the higher throughput and reduced cost of using siRNA pools generally outweigh the potential for false negatives compared with testing individual siRNAs.

8.4 siRNA DELIVERY AND TARGETING

As noted, the successful use of synthetic siRNAs depends on efficient delivery into cells. A range of commercially available lipid- and peptide-based transfection reagents are available that generally are useful for optimizing delivery to most transformed cell lines. Due to the instability and negative charge of siRNA, effective cellular delivery and uptake can be challenging. A number of barriers exist for efficient siRNA delivery *in vivo*. These include enzymatic degradation before reaching target cells, the need to penetrate the target cell membrane to gain access to the RISC complex in the cytoplasm, and the need to deliver a relatively high dose of siRNA required for gene silencing. These features must be achieved without substantial cell toxicity, off-target effects, and induction of inflammatory cytokines or interferon responses induced by the siRNA and/or carrier.

Bioconjugation of one or both siRNA strands with lipids or polymers has been used in an attempt to increase nuclease stability and improve biodistribution or cell-specific targeting. Conjugation with lipids may enhance siRNA uptake via receptor-mediated endocytosis or by an increased membrane permeability of the otherwise negatively charged RNA. For example, siRNAs have been conjugated to cholesterol to enhance cellular uptake because cholesterol increases the hydrophobicity [82]. Cholesterol conjugation has been shown to increase the cellular uptake of siRNAs in liver cells without use of any transfection reagent; however, this method has not been shown to increase the efficacy of siRNA delivery to other organs such as the lung. Thus, cholesterol-conjugated siRNAs may be useful to target viruses with liver cell tropism, for example, hepatitis virus [82, 157], but would offer little benefit for respiratory viruses that primarily replicate in respiratory epithelial cells. To overcome this limitation, membrane permeant peptides (MPPs) are being investigated for their ability to translocate siRNAs across cell membranes. MPPs consist of positively charged amino acids, for example, arginine and/or lysine that can transfect different cell types with very high efficiency and rapid uptake kinetics [158]. Similarly, different cationic lipid formulations are being been tested for *in vivo* transfection of siRNAs, as these agents offer a flexible design and have shown efficacy [55, 61, 77, 78]. The caveat of cationic lipid formulations is that formulation with siRNAs is an uncontrolled process leading to incomplete encapsulation of siRNA molecules, which may expose siRNAs to enzymatic degradation prior to delivery to cells. Optimally, to enhance siRNA delivery and uptake, transfection reagents should be stable, diffusible across the cell membrane and offer a cell targeting approach. Recent studies suggest that stable nucleic acid lipid particles (SNALPs) may enable such features [159]. For example, it has been shown that chemically modified siRNAs targeting hepatitis B virus (HBV), which were incorporated into SNALPs and administered intravenously into mice, improved efficacy of siRNA efficacy by increasing the pharmacokinetics compared with unformu-lated siRNA [103, 160]. To target siRNAs to hepatocytes, investigators have used ligands that bind to asialoglycoprotein receptors on hepatocytes [161]. To more specifically target siRNAs, monoclonal antibodies have been used to direct siRNAs carried inside liposomes to specific cell types [162]. It has also been shown that antibody fusion proteins may potentially mediate both systemic and cell-type-specific delivery of siRNAs [117].

8.5 PROOFS OF CONCEPT FOR THERAPEUTIC RNAi TREATMENT OF VIRUS INFECTION

Shortly after the first descriptions of gene silencing in plants and nematodes by RNAi, scientists began to explore the potential to silence host cell and viral gene targets. Subsequently, studies demonstrated that RNAi can significantly suppress gene expression when delivered into mammalian cells [163, 164]. These findings provided an avenue for developing RNAi-based drugs to inhibit viral gene expression, to protect mammalian cells, and potentially protect hosts from viral infection and disease.

The first demonstrations of targeted inhibition of virus replication in mam-malian cells were for a cytopathic RNA virus and a retrovirus, that is, po-liovirus and HIV. In these studies, a polymerase (pol) II promoter system was used to express rev-specific shRNAs where treatment mediated a 4-log reduction of DNA expression *in vitro* [165]. Using an siRNA specific for the capsid gene of poliovirus, it was shown that treatment reduced virus titers in both murine and human cells [166]. Similarly, it was shown that HIV repli-cation *in vitro* was inhibited by targeting Gag or the host receptor, CD4, with siRNAs [167], and that siRNAs and shRNAs targeting vif, nef, or the LTR for degrading viral RNA prevented HIV replication [168]. The potential for viral gene silencing by RNAi in an infected host was also described in a murine model of Hepatitis C virus (HCV) infection in which siRNAs and shRNA-expressing plasmids were used to inhibit HCV gene transcripts in adult mice [169]. In these studies, the proof-of-concept of *in vivo* gene silencing using hydrodynamic delivery of an RNAi payload was a major advancement in the field. These successes showed that RNAi could be used for targeting a spectrum of RNA and DNA viruses, and suggested that direct delivery of synthetic siRNAs targeting specific virus genes could protect a host against viral infection. Importantly, by identifying the viral genome as the drug target, RNAi provided an opportunity to develop antiviral compounds for pathogens that were previously considered not druggable.

Gammaherpesvirus, influenza virus, HBV, and West Nile virus (WNV) were the next viruses targeted for RNAi. siRNAs specific for Rta and ORF 45 of the gammaherpesvirus MHV68 were shown to suppress viral replication *in vitro* [170]. The first DNA virus to be successfully targeted for gene silencing by RNAi was HBV. shRNAs specific for the core or X ORF of HBV under control of a pol III promoter were demonstrated to suppress viral gene expression in *in vitro* cultures [171]. siRNAs expressed under the control of an RNA polymerase I promoter system were used to target gene expression of influenza A and WNV [172]. shRNAs targeting WNV capsid or NS5 genes reduced both genomic RNA and infectious virus levels and targeted M gene mRNA to reduce

Synthetic siRNAs have also been used to inhibit influenza A virus *in vitro* and *in vivo* [173]. siRNAs targeting each of the gene segments encoding internal viral antigens (acidic polymerase, PA; basic polymerases 1 and 2, PB1 and PB2; matrix, M; and nucleocapsid protein, NP) all reduced virus titers with siRNAs targeting NP, PA, and PB1 being most effective. Interestingly, it was shown that an siRNA targeting the M gene segment reduced not only M RNA but also viral and complementary RNAs despite the fact that influenza is a negative strand RNA virus, which uses specific nuclear targeting sequences in the NP protein to translocate the nucleocapsid into the nucleus. Moreover, an siRNA targeting the NP gene segment reduced all viral transcripts. This work was closely followed by two reports demonstrating effective knockdown of influenza virus replication *in vivo* using murine models of virus infection [144, 174]. Importantly, these were the first studies demonstrating a reduction of infectious virus titer and protection against a lethal virus challenge. The great promise of RNAi and the ability to target highly conserved regions of critical viral genes, a holy grail in a field where the pathogens are constantly mutating, was highlighted by a study showing inhibition of a spectrum of unrelated highly pathogenic avian influenza viruses using the same specific siRNAs, reducing viral titers, and protecting against a lethal challenge [144]. Subsequently, numerous studies have shown inhibition of replication of a spectrum of both DNA and RNA viruses *in vitro* and *in vivo*. To date, more than 30 RNA and DNA viruses have been successfully silenced using siRNAs and/or shRNAs (summarized in Table 8.2).

Using a mouse model of RSV infection, pulmonary RSV titers were reduced by >95% following intranasal prophylactic delivery of siRNAs specific to the P gene using a cationic polymer-based transfection reagent [198]. Similar delivery of siRNA targeting parainfluenza virus was also effective at reducing lung virus tiers [198]. Importantly, prophylactic siRNA treatment

TABLE 8.2 Viral Infections Inhibited by RNA Interference

Virus	Target(s)	Substrate	Model	References
RNA				
Poliovirus	Capsid, pol3	siRNAS3	HeLa	166
Coxsackievirus B3	3D, 2A	siRNA, shRNA	HeLa, mouse	175–177
Enterovirus 71	3'UTR, 2C, 3C, 3D	siRNA, shRNA	RD	178, 179
Foot-and-mouth disease virus	1D, 2B, 3B, 3D	siRNA, shRNA	BHK-21, IBRS-2, mouse, guinea pig, swine	180–183)
Bovine viral diarrhea virus	core, NS4B, NS5A	siRNA, shRNA	MDBK	184
Hepatitis delta virus	mRNA, genomic, antigenomic	siRNA	Huh-7	185
Rhinovirus	2C, 3D	siRNA	HeLa	186
Hepatitis C virus	5' NTR, core, NS3, NS5B	siRNA, shRNA	Huh-7, mouse	169, 187–190
Hepatitis A virus	2C	siRNA	Huh-7	191
Influenza A virus	NP, PA, PB1, PB2, M	siRNA, shRNA	MDCK, Vero, 293T, ECE, mouse	144, 172–174
SARS CoV	Rep 1A/1B, S, leader, N, 3' UTR	siRNA, shRNA	Frhk-4, 293T, Vero E6	192–197
Respiratory syncytial virus	P, F, SH	siRNA	Vero, A549, mice	198, 199
Bovine ephemeral fever virus	G	siRNA	BHK-21	200
Porcine reproductive and respiratory syndrome virus	GP5, N	shRNA	MARC-145	201, 202
Ebola virus	L	siRNA	Vero, guinea pig	159
Marburg virus	NP, VP35, VP30	siRNA	Vero	203

(Continued)

TABLE 8.2 Viral Infections Inhibited by RNA Interference (*Continued*)

Virus	Target(s)	Substrate	Model	References
Measles virus	L	siRNA, shRNA	Vero/SLAM	204
Reovirus	μ2, μNS, NS	shRNA	293T	205
Rotavirus	NSP5	siRNA	MA104	206
Venezuelan equine encephalitis virus	NSP1	siRNA	BHK-21	207
West Nile virus	Capsid, NS5, Env	siRNA, shRNA	293T, Vero	172, 208, 209
Retrovirus				
Porcine endogenous retrovirus	Gag, pol, env	siRNA, shRNA	293, PK15, porcine fetal fibroblast cultures	210, 211
Avian leukosis virus	env(B)	shRNA	DF-1	212
HIV	Rev, Gag, Tet, etc.	siRNA, shRNA, etc.	HeLa, 293, PBMCs, etc.	165, 167, 168 Reviewed in Reference [213]
DNA				
JC virus	T antigen, agnoprotein, VP1	siRNA	Primary hu astrocytes, transformed hu fetal glial cells	214, 215
Epstein-Barr virus	Lmp-1, Zta, EBNA1	siRNA, shRNA	NPC cell lines, 293, Raji, HeLa	216–219
Human papilloma virus	E6, E7	siRNA, shRNA	HeLa, CaSki, mouse	220–222
Hepatitis B virus	Core, pol, HBsAg, etc.	siRNA, shRNA	Huh-7, 2.2.15 cells, HepG2, mouse	171) Reviewed in [223]
Herpes simplex virus	gE, UL27, UL29	siRNA	HaCaT, Vero, NIH3T3, mouse	224, 225
Porcine circovirus 2	ORF1, ORF2	ShRNA	PK15, mouse	226

targeting RSV also reduced some parameters of pulmonary pathology as assessed by respiratory rate, leukotriene induction, and inflammation. While not the first demonstration of control of a viral infection by siRNA treatment, these studies demonstrated a reasonable drug delivery approach (intranasal) for siRNAs directed at respiratory virus infections. These findings provided a foundation for RNAi antiviral therapeutics for respiratory viruses, and are consistent with proprietary studies at the University of Georgia that led to the development of RNAi therapeutic strategies targeting RSV now in Phase II/III clinical trials by Alnylam Pharmaceuticals.

Over the past several years, a number of studies have been published that show RNAi-mediated silencing of viral genes and related disease by systemic or topical administration of siRNAs. Viruses targeted include Ebola virus [159], HBV [103, 227], influenza virus [144, 174], HCV [228], human papillomavirus [220], coxsackievirus [175], foot-and-mouth disease virus [180], and herpes simplex virus [224]. Critical to the success of these studies has been the use of chemical modifications or delivery formulations that impart desirable pharmacokinetic properties to the siRNA duplex and that also promote cellular uptake in tissues. These formulations are critical to both the synthesized siRNAs and plasmid-based shRNA expression vectors.

Other RNAi delivery studies have been forthcoming. Adenovirus and Ad-associated virus vectors have been successfully utilized to inhibit a number of viruses *in vivo*, including HBV [229–231] and foot-and-mouth disease virus [181]. These systems, while effective at specific transfection of difficult tissue or cell types, may have limited applications due to preexisting host immunity to the adenovirus delivery vectors and because of potential safety issues. Lentiviral vectors have also been used for shRNA gene delivery in *ex vivo* systems. This application shows particular promise for treatment of HIV patients. For example, peripheral blood stem cells from HIV-infected patients have been infected with lentiviral delivery systems carrying multiple expression cassettes containing HIV tat and rev specific shRNAs as well as ribozyme and decoy construct (reviewed in [232].

8.6 VIRAL COUNTERMEASURES FOR RNAi

While the first reports of mammalian virus silencing were being released, potential limits were also being described. As a general rule, DNA viruses replicate in the nucleus, while RNA viruses replicate in the cytoplasm. Early work to elucidate the mechanism of dsRNA-mediated gene silencing demonstrated that RNA sequestered in the nucleus is resistant to RNAi, while cytoplasmic RNAs and RNAs undergoing nuclear export are sensitive to silencing [232]. This raised the possibility that some viruses, particularly those that sequester viral nucleic acids from the cell, may not be susceptible to RNAi-based drugs [234].

A variety of earlier studies have demonstrated inhibition of posttranslational gene silencing in plants [235]. There is now evidence that some viruses encode proteins that specifically act to inhibit the RNAi machinery. For example, flock house virus encodes a protein, B2, that was shown to suppress RNAi in *Drosophila* cells and this activity was shown to be critical for virus replication [236]. The interferon agonist proteins, NS1 and E3L of influenza, and vaccinia virus, respectively, were shown to inhibit RNAi in *Drosophila* reporter assays [237]. However, both influenza A and vaccinia virus replication been successfully inhibited by siRNAs and shRNAs suggesting that the mechanism of action may not translate to mammalian systems or that the block is upstream of the entry of siRNAs in to the RNAi pathway. More recently inhibitors of RNAi have also been identified in La Crosse virus [238] and Nodamura virus [239]. The nonstructural protein of La Crosse virus, NSs, inhibited RNAi in 293T cells, however, siRNAs specific for the viral genome were still able to inhibit viral replication *in vitro* [238]. Nodamura virus encodes a B2 protein similar to the flock house virus B2 protein and inhibits RNAi in mammalian cells [239]. In both cases, while there was an inhibition in RNAi activity, the impact on viral infection and replication was unclear.

It is clear from the literature that viruses and RNA viruses in particular are prone to mutation. This is potentially a caveat of RNAi therapeutic approaches. The RNA-dependent RNA polymerases utilized by RNA viruses are error prone, with error rates up to 1 incorrect nucleotide per 10,000 nt copied. This extremely high error rate often results in dramatic mutation in permissive proteins. While some proteins and regions of proteins are refractory to mutation and generally highly conserved; even these regions have variability that could allow virus mutants that are resistant to specific siRNA drugs. Moreover, this new class of sequence-specific drugs may apply a new selective pressure to replicating viruses. Highly conserved regions of viral genomes may tolerate mutation to enable replication, and like traditional antiviral drugs, siRNA treatment may be capable of generating viral escape mutants. It may be possible to prevent RNAi-based drug resistance by targeting multiple viral genes and/or multiple sites although this area has yet to be fully explored.

8.7   TRANSLATING siRNA DELIVERY TO THE CLINIC

Numerous viruses have been successfully silenced by RNAi both *in vitro* and *in vivo*. Moreover, animal models are no longer limited to mice and efficacious RNAi treatment has been demonstrated in nonhuman primates and in some clinical trials. However, effective and targeted delivery is still the most challenging consideration for successful translation of RNAi to the clinic and to broad use in patients.

Given the high specificity of siRNAs for their viral target, exposure of nontargeted genes to siRNA drugs is not generally an issue; however, the induction of innate immune responses and off-target effects have been described [240, 241]. Chemical modifications of the siRNA backbones have been helpful to reduce nonspecific effects, and the increased understanding of microRNA structure and function has also clarified the design of siRNAs to avoid encoding the 6–8 nt touchdown site responsible for miRNA activity [242, 243].

For siRNA delivery there are generally two options: systemic delivery (e.g., intravenous) or localized delivery (e.g., topical, aerosol, direct tissue injection, etc.). Some of the considerations for selecting local versus systemic siRNA administration are the doses needed to achieve sufficient drug concentration in the target tissue or cell, and the effects of exposure of nontargeted tissues or cells to the drug. While most RNAi antiviral drug targets focus on virally encoded genes, a few reports have targeted host genes that are required for virus infection or replication [232, 244]. In these cases, systemic delivery of host-specific siRNAs could have high toxicity and so localized delivery is preferred. As previously noted, the *ex vivo* transduction of peripheral blood stem cells has successfully delivered gene suppression therapies for HIV infection [232].

In the case of respiratory targets, inhaled delivery of naked, modified, and complexed siRNAs have shown efficacy [174, 198]. In the case of RSV, topical and aerosol delivery of chemically modified siRNAs have shown efficacy in animal disease models, are well tolerated, and are now entering phase II/III clinical trials at Alnylam Pharmaceuticals.

While delivery of naked siRNAs is appealing, delivery agents have a number of advantages. Delivery formulations may provide more robust siRNA efficacy with doses of siRNA that are substantially lower, require less frequent treatment, or both. Moreover, carriers may enable target delivery while enhancing uptake. One system has utilized a protamine-monoclonal antibody fusion to deliver siRNAs to HIV-infected tissues *in vitro* and *in vivo* [119]. In this study, the single-chain antibody recognized the HIV envelope protein while the protamine bound the siRNAs. Intravenous deliver of HIV-specific siRNAs using this carrier specifically targeted the siRNA payload to envelope-expressing cells and blocked HIV production *in vitro*.

Less-specific delivery agents such as cationic lipids have been widely used in cell culture systems and can enhance siRNA uptake by a variety of cell types. Early *in vivo* efforts at systemic and topical siRNA delivery using these agents revealed that such formulations can have cytotoxic effects, a feature that limits their use *in vivo* for disease indications and dosing paradigms. A variety of proprietary formulations are being developed; however, a multipurpose *in vivo* delivery formulation is not yet available.

8.8 RNAi VERSUS TRADITIONAL ANTIVIRAL DRUGS

A principal advantage of siRNA drug candidates over traditional antiviral therapeutics is that "nondruggable" viral gene targets can be targeted. To date, most RNA viruses targeted for RNAi silencing have been successfully inhibited or the viral gene products inhibited *in vitro*. While viruses may encode RNAi-inhibitory proteins, these proteins appear to have limited efficacy possibly because of the RNAi drug concentrations delivered and/or because the RNAi inhibitory mechanism acts upstream of where delivered siRNAs enter the RNAi machinery.

Another important advantage of RNAi-based therapeutics is that the design algorithms are nearly identical for any pathogen. The target is always RNA and the same target selection process is generally applied for each gene or mRNA. Thus, lead siRNA drugs can be rapidly designed, developed, and tested. Moreover, from a chemistry standpoint, synthetic siRNAs are relatively easy to produce and purify, whereas traditional small molecule compounds may require extensive and expensive processing. Although viruses are prone to develop resistance to antiviral drugs and could mutate to become resistant to specific siRNAs, a modified siRNA targeting a new sequence could rapidly be designed, or multiple siRNAs targeting different genes or multiple sites could be employed. It is also important to note that the RNAi activity is mediated by the host cell machinery; thus, it is very unlikely that the virus could mutate to avoid the activity of RISC.

For example, in the case of siRNA drug development for influenza virus, the identification of highly selective and potent sequences required only identification of genomic sequences and candidate RNAi drugs were completed in months. In contrast, design and development of oseltamavir (Tamiflu), a neuraminidase inhibitor approved for prophylaxis, and treatment of influenza virus infection required crystallization of neuramindase (first published in 1983) and then years of drug development before approval in 1996 [245]. Unfortunately, oseltamavir resistant influenza viruses have been reported [246], and modification of oseltamavir to address drug resistant mutant viruses requires substantial time and effort that may not yield a potent inhibitor. In contrast, if an siRNA resistant influenza virus emerged, the virus could be treated with a cocktail of siRNAs targeting multiple genes or targets within genes. Alternatively, new gene targets could be readily identified, synthesized, and tested against the mutant virus in a very short time.

Lastly, while delivery formulations may vary, chemically synthesized siRNAs are all produced in a similar fashion and have similar chemical properties. Because of this, once testing and approval of the first siRNA therapeutic has been realized, it is hopeful that future siRNA investigational new drugs will be supported by safety data from earlier studies and allows a streamlined approval process.

8.9 CONCLUSIONS

Significant progress has been made in advancing RNAi therapeutics in a remarkably short period of time. Numerous viruses have been successfully silenced *in vitro* and *in vivo* using siRNAs and shRNAs. However, there are a variety of obstacles that must still be overcome between proofs of concept and patient application. While many viruses have been successfully silenced, a variety of viruses has demonstrated mechanisms to inhibit or avoid RNAi. Moreover, the constant evolution of viruses can also lead to escape mutants. Finally, delivery of siRNAs or RNAi expression systems continues to be the greatest challenge for translation of these drugs to the clinic. Despite these barriers, RNAi-based therapies are poised as the next generation of antiviral and disease intervention drugs that hold great promise.

REFERENCES

1. Fire, A., Xu, S., Montgomery, M. K., Kostas, S. A., Driver, S. E., and Mello, C. C. (1998). Potent and specific genetic interference by double-stranded RNA in *Caenorhabditis elegans*. *Nature* **391**: 806–11.

2. Montgomery, M. K., Xu, S., and Fire, A. (1998). RNA as a target of double-stranded RNA-mediated genetic interference in *Caenorhabditis elegans*. *Proc Natl Acad Sci U S A* **95**: 15502–7.

3. Zamore, P. D. (2001). RNA interference: listening to the sound of silence. *Nat Struct Biol* **8**: 746–50.

4. Baulcombe, D. (2004). RNA silencing in plants. *Nature* **431**: 356–63.

5. Mello, C. C. and Conte, D., Jr. (2004). Revealing the world of RNA interference. *Nature* **431**: 338–42.

6. Hannon, G. J. (2002). RNA interference. *Nature* **418**: 244–51.

7. Kim, D. H. and Rossi, J. J. (2007). Strategies for silencing human disease using RNA interference. *Nat Rev Genet* **8**: 173–84.

8. Bumcrot, D., Manoharan, M., Koteliansky, V., and Sah, D. W. (2006). RNAi therapeutics: a potential new class of pharmaceutical drugs. *Nat Chem Biol* **2**: 711–19.

9. Barik, S. and Bitko, V. (2006). Prospects of RNA interference therapy in respiratory viral diseases: update 2006. *Expert Opin Biol Ther* **6**: 1151–60.

10. Snove, O., Jr., and Rossi, J. J. (2006). Expressing short hairpin RNAs in vivo. *Nat Methods* **3**: 689–95.

11. Morris, K. V. and Rossi, J. J. (2006). Lentivirus-mediated RNA interference therapy for human immunodeficiency virus type 1 infection. *Hum Gene Ther* **17**: 479–86.

12. Pan, W. H. and Clawson, G. A. (2006). Antisense applications for biological control. *J Cell Biochem* **98**: 14–35.

13. Sandy, P., Ventura, A., and Jacks, T. (2005). Mammalian RNAi: a practical guide. *Biotechniques* **39**: 215–24.

14. Devroe, E. and Silver, P. A. (2004). Therapeutic potential of retroviral RNAi vectors. *Expert Opin Biol Ther* **4**: 319–27.

15. Scherer, L. J. and Rossi, J. J. (2003). Approaches for the sequence-specific knockdown of mRNA. *Nat Biotechnol* **21**: 1457–65.

16. Heale, B. S., Soifer, H. S., Bowers, C., and Rossi, J. J. (2005). siRNA target site secondary structure predictions using local stable substructures. *Nucleic Acids Res* **33**: e30.

17. Saetrom, P. and Snove, O., Jr. (2004). A comparison of siRNA efficacy predictors. *Biochem Biophys Res Commun* **321**: 247–53.

18. Ding, Y., Chan, C. Y., and Lawrence, C. E. (2004). Sfold web server for statistical folding and rational design of nucleic acids. *Nucleic Acids Res* **32**: W135–41.

19. Yuan, B., Latek, R., Hossbach, M., Tuschl, T., and Lewitter, F. (2004). siRNA selection server: an automated siRNA oligonucleotide prediction server. *Nucleic Acids Res* **32**: W130–34.

20. Amarzguioui, M., Rossi, J. J., and Kim, D. (2005). Approaches for chemically synthesized siRNA and vector-mediated RNAi. *FEBS Lett* **579**: 5974–81.

21. Spankuch, B. and Strebhardt, K. (2005). RNA interference-based gene silencing in mice: the development of a novel therapeutical strategy. *Curr Pharm Des* **11**: 3405–19.

22. Banan, M. and Puri, N. (2004). The ins and outs of RNAi in mammalian cells. *Curr Pharm Biotechnol* **5**: 441–50.

23. Wadhwa, R., Kaul, S. C., Miyagishi, M., and Taira, K. (2004). Know-how of RNA interference and its applications in research and therapy. *Mutat Res* **567**: 71–84.

24. Scherer, L. and Rossi, J. J. (2004). Recent applications of RNAi in mammalian systems. *Curr Pharm Biotechnol* **5**: 355–60.

25. Hammond, S. M. (2005). Dicing and slicing: the core machinery of the RNA interference pathway. *FEBS Lett* **579**: 5822–9.

26. Tijsterman, M. and Plasterk, R. H. (2004). Dicers at RISC; the mechanism of RNAi. *Cell* **117**: 1–3.

27. Manoharan, M. (2004). RNA interference and chemically modified small interfering RNAs. *Curr Opin Chem Biol* **8**: 570–9.

28. Kim, D. H., Behlke, M. A., Rose, S. D., Chang, M. S., Choi, S., and Rossi, J. J. (2005). Synthetic dsRNA Dicer substrates enhance RNAi potency and efficacy. *Nat Biotechnol* **23**: 222–6.

29. Shah, J. K., Garner, H. R., White, M. A., Shames, D. S., and Minna, J. D. (2007). sIR: siRNA Information Resource, a web-based tool for siRNA sequence design and analysis and an open access siRNA database. *BMC Bioinformatics* **8**: 178.

30. Elbashir, S. M., Harborth, J., Lendeckel, W., Yalcin, A., Weber, K., and Tuschl, T. (2001). Duplexes of 21-nucleotide RNAs mediate RNA interference in cultured mammalian cells. *Nature* **411**: 494–8.

31. Elbashir, S. M., Lendeckel, W., and Tuschl, T. (2001). RNA interference is mediated by 21- and 22-nucleotide RNAs. *Genes Dev* **15**: 188–200.

32. Zhang, L., Peeples, M. E., Boucher, R. C., Collins, P. L., and Pickles, R. J. (2002). Respiratory syncytial virus infection of human airway epithelial cells is polarized, specific to ciliated cells, and without obvious cytopathology. *J Virol* **76**: 5654-66.

33. Tristram, D. A., Hicks, W., Jr., and Hard, R. (1998). Respiratory syncytial virus and human bronchial epithelium. *Arch Otolaryngol Head Neck Surg* **124**: 777–83.

34. Braasch, D. A., Jensen, S., Liu, Y., Kaur, K., Arar, K., White, M. A., and Corey, D. R. (2003). RNA interference in mammalian cells by chemically-modified RNA. *Biochemistry* **42**: 7967–75.

35. Choung, S., Kim, Y. J., Kim, S., Park, H. O., and Choi, Y. C. (2006). Chemical modification of siRNAs to improve serum stability without loss of efficacy. *Biochem Biophys Res Commun* **342**: 919–27.

36. Czauderna, F., Fechtner, M., Dames, S., Aygun, H., Klippel, A., Pronk, G. J., Giese, K., and Kaufmann, J. (2003). Structural variations and stabilising modifications of synthetic siRNAs in mammalian cells. *Nucleic Acids Res* **31**: 2705–16.

37. Kurreck, J. (2003). Antisense technologies. Improvement through novel chemical modifications. *Eur J Biochem* **270**: 1628–44.

38. Zhang, H. Y., Du, Q., Wahlestedt, C., and Liang, Z. (2006). RNA Interference with chemically modified siRNA. *Curr Top Med Chem* **6**: 893–900.

39. Chen, X., Dudgeon, N., Shen, L., and Wang, J. H. (2005). Chemical modification of gene silencing oligonucleotides for drug discovery and development. *Drug Discov Today* **10**: 587–93.

40. Puri, N., Majumdar, A., Cuenoud, B., Natt, F., Martin, P., Boyd, A., Miller, P. S., and Seidman, M. M. (2001). Targeted gene knockout by 2'-O-aminoethyl modified triplex forming oligonucleotides. *J Biol Chem* **276**: 28991–8.

41. Rozners, E., Katkevica, D., Bizdena, E., and Stromberg, R. (2003). Synthesis and properties of RNA analogues having amides as interuridine linkages at selected positions. *J Am Chem Soc* **125**: 12125–36.

42. Amarzguioui, M., Lundberg, P., Cantin, E., Hagstrom, J., Behlke, M. A., and Rossi, J. J. (2006). Rational design and in vitro and in vivo delivery of Dicer substrate siRNA. *Nat Protoc* **1**: 508–17.

43. Vermeulen, A., Behlen, L., Reynolds, A., Wolfson, A., Marshall, W. S., Karpilow, J., and Khvorova, A. (2005). The contributions of dsRNA structure to Dicer specificity and efficiency. *Rna* **11**: 674–82.

44. Rose, S. D., Kim, D. H., Amarzguioui, M., Heidel, J. D., Collingwood, M. A., Davis, M. E., Rossi, J. J., and Behlke, M. A. (2005). Functional polarity is introduced by Dicer processing of short substrate RNAs. *Nucleic Acids Res* **33**: 4140–56.

45. Maniataki, E. and Mourelatos, Z. (2005). A human, ATP-independent, RISC assembly machine fueled by pre-miRNA. *Genes Dev* **19**: 2979–90.

46. Ma, J. B., Ye, K., and Patel, D. J. (2004). Structural basis for overhang-specific small interfering RNA recognition by the PAZ domain. *Nature* **429**: 318–22.

47. Zhang, H., Kolb, F. A., Brondani, V., Billy, E., and Filipowicz, W. (2002). Human Dicer preferentially cleaves dsRNAs at their termini without a requirement for ATP. *Embo J* **21**: 5875–85.

48. Jaronczyk, K., Carmichael, J. B., and Hobman, T. C. (2005). Exploring the functions of RNA interference pathway proteins: some functions are more RISCy than others? *Biochem J* **387**: 561–71.

49. Carmell, M. A. and Hannon, G. J. (2004). RNase III enzymes and the initiation of gene silencing. *Nat Struct Mol Biol* **11**: 214–18.

50. Kittler, R., Putz, G., Pelletier, L., Poser, I., Heninger, A. K., Drechsel, D., Fischer, S., Konstantinova, I., Habermann, B., Grabner, H., Yaspo, M. L., Himmelbauer, H., Korn, B., Neugebauer, K., Pisabarro, M. T., and Buchholz, F. (2004). An endoribonuclease-prepared siRNA screen in human cells identifies genes essential for cell division. *Nature* **432**: 1036–40.

51. Kittler, R., Surendranath, V., Heninger, A. K., Slabicki, M., Theis, M., Putz, G., Franke, K., Caldarelli, A., Grabner, H., Kozak, K., Wagner, J., Rees, E., Korn, B., Frenzel, C., Sachse, C., Sonnichsen, B., Guo, J., Schelter, J., Burchard, J., Linsley, P. S., Jackson, A. L., Habermann, B., and Buchholz, F. (2007). Genome-wide resources of endoribonuclease-prepared short interfering RNAs for specific loss-of-function studies. *Nat Methods* **4**: 337–44.

52. Xuan, B., Qian, Z., Tan, C., Min, T., Shen, S., and Huang, W. (2005). esiRNAs purified with chromatography suppress homologous gene expression with high efficiency and specificity. *Mol Biotechnol* **31**: 203–9.

53. Yang, D., Buchholz, F., Huang, Z., Goga, A., Chen, C. Y., Brodsky, F. M., and Bishop, J. M. (2002). Short RNA duplexes produced by hydrolysis with *Escherichia coli* RNase III mediate effective RNA interference in mammalian cells. *Proc Natl Acad Sci U S A* **99**: 9942–7.

54. Hagemann, C., Meyer, C., Stojic, J., Eicker, S., Gerngras, S., Kuhnel, S., Roosen, K., and Vince, G. H. (2006). High efficiency transfection of glioma cell lines and primary cells for overexpression and RNAi experiments. *J Neurosci Methods* **156**: 194–2.

55. Nicholson, L. J., Philippe, M., Paine, A. J., Mann, D. A., and Dolphin, C. T. (2005). RNA interference mediated in human primary cells via recombinant baculoviral vectors. *Mol Ther* **11**: 638–44.

56. Dalby, B., Cates, S., Harris, A., Ohki, E. C., Tilkins, M. L., Price, P. J., and Ciccarone, V. C. (2004). Advanced transfection with Lipofectamine 2000 reagent: primary neurons, siRNA, and high-throughput applications. *Methods* **33**: 95–103.

57. Gilmore, I. R., Fox, S. P., Hollins, A. J., and Akhtar, S. (2006). Delivery strategies for siRNA-mediated gene silencing. *Curr Drug Deliv* **3**: 147–145.

58. Paroo, Z. and Corey, D. R. (2004). Challenges for RNAi in vivo. *Trends Biotechnol* **22**: 390–94.

59. Vanhecke, D., and Janitz, M. (2004). High-throughput gene silencing using cell arrays. *Oncogene* **23**: 8353–8.

60. Gresch, O., Engel, F. B., Nesic, D., Tran, T. T., England, H. M., Hickman, E. S., Korner, I., Gan, L., Chen, S., Castro-Obregon, S., Hammermann, R., Wolf, J., Muller-Hartmann, H., Nix, M., Siebenkotten, G., Kraus, G., and Lun, K. (2004). New non-viral method for gene transfer into primary cells. *Methods* **33**: 151–63.

61. Zuhorn, I. S., Engberts, J. B., and Hoekstra, D. (2007). Gene delivery by cationic lipid vectors: overcoming cellular barriers. *Eur Biophys J* **36**: 349–62.

62. Courtete, J., Sibler, A. P., Zeder-Lutz, G., Dalkara, D., Oulad-Abdelghani, M., Zuber, G., and Weiss, E. (2007). Suppression of cervical carcinoma cell growth by intracytoplasmic codelivery of anti-oncoprotein E6 antibody and small interfering RNA. *Mol Cancer Ther* **6**: 1728–35.

63. Guissouma, H., Froidevaux, M. S., Hassani, Z., and Demeneix, B. A. (2006). In vivo siRNA delivery to the mouse hypothalamus confirms distinct roles of TR beta isoforms in regulating TRH transcription. *Neurosci Lett* **406**: 240–43.

64. Bollerot, K., Sugiyama, D., Escriou, V., Gautier, R., Tozer, S., Scherman, D., and Jaffredo, T. (2006). Widespread lipoplex-mediated gene transfer to vascular endothelial cells and hemangioblasts in the vertebrate embryo. *Dev Dyn* **235**: 105–14.

65. Luo, M. C., Zhang, D. Q., Ma, S. W., Huang, Y. Y., Shuster, S. J., Porreca, F., and Lai, J. (2005). An efficient intrathecal delivery of small interfering RNA to the spinal cord and peripheral neurons. *Mol Pain* **1**: 29.

66. Pal, A., Ahmad, A., Khan, S., Sakabe, I., Zhang, C., Kasid, U. N., and Ahmad, I. (2005). Systemic delivery of RafsiRNA using cationic cardiolipin liposomes silences Raf-1 expression and inhibits tumor growth in xenograft model of human prostate cancer. *Int J Oncol* **26**: 1087–91.

67. Brazas, R. M. and Hagstrom, J. E. (2005). Delivery of small interfering RNA to mammalian cells in culture by using cationic lipid/polymer-based transfection reagents. *Methods Enzymol* **392**: 112–24.

68. Chien, P. Y., Wang, J., Carbonaro, D., Lei, S., Miller, B., Sheikh, S., Ali, S. M., Ahmad, M. U., and Ahmad, I. (2005). Novel cationic cardiolipin analogue-based liposome for efficient DNA and small interfering RNA delivery in vitro and in vivo. *Cancer Gene Ther* **12**: 321–8.

69. Spagnou, S., Miller, A. D., and Keller, M. (2004). Lipidic carriers of siRNA: differences in the formulation, cellular uptake, and delivery with plasmid DNA. *Biochemistry* **43**: 13348–56.

70. Beale, G., Hollins, A. J., Benboubetra, M., Sohail, M., Fox, S. P., Benter, I., and Akhtar, S. (2003). Gene silencing nucleic acids designed by scanning arrays: anti-EGFR activity of siRNA, ribozyme and DNA enzymes targeting a single hybridization-accessible region using the same delivery system. *J Drug Target* **11**: 449–56.

71. Sioud, M., and Sorensen, D. R. (2003). Cationic liposome-mediated delivery of siRNAs in adult mice. *Biochem Biophys Res Commun* **312**: 1220–25.

72. Sorensen, D. R., Leirdal, M., and Sioud, M. (2003). Gene silencing by systemic delivery of synthetic siRNAs in adult mice. *J Mol Biol* **327**: 761–6.

73. Yan, W., Chen, W., and Huang, L. (2007). Mechanism of adjuvant activity of cationic liposome: phosphorylation of a MAP kinase, ERK and induction of chemokines. *Mol Immunol* **44**: 3672–81.

74. Cardoso, A. L., Simoes, S., de Almeida, L. P., Pelisek, J., Culmsee, C., Wagner, E., and Pedroso de Lima, M. C. (2007). siRNA delivery by a transferrin-associated lipid-based vector: a non-viral strategy to mediate gene silencing. *J Gene Med* **9**: 170–83.

75. Li, S. D., and Huang, L. (2006). Targeted delivery of antisense oligodeoxynucleotide and small interference RNA into lung cancer cells. *Mol Pharm* **3**: 579–88.

76. Bouxsein, N. F., McAllister, C. S., Ewert, K. K., Samuel, C. E., and Safinya, C. R. (2007). Structure and gene silencing activities of monovalent and pentavalent cationic lipid vectors complexed with siRNA. *Biochemistry* **46**: 4785–92.

77. Huckriede, A., De Jonge, J., Holtrop, M., and Wilschut, J. (2007). Cellular delivery of siRNA mediated by fusion-active virosomes. *J Liposome Res* **17**: 39–47.

78. de Jonge, J., Holtrop, M., Wilschut, J., and Huckriede, A. (2006). Reconstituted influenza virus envelopes as an efficient carrier system for cellular delivery of small-interfering RNAs. *Gene Ther* **13**: 400–411.

79. Tonges, L., Lingor, P., Egle, R., Dietz, G. P., Fahr, A., and Bahr, M. (2006). Stearylated octaarginine and artificial virus-like particles for transfection of siRNA into primary rat neurons. *Rna* **12**: 1431–8.

80. Adams, C. M., Reitz, J., De Brabander, J. K., Feramisco, J. D., Li, L., Brown, M. S., and Goldstein, J. L. (2004). Cholesterol and 25-hydroxycholesterol

inhibit activation of SREBPs by different mechanisms, both involving SCAP and Insigs. *J Biol Chem* **279**: 52772–80.

81. Lorenz, C., Hadwiger, P., John, M., Vornlocher, H. P., and Unverzagt, C. (2004). Steroid and lipid conjugates of siRNAs to enhance cellular uptake and gene silencing in liver cells. *Bioorg Med Chem Lett* **14**: 4975–7.

82. Kim, S. I., Shin, D., Choi, T. H., Lee, J. C., Cheon, G. J., Kim, K. Y., Park, M., and Kim, M. (2007). Systemic and specific delivery of small interfering RNAs to the liver mediated by apolipoprotein A-I. *Mol Ther* **15**: 1145–52.

83. Li, W. and Szoka, F. C., Jr. (2007). Lipid-based nanoparticles for nucleic acid delivery. *Pharm Res* **24**: 438–49.

84. Baigude, H., McCarroll, J., Yang, C. S., Swain, P. M., and Rana, T. M. (2007). Design and creation of new nanomaterials for therapeutic RNAi. *ACS Chem Biol* **2**: 237–41.

85. Aigner, A. (2007). Applications of RNA interference: current state and prospects for siRNA-based strategies in vivo. *Appl Microbiol Biotechnol* **76**: 9–21.

86. Heidel, J. D., Yu, Z., Liu, J. Y., Rele, S. M., Liang, Y., Zeidan, R. K., Kornbrust, D. J., and Davis, M. E. (2007). Administration in non-human primates of escalating intravenous doses of targeted nanoparticles containing ribonucleotide reductase subunit M2 siRNA. *Proc Natl Acad Sci U S A* **104**: 5715–21.

87. Bartlett, D. W. and Davis, M. E. (2007). Physicochemical and biological characterization of targeted, nucleic acid-containing nanoparticles. *Bioconjug Chem* **18**: 456–68.

88. Medarova, Z., Pham, W., Farrar, C., Petkova, V., and Moore, A. (2007). In vivo imaging of siRNA delivery and silencing in tumors. *Nat Med* **13**: 372–7.

89. Tan, W. B., Jiang, S., and Zhang, Y. (2007). Quantum-dot based nanoparticles for targeted silencing of HER2/neu gene via RNA interference. *Biomaterials* **28**: 1565–71.

90. Yuan, X., Li, L., Rathinavelu, A., Hao, J., Narasimhan, M., He, M., Heitlage, V., Tam, L., Viqar, S., and Salehi, M. (2006). siRNA drug delivery by biodegradable polymeric nanoparticles. *J Nanosci Nanotechnol* **6**: 2821–8.

91. Li, C. X., Parker, A., Menocal, E., Xiang, S., Borodyansky, L., and Fruehauf, J. H. (2006). Delivery of RNA interference. *Cell Cycle* **5**: 2103–9.

92. Pille, J. Y., Li, H., Blot, E., Bertrand, J. R., Pritchard, L. L., Opolon, P., Maksimenko, A., Lu, H., Vannier, J. P., Soria, J., Malvy, C., and Soria, C. (2006). Intravenous delivery of anti-RhoA small interfering RNA loaded in nanoparticles of chitosan in mice: safety and efficacy in xenografted aggressive breast cancer. *Hum Gene Ther* **17**: 1019–26.

93. Wang, Y., Gao, S., Ye, W. H., Yoon, H. S., and Yang, Y. Y. (2006). Co-delivery of drugs and DNA from cationic core-shell nanoparticles self-assembled from a biodegradable copolymer. *Nat Mater* **5**: 791–6.

94. Katas, H. and Alpar, H. O. (2006). Development and characterisation of chitosan nanoparticles for siRNA delivery. *J Control Release* **115**: 216–25.

95. Toub, N., Malvy, C., Fattal, E., and Couvreur, P. (2006). Innovative nanotechnologies for the delivery of oligonucleotides and siRNA. *Biomed Pharmacother* **60**: 607–20.

96. Howard, K. A., Rahbek, U. L., Liu, X., Damgaard, C. K., Glud, S. Z., Andersen, M. O., Hovgaard, M. B., Schmitz, A., Nyengaard, J. R., Besenbacher, F., and Kjems, J. (2006). RNA interference in vitro and in vivo using a novel chitosan/siRNA nanoparticle system. *Mol Ther* **14**: 476–84.

97. Khaled, A., Guo, S., Li, F., and Guo, P. (2005). Controllable self-assembly of nanoparticles for specific delivery of multiple therapeutic molecules to cancer cells using RNA nanotechnology. *Nano Lett* **5**: 1797–808.

98. Shekunov, B. (2005). Nanoparticle technology for drug delivery: from nanoparticles to cutting-edge delivery strategies—part I. *IDrugs* **8**: 399–401.

99. Lochmann, D., Weyermann, J., Georgens, C., Prassl, R., and Zimmer, A. (2005). Albumin-protamine-oligonucleotide nanoparticles as a new antisense delivery system. Part 1: physicochemical characterization. *Eur J Pharm Biopharm* **59**: 419–29.

100. Juliano, R. L. (2006). Intracellular delivery of oligonucleotide conjugates and dendrimer complexes. *Ann N Y Acad Sci* **1082**: 18–26.

101. Utku, Y., Dehan, E., Ouerfelli, O., Piano, F., Zuckermann, R. N., Pagano, M., and Kirshenbaum, K. (2006). A peptidomimetic siRNA transfection reagent for highly effective gene silencing. *Mol Biosyst* **2**: 312–17.

102. El-Andaloussi, S., Holm, T., and Langel, U. (2005). Cell-penetrating peptides: mechanisms and applications. *Curr Pharm Des* **11**: 3597–611.

103. Morrissey, D. V., Lockridge, J. A., Shaw, L., Blanchard, K., Jensen, K., Breen, W., Hartsough, K., Machemer, L., Radka, S., Jadhav, V., Vaish, N., Zinnen, S., Vargeese, C., Bowman, K., Shaffer, C. S., Jeffs, L. B., Judge, A., MacLachlan, I., and Polisky, B. (2005). Potent and persistent in vivo anti-HBV activity of chemically modified siRNAs. *Nat Biotechnol* **23**: 1002–7.

104. Heyes, J., Palmer, L., Bremner, K., and MacLachlan, I. (2005). Cationic lipid saturation influences intracellular delivery of encapsulated nucleic acids. *J Control Release* **107**: 276–87.

105. Zimmermann, T. S., Lee, A. C., Akinc, A., Bramlage, B., Bumcrot, D., Fedoruk, M. N., Harborth, J., Heyes, J. A., Jeffs, L. B., John, M., Judge, A. D., Lam, K., McClintock, K., Nechev, L. V., Palmer, L. R., Racie, T., Rohl, I., Seiffert, S., Shanmugam, S., Sood, V., Soutschek, J., Toudjarska, I., Wheat, A. J., Yaworski, E., Zedalis, W., Koteliansky, V., Manoharan, M., Vornlocher, H. P., and MacLachlan, I. (2006). RNAi-mediated gene silencing in non-human primates. *Nature* **441**: 111–14.

106. Hassani, Z., Lemkine, G. F., Erbacher, P., Palmier, K., Alfama, G., Giovannangeli, C., Behr, J. P., and Demeneix, B. A. (2005). Lipid-mediated siRNA delivery down-regulates exogenous gene expression in the mouse brain at picomolar levels. *J Gene Med* **7**: 198–207.

107. Wang, X. L., Jensen, R., and Lu, Z. R. (2007). A novel environment-sensitive biodegradable polydisulfide with protonatable pendants for nucleic acid delivery. *J Control Release* **120**: 250–58.

108. Park, I. K., Lasiene, J., Chou, S. H., Horner, P. J., and Pun, S. H. (2007). Neuron-specific delivery of nucleic acids mediated by Tet1-modified poly(ethylenimine). *J Gene Med*

109. Tarcha, P. J., Pelisek, J., Merdan, T., Waters, J., Cheung, K., von Gersdorff, K., Culmsee, C., and Wagner, E. (2007). Synthesis and characterization of chemically condensed oligoethylenimine containing beta-aminopropionamide linkages for siRNA delivery. *Biomaterials* **28**: 3731–40.

110. An, D. S., Qin, F. X., Auyeung, V. C., Mao, S. H., Kung, S. K., Baltimore, D., and Chen, I. S. (2006). Optimization and functional effects of stable short hairpin RNA expression in primary human lymphocytes via lentiviral vectors. *Mol Ther* **14**: 494–504.

111. Patnaik, S., Aggarwal, A., Nimesh, S., Goel, A., Ganguli, M., Saini, N., Singh, Y., and Gupta, K. C. (2006). PEI-alginate nanocomposites as efficient in vitro gene transfection agents. *J Control Release* **114**: 398–409.

112. Grayson, A. C., Doody, A. M., and Putnam, D. (2006). Biophysical and structural characterization of polyethylenimine-mediated siRNA delivery in vitro. *Pharm Res* **23**: 1868–76.

113. Grzelinski, M., Urban-Klein, B., Martens, T., Lamszus, K., Bakowsky, U., Hobel, S., Czubayko, F., and Aigner, A. (2006). RNA interference-mediated gene silencing of pleiotrophin through polyethylenimine-complexed small interfering RNAs in vivo exerts antitumoral effects in glioblastoma xenografts. *Hum Gene Ther* **17**: 751–66.

114. Aigner, A. (2006). Gene silencing through RNA interference (RNAi) in vivo: strategies based on the direct application of siRNAs. *J Biotechnol* **124**: 12–25.

115. Hwa Kim, S., Hoon Jeong, J., Chul Cho, K., Wan Kim, S., and Gwan Park, T. (2005). Target-specific gene silencing by siRNA plasmid DNA complexed with folate-modified poly(ethylenimine). *J Control Release* **104**: 223–32.

116. Urban-Klein, B., Werth, S., Abuharbeid, S., Czubayko, F., and Aigner, A. (2005). RNAi-mediated gene-targeting through systemic application of polyethylenimine (PEI)-complexed siRNA in vivo. *Gene Ther* **12**: 461–6.

117. Peer, D., Zhu, P., Carman, C. V., Lieberman, J., and Shimaoka, M. (2007). Selective gene silencing in activated leukocytes by targeting siRNAs to the integrin lymphocyte function-associated antigen-1. *Proc Natl Acad Sci U S A* **104**: 4095–4100.

118. Song, E., Zhu, P., Lee, S. K., Chowdhury, D., Kussman, S., Dykxhoorn, D. M., Feng, Y., Palliser, D., Weiner, D. B., Shankar, P., Marasco, W. A., and Lieberman, J. (2005). Antibody mediated in vivo delivery of small interfering RNAs via cell-surface receptors. *Nat Biotechnol* **23**: 709–17.

119. Shao, K., Hou, Q., Go, M. L., Duan, W., Cheung, N. S., Feng, S. S., Wong, K. P., Yoram, A., Zhang, W., Huang, Z., and Li, Q. T. (2007). Sulfatide-tenascin

interaction mediates binding to the extracellular matrix and endocytic uptake of liposomes in glioma cells. *Cell Mol Life Sci* **64**: 506–15.

120. Furset, G. and Sioud, M. (2007). Design of bifunctional siRNAs: combining immunostimulation and gene-silencing in one single siRNA molecule. *Biochem Biophys Res Commun* **352**: 642–9.

121. Chu, T. C., Twu, K. Y., Ellington, A. D., and Levy, M. (2006). Aptamer mediated siRNA delivery. *Nucleic Acids Res* **34**: e73.

122. Wen, W. H., Liu, J. Y., Qin, W. J., Zhao, J., Wang, T., Jia, L. T., Meng, Y. L., Gao, H., Xue, C. F., Jin, B. Q., Yao, L. B., Chen, S. Y., and Yang, A. G. (2007). Targeted inhibition of HBV gene expression by single-chain antibody mediated small interfering RNA delivery. *Hepatology* **46**: 84–94.

123. Hogrefe, R. I., Lebedev, A. V., Zon, G., Pirollo, K. F., Rait, A., Zhou, Q., Yu, W., and Chang, E. H. (2006). Chemically modified short interfering hybrids (siHYBRIDS): nanoimmunoliposome delivery in vitro and in vivo for RNAi of HER-2. *Nucleosides Nucleotides Nucleic Acids* **25**: 889–907.

124. Ikeda, Y., and Taira, K. (2006). Ligand-targeted delivery of therapeutic siRNA. *Pharm Res* **23**: 1631–40.

125. Oliveira, S., Fretz, M. M., Hogset, A., Storm, G., and Schiffelers, R. M. (2007). Photochemical internalization enhances silencing of epidermal growth factor receptor through improved endosomal escape of siRNA. *Biochim Biophys Acta* **1768**: 1211–17.

126. Aoki, M., Ishii, T., Kanaoka, M., and Kimura, T. (2006). RNA interference in immune cells by use of osmotic delivery of siRNA. *Biochem Biophys Res Commun* **341**: 326–33.

127. Mook, O. R., Baas, F., de Wissel, M. B., and Fluiter, K. (2007). Evaluation of locked nucleic acid-modified small interfering RNA in vitro and in vivo. *Mol Cancer Ther* **6**: 833–43.

128. Hanai, K., Takeshita, F., Honma, K., Nagahara, S., Maeda, M., Minakuchi, Y., Sano, A., and Ochiya, T. (2006). Atelocollagen-mediated systemic DDS for nucleic acid medicines. *Ann N Y Acad Sci* **1082**: 9–17.

129. Banno, H., Takei, Y., Muramatsu, T., Komori, K., and Kadomatsu, K. (2006). Controlled release of small interfering RNA targeting midkine attenuates intimal hyperplasia in vein grafts. *J Vasc Surg* **44**: 633–41.

130. Honma, K., Miyata, T., and Ochiya, T. (2004). The role of atelocollagen-based cell transfection array in high-throughput screening of gene functions and in drug discovery. *Curr Drug Discov Technol* **1**: 287–94.

131. Takeshita, F., Minakuchi, Y., Nagahara, S., Honma, K., Sasaki, H., Hirai, K., Teratani, T., Namatame, N., Yamamoto, Y., Hanai, K., Kato, T., Sano, A., and Ochiya, T. (2005). Efficient delivery of small interfering RNA to bone-metastatic tumors by using atelocollagen in vivo. *Proc Natl Acad Sci U S A* **102**: 12177–82.

132. Minakuchi, Y., Takeshita, F., Kosaka, N., Sasaki, H., Yamamoto, Y., Kouno, M., Honma, K., Nagahara, S., Hanai, K., Sano, A., Kato, T., Terada, M., and

Ochiya, T. (2004). Atelocollagen-mediated synthetic small interfering RNA delivery for effective gene silencing in vitro and in vivo. *Nucleic Acids Res* **32**: e109.

133. Geiss, B. J., Pierson, T. C., and Diamond, M. S. (2005). Actively replicating West Nile virus is resistant to cytoplasmic delivery of siRNA. *Virol J* **2**: 53.

134. Krautz-Peterson, G., Radwanska, M., Ndegwa, D., Shoemaker, C. B., and Skelly, P. J. (2007). Optimizing gene suppression in schistosomes using RNA interference. *Mol Biochem Parasitol* **153**: 194–202.

135. Bejjani, R. A., Andrieu, C., Bloquel, C., Berdugo, M., BenEzra, D., and Behar-Cohen, F. (2007). Electrically assisted ocular gene therapy. *Surv Ophthalmol* **52**: 196–208.

136. Golzio, M., Mazzolini, L., Ledoux, A., Paganin, A., Izard, M., Hellaudais, L., Bieth, A., Pillaire, M. J., Cazaux, C., Hoffmann, J. S., Couderc, B., and Teissie, J. (2007). In vivo gene silencing in solid tumors by targeted electrically mediated siRNA delivery. *Gene Ther* **14**: 752–9.

137. Merkerova, M., Klamova, H., Brdicka, R., and Bruchova, H. (2007). Targeting of gene expression by siRNA in CML primary cells. *Mol Biol Rep* **34**: 27–33.

138. Prud'homme, G. J., Glinka, Y., Khan, A. S., and Draghia-Akli, R. (2006). Electroporation-enhanced nonviral gene transfer for the prevention or treatment of immunological, endocrine and neoplastic diseases. *Curr Gene Ther* **6**: 243–73.

139. Inoue, A., Takahashi, K. A., Mazda, O., Terauchi, R., Arai, Y., Kishida, T., Shin-Ya, M., Asada, H., Morihara, T., Tonomura, H., Ohashi, S., Kajikawa, Y., Kawahito, Y., Imanishi, J., Kawata, M., and Kubo, T. (2005). Electro-transfer of small interfering RNA ameliorated arthritis in rats. *Biochem Biophys Res Commun* **336**: 903–8.

140. Issa, Z., Grant, W. N., Stasiuk, S., and Shoemaker, C. B. (2005). Development of methods for RNA interference in the sheep gastrointestinal parasite, *Trichostrongylus colubriformis*. *Int J Parasitol* **35**: 935–40.

141. Takahashi, Y., Nishikawa, M., Kobayashi, N., and Takakura, Y. (2005). Gene silencing in primary and metastatic tumors by small interfering RNA delivery in mice: quantitative analysis using melanoma cells expressing firefly and sea pansy luciferases. *J Control Release* **105**: 332–43.

142. Takabatake, Y., Isaka, Y., Mizui, M., Kawachi, H., Shimizu, F., Ito, T., Hori, M., and Imai, E. (2005). Exploring RNA interference as a therapeutic strategy for renal disease. *Gene Ther* **12**: 965–73.

143. Herweijer, H. and Wolff, J. A. (2003). Progress and prospects: naked DNA gene transfer and therapy. *Gene Ther* **10**: 453–8.

144. Tompkins, S. M., Lo, C. Y., Tumpey, T. M., and Epstein, S. L. (2004). Protection against lethal influenza virus challenge by RNA interference in vivo. *Proc Natl Acad Sci U S A* **101**: 8682–6.

145. Lewis, D. L. and Wolff, J. A. (2007). Systemic siRNA delivery via hydrodynamic intravascular injection. *Adv Drug Deliv Rev* **59**: 115–23.

146. Zender, L. and Kubicka, S. (2007). Suppression of apoptosis in the liver by systemic and local delivery of small-interfering RNAs. *Methods Mol Biol* **361**: 217–26.

147. Herweijer, H. and Wolff, J. A. (2007). Gene therapy progress and prospects: hydrodynamic gene delivery. *Gene Ther* **14**: 99–107.

148. Hino, T., Yokota, T., Ito, S., Nishina, K., Kang, Y. S., Mori, S., Hori, S., Kanda, T., Terasaki, T., and Mizusawa, H. (2006). In vivo delivery of small interfering RNA targeting brain capillary endothelial cells. *Biochem Biophys Res Commun* **340**: 263–7.

149. Bradley, S. P., Rastellini, C., da Costa, M. A., Kowalik, T. F., Bloomenthal, A. B., Brown, M., Cicalese, L., Basadonna, G. P., and Uknis, M. E. (2005). Gene silencing in the endocrine pancreas mediated by short-interfering RNA. *Pancreas* **31**: 373–9.

150. Lewis, D. L. and Wolff, J. A. (2005). Delivery of siRNA and siRNA expression constructs to adult mammals by hydrodynamic intravascular injection. *Methods Enzymol* **392**: 336–50.

151. McNamara, J. O., 2nd, Andrechek, E. R., Wang, Y., Viles, K. D., Rempel, R. E., Gilboa, E., Sullenger, B. A., and Giangrande, P. H. (2006). Cell type-specific delivery of siRNAs with aptamer-siRNA chimeras. *Nat Biotechnol* **24**: 1005–15.

152. Guo, P. (2005). RNA nanotechnology: engineering, assembly and applications in detection, gene delivery and therapy. *J Nanosci Nanotechnol* **5**: 1964–82.

153. Guo, S., Tschammer, N., Mohammed, S., and Guo, P. (2005). Specific delivery of therapeutic RNAs to cancer cells via the dimerization mechanism of phi29 motor pRNA. *Hum Gene Ther* **16**: 1097–1109.

154. Gomez, J., Nadal, A., Sabariegos, R., Beguiristain, N., Martell, M., and Piron, M. (2004). Three properties of the hepatitis C virus RNA genome related to antiviral strategies based on RNA-therapeutics: variability, structural conformation and tRNA mimicry. *Curr Pharm Des* **10**: 3741–56.

155. Nakahara, K., and Carthew, R. W. (2004). Expanding roles for miRNAs and siRNAs in cell regulation. *Curr Opin Cell Biol* **16**: 127–33.

156. Pancoska, P., Moravek, Z., and Moll, U. M. (2004). Efficient RNA interference depends on global context of the target sequence: quantitative analysis of silencing efficiency using Eulerian graph representation of siRNA. *Nucleic Acids Res* **32**: 1469–79.

157. Rakic, B., Sagan, S. M., Noestheden, M., Belanger, S., Nan, X., Evans, C. L., Xie, X. S., and Pezacki, J. P. (2006). Peroxisome proliferator-activated receptor alpha antagonism inhibits hepatitis C virus replication. *Chem Biol* **13**: 23–30.

158. Muratovska, A. and Eccles, M. R. (2004). Conjugate for efficient delivery of short interfering RNA (siRNA) into mammalian cells. *FEBS Lett* **558**: 63–68.

159. Geisbert, T. W., Hensley, L. E., Kagan, E., Yu, E. Z., Geisbert, J. B., Daddario-DiCaprio, K., Fritz, E. A., Jahrling, P. B., McClintock, K., Phelps, J. R., Lee, A. C., Judge, A., Jeffs, L. B., and MacLachlan, I. (2006). Postexposure protection

of guinea pigs against a lethal Ebola virus challenge is conferred by RNA interference. *J Infect Dis* **193**: 1650–1657.

160. Morrissey, D. V., Blanchard, K., Shaw, L., Jensen, K., Lockridge, J. A., Dickinson, B., McSwiggen, J. A., Vargeese, C., Bowman, K., Shaffer, C. S., Polisky, B. A., and Zinnen, S. (2005). Activity of stabilized short interfering RNA in a mouse model of hepatitis B virus replication. *Hepatology* **41**: 1349–56.

161. Kim, E. M., Jeong, H. J., Park, I. K., Cho, C. S., Moon, H. B., Yu, D. Y., Bom, H. S., Sohn, M. H., and Oh, I. J. (2005). Asialoglycoprotein receptor targeted gene delivery using galactosylated polyethylenimine-graft-poly(ethylene glycol): in vitro and in vivo studies. *J Control Release* **108**: 557–67.

162. Pirollo, K. F., Zon, G., Rait, A., Zhou, Q., Yu, W., Hogrefe, R., and Chang, E. H. (2006). Tumor-targeting nanoimmunoliposome complex for short interfering RNA delivery. *Hum Gene Ther* **17**: 117–24.

163. Dykxhoorn, D. M., Novina, C. D., and Sharp, P. A. (2003). Killing the messenger: short RNAs that silence gene expression. *Nat Rev Mol Cell Biol* **4**: 457–67.

164. McManus, M. T., and Sharp, P. A. (2002). Gene silencing in mammals by small interfering RNAs. *Nat Rev Genet* **3**: 737–47.

165. Lee, N. S., Dohjima, T., Bauer, G., Li, H., Li, M.-J., Ehsani, A., Salvaterra, P., and Rossi, J. (2002). Expression of small interfering RNAs targeted against HIV-1 rev transcripts in human cells. *Nat Biotech* **20**: 500–505.

166. Gitlin, L., Karelsky, S., and Andino, R. (2002). Short interfering RNA confers intracellular antiviral immunity in human cells. *Nature* **418**: 430–34.

167. Novina, C. D., Murray, M. F., Dykxhoorn, D. M., Beresford, P. J., Riess, J., Lee, S. K., Collman, R. G., Lieberman, J., Shankar, P., and Sharp, P. A. (2002). siRNA-directed inhibition of HIV-1 infection. *Nat Med* **8**: 681–6.

168. Jacque, J. M., Triques, K., and Stevenson, M. (2002). Modulation of HIV-1 replication by RNA interference. *Nature* **418**: 435–8.

169. McCaffrey, A. P., Meuse, L., Pham, T.-T. T., Conklin, D. S., Hannon, G. J., and Kay, M. A. (2002). Gene expression: RNA interference in adult mice. *Nature* **418**: 38–39.

170. Jia, Q., and Sun, R. (2003). Inhibition of gammaherpesvirus replication by RNA interference. *J. Virol.* **77**: 3301–6.

171. Shlomai, A. and Shaul, Y. (2003). Inhibition of hepatitis B virus expression and replication by RNA interference. *Hepatology* **37**: 764–70.

172. McCown, M., Diamond, M. S., and Pekosz, A. (2003). The utility of siRNA transcripts produced by RNA polymerase I in down regulating viral gene expression and replication of negative- and positive-strand RNA viruses. *Virology* **313**: 514–24.

173. Ge, Q., McManus, M. T., Nguyen, T., Shen, C. H., Sharp, P. A., Eisen, H. N., and Chen, J. (2003). RNA interference of influenza virus production by directly targeting mRNA for degradation and indirectly inhibiting all viral RNA transcription. *Proc Natl Acad Sci U S A* **100**: 2718–23.

174. Ge, Q., Filip, L., Bai, A., Nguyen, T., Eisen, H. N., and Chen, J. (2004). Inhibition of influenza virus production in virus-infected mice by RNA interference. *Proc Natl Acad Sci U S A* **101**: 8676–81.

175. Merl, S., Michaelis, C., Jaschke, B., Vorpahl, M., Seidl, S., and Wessely, R. (2005). Targeting 2A protease by RNA interference attenuates coxsackieviral cytopathogenicity and promotes survival in highly susceptible mice. *Circulation* **111**: 1583–92.

176. Schubert, S., Grunert, H.-P., Zeichhardt, H., Werk, D., Erdmann, V. A., and Kurreck, J. (2005). Maintaining inhibition: siRNA double expression vectors against coxsackieviral RNAs. *J Mol Biol* **346**: 457–465.

177. Yuan, J., Cheung, P. K. M., Zhang, H. M., Chau, D., and Yang, D. (2005). Inhibition of coxsackievirus B3 replication by small interfering RNAs requires perfect sequence match in the central region of the viral positive strand. *J Virol* **79**: 2151–9.

178. Sim, A. C. N., Luhur, A., Tan, T. M. C., Chow, V. T. K., and Poh, C. L. (2005). RNA interference against enterovirus 71 infection. *Virology* **341**: 72–9.

179. Tan, E. L., Tan, T. M. C., Chow, V. T. K., and Poh, C. L. (2007). Enhanced potency and efficacy of 29-mer shRNAs in inhibition of enterovirus 71. *Antiviral Research* **74**: 9–15.

180. Chen, W., Yan, W., Du, Q., Fei, L., Liu, M., Ni, Z., Sheng, Z., and Zheng, Z. (2004). RNA interference targeting VP1 inhibits foot-and-mouth disease virus replication in BHK-21 cells and suckling mice. *J Virol* **78**: 6900–6907.

181. Chen, W., Liu, M., Jiao, Y., Yan, W., Wei, X., Chen, J., Fei, L., Liu, Y., Zuo, X., Yang, F., Lu, Y., and Zheng, Z. (2006). Adenovirus-mediated RNA interference against foot-and-mouth disease virus infection both in vitro and in vivo. *J Virol* **80**: 3559–66.

182. Kahana, R., Kuznetzova, L., Rogel, A., Shemesh, M., Hai, D., Yadin, H., and Stram, Y. (2004). Inhibition of foot-and-mouth disease virus replication by small interfering RNA. *J Gen Virol* **85**: 3213–17.

183. de los Santos, T., Wu, Q., de Avila Botton, S., and Grubman, M. J. (2005). Short hairpin RNA targeted to the highly conserved 2B nonstructural protein coding region inhibits replication of multiple serotypes of foot-and-mouth disease virus. *Virology* **335**: 222–31.

184. Lambeth, L. S., Moore, R. J., Muralitharan, M. S., and Doran, T. J. (2007). Suppression of bovine viral diarrhea virus replication by small interfering RNA and short hairpin RNA-mediated RNA interference. *Vet Microbiol* **119**: 132–43.

185. Chang, J. and Taylor, J. M. (2003). Susceptibility of human hepatitis delta virus RNAs to small interfering RNA action. *J Virol* **77**: 9728–31.

186. Phipps, K. M., Martinez, A., Lu, J., Heinz, B. A., and Zhao, G. (2004). Small interfering RNA molecules as potential anti-human rhinovirus agents: in vitro potency, specificity, and mechanism. *Antiviral Res* **61**: 49–55.

187. Seo, M. Y., Abrignani, S., Houghton, M., and Han, J. H. (2003). Small interfering RNA-mediated inhibition of hepatitis C virus replication in the human hepatoma cell line Huh-7. *J Virol* **77**: 810–12.

188. Randall, G., Grakoui, A., and Rice, C. M. (2003). Clearance of replicating hepatitis C virus replicon RNAs in cell culture by small interfering RNAs. *PNAS* **100**: 235–40.

189. Kapadia, S. B., Brideau-Andersen, A., and Chisari, F. V. (2003). Interference of hepatitis C virus RNA replication by short interfering RNAs. *PNAS* **100**: 2014–18.

190. Wilson, J. A., Jayasena, S., Khvorova, A., Sabatinos, S., Rodrigue-Gervais, I. G., Arya, S., Sarangi, F., Harris-Brandts, M., Beaulieu, S., and Richardson, C. D. (2003). RNA interference blocks gene expression and RNA synthesis from hepatitis C replicons propagated in human liver cells. *Proc Natl Acad Sci U S A* **100**: 2783–8.

191. Kusov, Y., Kanda, T., Palmenberg, A., Sgro, J.-Y., and Gauss-Muller, V. (2006). Silencing of hepatitis A virus infection by small interfering RNAs. *J Virol* **80**: 5599–5610.

192. He, M.-L., Zheng, B., Peng, Y., Peiris, J. S. M., Poon, L. L. M., Yuen, K. Y., Lin, M. C. M., Kung, H.-f., and Guan, Y. (2003). Inhibition of SARS-associated coronavirus infection and replication by RNA interference. *JAMA* **290**: 2665–6.

193. Zhang, Y., Li, T., Fu, L., Yu, C., Li, Y., Xu, X., Wang, Y., Ning, H., Zhang, S., Chen, W., Babiuk, L. A., and Chang, Z. (2004). Silencing SARS-CoV Spike protein expression in cultured cells by RNA interference. *FEBS Lett* **560**: 141–6.

194. Lu, A., Zhang, H., Zhang, X., Wang, H., Hu, Q., Shen, L., Schaffhausen, B. S., Hou, W., and Li, L. (2004). Attenuation of SARS coronavirus by a short hairpin RNA expression plasmid targeting RNA-dependent RNA polymerase. *Virology* **324**: 84–9.

195. Wang, Z., Ren, L., Zhao, X., Hung, T., Meng, A., Wang, J., and Chen, Y.-G. (2004). Inhibition of severe acute respiratory syndrome virus replication by small interfering RNAs in mammalian cells. *J Virol* **78**: 7523–7.

196. Wu, C.-J., Huang, H.-W., Liu, C.-Y., Hong, C.-F., and Chan, Y.-L. (2005). Inhibition of SARS-CoV replication by siRNA. *Antiviral Res* **65**: 45–8.

197. Li, T., Zhang, Y., Fu, L., Yu, C., Li, X., Li, Y., Zhang, X., Rong, Z., Wang, Y., Ning, H., Liang, R., Chen, W., Babiuk, L. A., and Chang, Z. (2005). siRNA targeting the Leader sequence of SARS-CoV inhibits virus replication. *Gene Ther* **12**: 751–61.

198. Bitko, V., Musiyenko, A., Shulyayeva, O., and Barik, S. (2005). Inhibition of respiratory viruses by nasally administered siRNA. *Nat Med* **11**: 50–55.

199. Barik, S. (2004). Control of nonsegmented negative-strand RNA virus replication by siRNA. *Virus Res* **102**: 27–35.

200. Chuang, S. T., Ji, W. T., Chen, Y. T., Lin, C. H., Hsieh, Y. C., and Liu, H. J. (2006). Suppression of bovine ephemeral fever virus by RNA interference. *J Virol Methods* **115**: 302–10.

201. Huang, J., Jiang, P., Li, Y., Xu, J., Jiang, W., and Wang, X. (2006). Inhibition of porcine reproductive and respiratory syndrome virus replication by short hairpin RNA in MARC-145 cells. *Vet Microbiol* **115**: 302–10.

202. He, Y.-x., Hua, R.-h., Zhou, Y.-j., Qiu, H.-j., and Tong, G.-z. (2007). Interference of porcine reproductive and respiratory syndrome virus replication on MARC-145 cells using DNA-based short interfering RNAs. *Antiviral Res* **74**: 83–91.

203. Fowler, T., Bamberg, S., Moller, P., Klenk, H.-D., Meyer, T. F., Becker, S., and Rudel, T. (2005). Inhibition of Marburg virus protein expression and viral release by RNA interference. *J Gen Virol* **86**: 1181–8.

204. Otaki, M., Sada, K., Kadoya, H., Nagano-Fujii, M., and Hotta, H. (2006). Inhibition of measles virus and subacute sclerosing panencephalitis virus by RNA interference. *Antiviral Res* **70**: 105–11.

205. Kobayashi, T., Chappell, J. D., Danthi, P., and Dermody, T. S. (2006). Gene-specific inhibition of reovirus replication by RNA interference. *J. Virol.* **80**: 9053–63.

206. Campagna, M., Eichwald, C., Vascotto, F., and Burrone, O. R. (2005). RNA interference of rotavirus segment 11 mRNA reveals the essential role of NSP5 in the virus replicative cycle. *J Gen Virol* **86**: 1481–7.

207. O'Brien, L. (2007). Inhibition of multiple strains of Venezuelan equine encephalitis virus by a pool of four short interfering RNAs. *Antiviral Res* **75**: 20–29.

208. Bai, F., Wang, T., Pal, U., Bao, F., Gould, L. H., and Fikrig, E. (2005). Use of RNA interference to prevent lethal murine West Nile virus infection. *J Infect Dis* **191**: 1148–54.

209. Ong, S. P., Choo, B. G. H., Chu, J. J. H., and Ng, M. L. (2006). Expression of vector-based small interfering RNA against West Nile virus effectively inhibits virus replication. *Antiviral Res* **72**: 216–23.

210. Karlas, A., Kurth, R., and Denner, J. (2004). Inhibition of porcine endogenous retroviruses by RNA interference: increasing the safety of xenotransplantation. *Virology* **325**: 18–23.

211. Dieckhoff, B., Karlas, A., Hofmann, A., Kues, W. A., Petersen, B., Pfeifer, A., Niemann, H., Kurth, R., and Denner, J. (2007). Inhibition of porcine endogenous retroviruses (PERVs) in primary porcine cells by RNA interference using lentiviral vectors. *Arch Virol* **152**: 629–34.

212. Chen, M., Granger, A. J., VanBrocklin, M. W., Payne, W. S., Hunt, H., Zhang, H., Dodgson, J. B., and Holmen, S. L. (2007). Inhibition of avian leukosis virus replication by vector-based RNA interference. *Virology* **365**: 464–472.

213. Rossi, J. J. (2006). RNAi as a treatment for HIV-1 infection. *Biotechniques* **Suppl**: 25–29.

214. Orba, Y., Sawa, H., Iwata, H., Tanaka, S., and Nagashima, K. (2004). Inhibition of virus production in JC virus-infected cells by postinfection RNA interference. *J Virol* **78**: 7270–73.

215. Radhakrishnan, S., Gordon, J., Del Valle, L., Cui, J., and Khalili, K. (2004). Intracellular approach for blocking JC virus gene expression by using RNA interference during viral infection. *J Virol* **78**: 7264–9.

216. Li, X.-P., Li, G., Peng, Y., Kung, H.-f., and Lin, M. C. (2004). Suppression of Epstein-Barr virus-encoded latent membrane protein-1 by RNA interference inhibits the metastatic potential of nasopharyngeal carcinoma cells. *Biochem Biophys Res Commun* **315**: 212–18.

217. Chang, Y., Chang, S.-S., Lee, H.-H., Doong, S.-L., Takada, K., and Tsai, C.-H. (2004). Inhibition of the Epstein-Barr virus lytic cycle by Zta-targeted RNA interference. *J Gen Virol* **85**: 1371–9.

218. Hong, M., Murai, Y., Kutsuna, T., Takahashi, H., Nomoto, K., Cheng, C. M., Ishizawa, S., Zhao, Q. L., Ogawa, R., Harmon, B. V., Tsuneyama, K., and Takano, Y. (2006). Suppression of Epstein-Barr nuclear antigen 1 (EBNA1) by RNA interference inhibits proliferation of EBV-positive Burkitt's lymphoma cells. *J Cancer Res Clin Oncol* **132**: 1–8.

219. Yin, Q. and Flemington, E. K. (2006). siRNAs against the Epstein Barr virus latency replication factor, EBNA1, inhibit its function and growth of EBV-dependent tumor cells. *Virology* **346**: 385–93.

220. Jiang, M. and Milner, J. (2005). Selective silencing of viral gene E6 and E7 expression in HPV-positive human cervical carcinoma cells using small interfering RNAs. *Methods Mol Biol* **292**: 401–20.

221. Niu, X. Y., Peng, Z. L., Duan, W. Q., Wang, H., and Wang, P. (2006). Inhibition of HPV 16 E6 oncogene expression by RNA interference in vitro and in vivo. *Int J Gynecol Cancer* **16**: 743–51.

222. Gu, W., Putral, L., Hengst, K., Minto, K., Saunders, N. A., Leggatt, G., and McMillan, N. A. J. (2006). Inhibition of cervical cancer cell growth in vitro and in vivo with lentiviral-vector delivered short hairpin RNA targeting human papillomavirus E6 and E7 oncogenes. *Cancer Gene Ther* **13**: 1023–32.

223. Grimm, D. and Kay, M. A. (2006). Therapeutic short hairpin RNA expression in the liver: viral targets and vectors. *Gene Ther* **13**: 563–75.

224. Palliser, D., Chowdhury, D., Wang, Q.-Y., Lee, S. J., Bronson, R. T., Knipe, D. M., and Lieberman, J. (2006). An siRNA-based microbicide protects mice from lethal herpes simplex virus 2 infection. *Nature* **439**: 89–94.

225. Bhuyan, P. K., Kariko, K., Capodici, J., Lubinski, J., Hook, L. M., Friedman, H. M., and Weissman, D. (2004). Short interfering RNA-mediated inhibition of herpes simplex virus type 1 gene expression and function during infection of human keratinocytes. *J Virol* **78**: 10276–81.

226. Liu, J., Chen, I., Chua, H., Du, Q., and Kwang, J. (2006). Inhibition of porcine circovirus type 2 replication in mice by RNA interference. *Virology* **347**: 422–33.

227. Giladi, H., Ketzinel-Gilad, M., Rivkin, L., Felig, Y., Nussbaum, O., and Galun, E. (2003). Small interfering RNA inhibits hepatitis B virus replication in mice. *Mol Ther* **8**: 769–776.

228. Kim, M., Shin, D., Kim, S. I., and Park, M. (2006). Inhibition of hepatitis C virus gene expression by small interfering RNAs using a tri-cistronic full-length viral replicon and a transient mouse model. *Virus Res* **122**: 1–10.

229. Uprichard, S. L., Boyd, B., Althage, A., and Chisari, F. V. (2005). Clearance of hepatitis B virus from the liver of transgenic mice by short hairpin RNAs. *Proc Natl Acad Sci U S A* **102**: 773–8.

230. Chen, C. C., Ko, T. M., Ma, H. I., Wu, H. L., Xiao, X., Li, J., Chang, C. M., Wu, P. Y., Chen, C. H., Han, J. M., Yu, C. P., Jeng, K. S., Hu, C. P., and Tao, M. H. (2007). Long-term inhibition of hepatitis B virus in transgenic mice by double-stranded adeno-associated virus 8-delivered short hairpin RNA. *Gene Ther* **14**: 11–19.

231. Ying, R. S., Zhu, C., Fan, X. G., Li, N., Tian, X. F., Liu, H. B., and Zhang, B. X. (2007). Hepatitis B virus is inhibited by RNA interference in cell culture and in mice. *Antiviral Res* **73**: 24–30.

232. Li, M., Li, H., and Rossi, J. J. (2006). RNAi in combination with a ribozyme and TAR decoy for treatment of HIV infection in hematopoietic cell gene therapy. *Ann N Y Acad Sci* **1082**: 172–9.

233. Zeng, Y., and Cullen, B. R. (2002). RNA interference in human cells is restricted to the cytoplasm. *RNA* **8**: 855–60.

234. Silva, J. M., Hammond, S. M., and Hannon, G. J. (2002). RNA interference: a promising approach to antiviral therapy? *Trends Mol Med* **8**: 505–8.

235. Voinnet, O., Pinto, Y. M., and Baulcombe, D. C. (1999). Suppression of gene silencing: A general strategy used by diverse DNA and RNA viruses of plants. *PNAS* **96**: 14147–52.

236. Li, H., Li, W. X., and Ding, S. W. (2002). Induction and suppression of RNA silencing by an animal virus. *Science* **296**: 1319–21.

237. Li, W.-X., Li, H., Lu, R., Li, F., Dus, M., Atkinson, P., Brydon, E. W. A., Johnson, K. L., Garcia-Sastre, A., Ball, L. A., Palese, P., and Ding, S.-W. (2004). Interferon antagonist proteins of influenza and vaccinia viruses are suppressors of RNA silencing. *PNAS* **101**: 1350–55.

238. Soldan, S. S., Plassmeyer, M. L., Matukonis, M. K., and Gonzalez-Scarano, F. (2005). La Crosse virus nonstructural protein NSs counteracts the effects of short interfering RNA. *J Virol* **79**: 234–44.

239. Sullivan, C. S. and Ganem, D. (2005). A virus-encoded inhibitor that blocks RNA interference in mammalian cells. *J Virol* **79**: 7371–9.

240. Judge, A. D., Sood, V., Shaw, J. R., Fang, D., McClintock, K., and MacLachlan, I. (2005). Sequence-dependent stimulation of the mammalian innate immune response by synthetic siRNA. *Nat Biotech* **23**: 457–462.

241. Qiu, S., Adema, C. M., and Lane, T. (2005). A computational study of off-target effects of RNA interference. *Nucl Acids Res* **33**: 1834–47.

242. Birmingham, A., Anderson, E. M., Reynolds, A., Ilsley-Tyree, D., Leake, D., Fedorov, Y., Baskerville, S., Maksimova, E., Robinson, K., Karpilow, J., Marshall, W. S., and Khvorova, A. (2006). 3[prime] UTR seed matches, but not overall identity, are associated with RNAi off-targets. *Nat Methods* **3**: 199–204.

243. Lin, X., Ruan, X., Anderson, M. G., McDowell, J. A., Kroeger, P. E., Fesik, S. W., and Shen, Y. (2005). siRNA-mediated off-target gene silencing triggered by a 7 nt complementation. *Nucl Acids Res* **33**: 4527–35.

244. Murray, J. L., Mavrakis, M., McDonald, N. J., Yilla, M., Sheng, J., Bellini, W. J., Zhao, L., Le Doux, J. M., Shaw, M. W., Luo, C.-C., Lippincott-Schwartz, J., Sanchez, A., Rubin, D. H., and Hodge, T. W. (2005). Rab9 GTPase is required for replication of human immunodeficiency virus type 1, filoviruses, and measles virus. *J Virol* **79**: 11742–51.

245. Wade, R. C. (1997). 'Flu' and structure-based drug design. *Structure* **5**: 1139–45.

246. Fiore, A. E., Shay, D. K., Haber, P., Iskander, J. K., Uyeki, T. M., Mootrey, G., Bresee, J. S., and Cox, N. J. (2007). Prevention and control of influenza. Recommendations of the Advisory Committee on Immunization Practices (ACIP), 2007. *MMWR Recomm Rep* **56**: 1–54.

INDEX

RNA Interference: Application to Drug Discovery and Challenges to Pharmaceutical Development, Edited by Paul H. Johnson
Copyright © 2011 John Wiley & Sons, Inc.